50% OFF Online NCMHCE Pre

Dear Customer,

We consider it an honor and a privilege that you chose our NCMHCE Study Guide. As a way of showing our appreciation and to help us better serve you, we have partnered with Mometrix Test Preparation to offer you **50% off their online NCMHCE Prep Course**. Many NCMHCE courses are needlessly expensive and don't deliver enough value. With their course, you get access to the best NCMHCE prep material, and **you only pay half price**.

Mometrix has structured their online course to perfectly complement your printed study guide. The NCMHCE Prep Course contains **in-depth lessons** that cover all the most important topics, **30+ video reviews** that explain difficult concepts, over **600 practice questions** to ensure you feel prepared, and more than **500 digital flashcards**, so you can study while you're on the go.

Online NCMHCE Prep Course

Topics Included:

- Professional Practice and Ethics
- Intake, Assessment, and Diagnosis
- Areas of Clinical Focus
- Treatment Planning
- Counseling Skills and Interventions
- Core Counseling Attributes

Course Features:

- NCMHCE Study Guide
  - Get content that complements our best-selling study guide.
- Full-Length Practice Tests
  - With over 600 practice questions, you can test yourself again and again.
- Mobile Friendly
  - If you need to study on the go, the course is easily accessible from your mobile device.
- NCMHCE Flashcards
  - Their course includes a flashcard mode with over 500 content cards to help you study.

To receive this discount, visit mometrix.com/university/NCMHCE or simply scan this QR code with your smartphone. At the checkout page, enter the discount code: **TPBNCMHCE50**

If you have any questions or concerns, please contact them at support@mometrix.com.

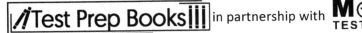 in partnership with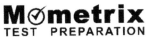

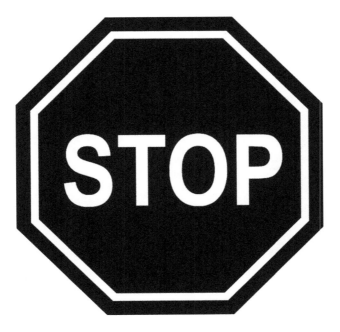

FREE Test Taking Tips Video/DVD Offer

To better serve you, we created videos covering test taking tips that we want to give you for FREE. **These videos cover world-class tips that will help you succeed on your test.**

We just ask that you send us feedback about this product. Please let us know what you thought about it—whether good, bad, or indifferent.

To get your **FREE videos**, you can use the QR code below or email freevideos@studyguideteam.com with "Free Videos" in the subject line and the following information in the body of the email:

- a. The title of your product
- b. Your product rating on a scale of 1-5, with 5 being the highest
- c. Your feedback about the product

If you have any questions or concerns, please don't hesitate to contact us at info@studyguideteam.com.

Thank you!

NCMHCE Study Guide

Test Prep and Practice Questions for the National Clinical Mental Health Counseling Examination [3rd Edition]

Joshua Rueda

Interested in buying more than 10 copies of our product? Contact us about bulk discounts:
bulkorders@studyguideteam.com

ISBN 13: 9781637750209
ISBN 10: 163775020X

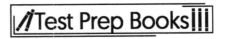

Table of Contents

Answer Explanations..**233**

Index **258**

Quick Overview

As you draw closer to taking your exam, effective preparation becomes more and more important. Thankfully, you have this study guide to help you get ready. Use this guide to help keep your studying on track and refer to it often.

This study guide contains several key sections that will help you be successful on your exam. The guide contains tips for what you should do the night before and the day of the test. Also included are test-taking tips. Knowing the right information is not always enough. Many well-prepared test takers struggle with exams. These tips will help equip you to accurately read, assess, and answer test questions.

A large part of the guide is devoted to showing you what content to expect on the exam and to helping you better understand that content. In this guide are practice test questions so that you can see how well you have grasped the content. Then, answer explanations are provided so that you can understand why you missed certain questions.

Don't try to cram the night before you take your exam. This is not a wise strategy for a few reasons. First, your retention of the information will be low. Your time would be better used by reviewing information you already know rather than trying to learn a lot of new information. Second, you will likely become stressed as you try to gain a large amount of knowledge in a short amount of time. Third, you will be depriving yourself of sleep. So be sure to go to bed at a reasonable time the night before. Being well-rested helps you focus and remain calm.

Be sure to eat a substantial breakfast the morning of the exam. If you are taking the exam in the afternoon, be sure to have a good lunch as well. Being hungry is distracting and can make it difficult to focus. You have hopefully spent lots of time preparing for the exam. Don't let an empty stomach get in the way of success!

When travelling to the testing center, leave earlier than needed. That way, you have a buffer in case you experience any delays. This will help you remain calm and will keep you from missing your appointment time at the testing center.

Be sure to pace yourself during the exam. Don't try to rush through the exam. There is no need to risk performing poorly on the exam just so you can leave the testing center early. Allow yourself to use all of the allotted time if needed.

Remain positive while taking the exam even if you feel like you are performing poorly. Thinking about the content you should have mastered will not help you perform better on the exam.

Once the exam is complete, take some time to relax. Even if you feel that you need to take the exam again, you will be well served by some down time before you begin studying again. It's often easier to convince yourself to study if you know that it will come with a reward!

Test-Taking Strategies

1. Predicting the Answer

When you feel confident in your preparation for a multiple-choice test, try predicting the answer before reading the answer choices. This is especially useful on questions that test objective factual knowledge. By predicting the answer before reading the available choices, you eliminate the possibility that you will be distracted or led astray by an incorrect answer choice. You will feel more confident in your selection if you read the question, predict the answer, and then find your prediction among the answer choices. After using this strategy, be sure to still read all of the answer choices carefully and completely. If you feel unprepared, you should not attempt to predict the answers. This would be a waste of time and an opportunity for your mind to wander in the wrong direction.

2. Reading the Whole Question

Too often, test takers scan a multiple-choice question, recognize a few familiar words, and immediately jump to the answer choices. Test authors are aware of this common impatience, and they will sometimes prey upon it. For instance, a test author might subtly turn the question into a negative, or he or she might redirect the focus of the question right at the end. The only way to avoid falling into these traps is to read the entirety of the question carefully before reading the answer choices.

3. Looking for Wrong Answers

Long and complicated multiple-choice questions can be intimidating. One way to simplify a difficult multiple-choice question is to eliminate all of the answer choices that are clearly wrong. In most sets of answers, there will be at least one selection that can be dismissed right away. If the test is administered on paper, the test taker could draw a line through it to indicate that it may be ignored; otherwise, the test taker will have to perform this operation mentally or on scratch paper. In either case, once the obviously incorrect answers have been eliminated, the remaining choices may be considered. Sometimes identifying the clearly wrong answers will give the test taker some information about the correct answer. For instance, if one of the remaining answer choices is a direct opposite of one of the eliminated answer choices, it may well be the correct answer. The opposite of obviously wrong is obviously right! Of course, this is not always the case. Some answers are obviously incorrect simply because they are irrelevant to the question being asked. Still, identifying and eliminating some incorrect answer choices is a good way to simplify a multiple-choice question.

4. Don't Overanalyze

Anxious test takers often overanalyze questions. When you are nervous, your brain will often run wild, causing you to make associations and discover clues that don't actually exist. If you feel that this may be a problem for you, do whatever you can to slow down during the test. Try taking a deep breath or counting to ten. As you read and consider the question, restrict yourself to the particular words used by the author. Avoid thought tangents about what the author *really* meant, or what he or she was *trying* to say. The only things that matter on a multiple-choice test are the words that are actually in the question. You must avoid reading too much into a multiple-choice question, or supposing that the writer meant something other than what he or she wrote.

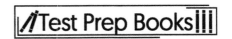

5. No Need for Panic

It is wise to learn as many strategies as possible before taking a multiple-choice test, but it is likely that you will come across a few questions for which you simply don't know the answer. In this situation, avoid panicking. Because most multiple-choice tests include dozens of questions, the relative value of a single wrong answer is small. As much as possible, you should compartmentalize each question on a multiple-choice test. In other words, you should not allow your feelings about one question to affect your success on the others. When you find a question that you either don't understand or don't know how to answer, just take a deep breath and do your best. Read the entire question slowly and carefully. Try rephrasing the question a couple of different ways. Then, read all of the answer choices carefully. After eliminating obviously wrong answers, make a selection and move on to the next question.

6. Confusing Answer Choices

When working on a difficult multiple-choice question, there may be a tendency to focus on the answer choices that are the easiest to understand. Many people, whether consciously or not, gravitate to the answer choices that require the least concentration, knowledge, and memory. This is a mistake. When you come across an answer choice that is confusing, you should give it extra attention. A question might be confusing because you do not know the subject matter to which it refers. If this is the case, don't eliminate the answer before you have affirmatively settled on another. When you come across an answer choice of this type, set it aside as you look at the remaining choices. If you can confidently assert that one of the other choices is correct, you can leave the confusing answer aside. Otherwise, you will need to take a moment to try to better understand the confusing answer choice. Rephrasing is one way to tease out the sense of a confusing answer choice.

7. Your First Instinct

Many people struggle with multiple-choice tests because they overthink the questions. If you have studied sufficiently for the test, you should be prepared to trust your first instinct once you have carefully and completely read the question and all of the answer choices. There is a great deal of research suggesting that the mind can come to the correct conclusion very quickly once it has obtained all of the relevant information. At times, it may seem to you as if your intuition is working faster even than your reasoning mind. This may in fact be true. The knowledge you obtain while studying may be retrieved from your subconscious before you have a chance to work out the associations that support it. Verify your instinct by working out the reasons that it should be trusted.

8. Key Words

Many test takers struggle with multiple-choice questions because they have poor reading comprehension skills. Quickly reading and understanding a multiple-choice question requires a mixture of skill and experience. To help with this, try jotting down a few key words and phrases on a piece of scrap paper. Doing this concentrates the process of reading and forces the mind to weigh the relative importance of the question's parts. In selecting words and phrases to write down, the test taker thinks about the question more deeply and carefully. This is especially true for multiple-choice questions that are preceded by a long prompt.

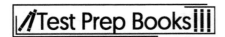

9. Subtle Negatives

One of the oldest tricks in the multiple-choice test writer's book is to subtly reverse the meaning of a question with a word like *not* or *except*. If you are not paying attention to each word in the question, you can easily be led astray by this trick. For instance, a common question format is, "Which of the following is…?" Obviously, if the question instead is, "Which of the following is not…?," then the answer will be quite different. Even worse, the test makers are aware of the potential for this mistake and will include one answer choice that would be correct if the question were not negated or reversed. A test taker who misses the reversal will find what he or she believes to be a correct answer and will be so confident that he or she will fail to reread the question and discover the original error. The only way to avoid this is to practice a wide variety of multiple-choice questions and to pay close attention to each and every word.

10. Reading Every Answer Choice

It may seem obvious, but you should always read every one of the answer choices! Too many test takers fall into the habit of scanning the question and assuming that they understand the question because they recognize a few key words. From there, they pick the first answer choice that answers the question they believe they have read. Test takers who read all of the answer choices might discover that one of the latter answer choices is actually *more* correct. Moreover, reading all of the answer choices can remind you of facts related to the question that can help you arrive at the correct answer. Sometimes, a misstatement or incorrect detail in one of the latter answer choices will trigger your memory of the subject and will enable you to find the right answer. Failing to read all of the answer choices is like not reading all of the items on a restaurant menu: you might miss out on the perfect choice.

11. Spot the Hedges

One of the keys to success on multiple-choice tests is paying close attention to every word. This is never truer than with words like almost, most, some, and sometimes. These words are called "hedges" because they indicate that a statement is not totally true or not true in every place and time. An absolute statement will contain no hedges, but in many subjects, the answers are not always straightforward or absolute. There are always exceptions to the rules in these subjects. For this reason, you should favor those multiple-choice questions that contain hedging language. The presence of qualifying words indicates that the author is taking special care with their words, which is certainly important when composing the right answer. After all, there are many ways to be wrong, but there is only one way to be right! For this reason, it is wise to avoid answers that are absolute when taking a multiple-choice test. An absolute answer is one that says things are either all one way or all another. They often include words like *every*, *always*, *best*, and *never*. If you are taking a multiple-choice test in a subject that doesn't lend itself to absolute answers, be on your guard if you see any of these words.

12. Long Answers

In many subject areas, the answers are not simple. As already mentioned, the right answer often requires hedges. Another common feature of the answers to a complex or subjective question are qualifying clauses, which are groups of words that subtly modify the meaning of the sentence. If the question or answer choice describes a rule to which there are exceptions or the subject matter is complicated, ambiguous, or confusing, the correct answer will require many words in order to be expressed clearly and accurately. In essence, you should not be deterred by answer choices that seem

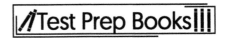

excessively long. Oftentimes, the author of the text will not be able to write the correct answer without offering some qualifications and modifications. Your job is to read the answer choices thoroughly and completely and to select the one that most accurately and precisely answers the question.

13. Restating to Understand

Sometimes, a question on a multiple-choice test is difficult not because of what it asks but because of how it is written. If this is the case, restate the question or answer choice in different words. This process serves a couple of important purposes. First, it forces you to concentrate on the core of the question. In order to rephrase the question accurately, you have to understand it well. Rephrasing the question will concentrate your mind on the key words and ideas. Second, it will present the information to your mind in a fresh way. This process may trigger your memory and render some useful scrap of information picked up while studying.

14. True Statements

Sometimes an answer choice will be true in itself, but it does not answer the question. This is one of the main reasons why it is essential to read the question carefully and completely before proceeding to the answer choices. Too often, test takers skip ahead to the answer choices and look for true statements. Having found one of these, they are content to select it without reference to the question above. Obviously, this provides an easy way for test makers to play tricks. The savvy test taker will always read the entire question before turning to the answer choices. Then, having settled on a correct answer choice, he or she will refer to the original question and ensure that the selected answer is relevant. The mistake of choosing a correct-but-irrelevant answer choice is especially common on questions related to specific pieces of objective knowledge. A prepared test taker will have a wealth of factual knowledge at their disposal, and should not be careless in its application.

15. No Patterns

One of the more dangerous ideas that circulates about multiple-choice tests is that the correct answers tend to fall into patterns. These erroneous ideas range from a belief that B and C are the most common right answers, to the idea that an unprepared test-taker should answer "A-B-A-C-A-D-A-B-A." It cannot be emphasized enough that pattern-seeking of this type is exactly the WRONG way to approach a multiple-choice test. To begin with, it is highly unlikely that the test maker will plot the correct answers according to some predetermined pattern. The questions are scrambled and delivered in a random order. Furthermore, even if the test maker was following a pattern in the assignation of correct answers, there is no reason why the test taker would know which pattern he or she was using. Any attempt to discern a pattern in the answer choices is a waste of time and a distraction from the real work of taking the test. A test taker would be much better served by extra preparation before the test than by reliance on a pattern in the answers.

FREE DVD OFFER

Don't forget that doing well on your exam includes both understanding the test content and understanding how to use what you know to do well on the test. We offer a completely FREE Test Taking Tips DVD that covers world class test taking tips that you can use to be even more successful when you are taking your test.

All that we ask is that you email us your feedback about your study guide. To get your **FREE Test Taking Tips DVD**, email freedvd@studyguideteam.com with "FREE DVD" in the subject line and the following information in the body of the email:

- The title of your study guide.
- Your product rating on a scale of 1-5, with 5 being the highest rating.
- Your feedback about the study guide. What did you think of it?
- Your full name and shipping address to send your free DVD.

Introduction to the NCMHCE

Function of the Test

The National Clinical Mental Health Counseling Examination (NCMHCE) is a required nationwide exam taken by recent graduates who apply for national Certified Clinical Mental Health Counselor (CCMHC) certification. The exam can also be used to gain a state license. The NCMHCE is used to gauge the candidate's application of counseling skills and theories. Candidates must hold the NCC certification in order to be eligible to take the NCMHCE. There are additional educational requirements that can be found on the NBCC's CCMHC certification eligibility webpage.

Test Registration and Administration

In order to register for and schedule an examination for the NCMHCE, the test candidate must first fill out the national certification application. After NBCC has approved the application, Pearson VUE will notify the applicant via email with information to schedule the exam. Scheduling of the exam can occur either online or by phone. Fees can be paid separately for the application and for exam registration, or the fees can be combined in one payment.

The NCMHCE is given twice a year (April and October) through approximately 900 Pearson VUE testing centers. There is also the option of taking the exam at home through OnVUE. If a candidate receives a failing score, they can pay a reregistration fee and register to retake the exam during the next testing session. Using a single application, candidates can retake the exam two times within a two-year period.

Test Format

The NCMHCE is administered by computer at a testing center or at home. Candidates are given 225 minutes to complete the exam. Before beginning the sixth case study, candidates are allowed a fifteen-minute break. An additional fifteen minutes will be used before the exam begins to go over the disclosure agreement and a tutorial. Overall, 255 minutes of the candidate's time will be needed for the examination.

The exam consists of eleven case studies, each with thirteen multiple-choice questions, making a total of 143 questions. Each case study is divided into three sections, with the first being a summary of the initial intake and the next two sections being subsequent sessions. Each section is followed by exam questions. The domains covered in the exam are Professional Practice and Ethics; Intake, Assessment, and Diagnosis; Treatment Planning; Counseling Skills and Interventions; and Core Counseling Attributes.

Scoring

One hundred of the questions will count toward the candidate's score. One point will be given for each correct answer. Subject matter experts will evaluate the questions that are answered correctly and decide, based on how challenging the questions are, whether the candidate has scored enough points to pass the exam. The candidate will have a ProCounselor account in which their score will be shared approximately four to five weeks after completing the NCMHCE.

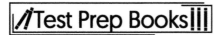

Recent/Future Developments

Starting in 2022, the NBCC has decided to change the educational requirements for national certification, stating that applicants must obtain a master's degree from a CACREP-accredited program. Note that this does not affect current NCCs or their certification.

Study Prep Plan for the NCMHCE

1 **Schedule -** Use one of our study schedules below or come up with one of your own.

2 **Relax -** Test anxiety can hurt even the best students. There are many ways to reduce stress. Find the one that works best for you.

3 **Execute -** Once you have a good plan in place, be sure to stick to it.

One Week Study Schedule	
Day 1	Professional Practice and Ethics
Day 2	Intake, Assessment, and Diagnosis
Day 3	Areas of Clinical Focus
Day 4	Counseling Skills and Interventions
Day 5	Case Studies and Practice Questions
Day 6	Answer Explanations
Day 7	Take Your Exam!

Two Week Study Schedule			
Day 1	Professional Practice and Ethics	Day 8	Treatment Planning
Day 2	Clients' Rights and Responsibilities	Day 9	Counseling Skills and Interventions
Day 3	Intake, Assessment, and Diagnosis	Day 10	Facilitating Clients' Motivation to Make...
Day 4	Obsessive-Compulsive and Related Disorders	Day 11	Core Counseling Attributes
Day 5	Evaluating an Individual's Level...	Day 12	Case Studies and Practice Questions
Day 6	Areas of Clinical Focus	Day 13	Answer Explanations
Day 7	Stress Management	Day 14	Take Your Exam!

9

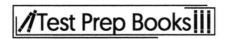

One Month Study Schedule						
Day 1	Professional Practice and Ethics	Day 11	Evaluating an Individual's Level of Mental...	Day 21	Counseling Skills and Interventions
Day 2	Legal and Ethical Counseling	Day 12	Assessing for Trauma	Day 22	Family Composition and Cultural Considerations
Day 3	Clarifying Counselor/ Client Roles	Day 13	Interactional Dynamics	Day 23	Guiding Clients in the Development of Skills...
Day 4	Payment, Fees, and Insurance Benefits	Day 14	Areas of Clinical Focus	Day 24	Helping Clients Develop Support Systems
Day 5	Providing Information to Third Parties	Day 15	Grief and Loss	Day 25	Developing and Facilitating Conflict...
Day 6	Intake, Assessment, and Diagnosis	Day 16	Occupation and Career Development	Day 26	Phases in the Group Process
Day 7	Determining Diagnosis	Day 17	Sexual Functioning Concerns	Day 27	Core Counseling Attributes
Day 8	Depressive Disorders	Day 18	Dating and Relationship Problems	Day 28	Case Studies and Practice Questions
Day 9	Feeding and Eating Disorders	Day 19	Treatment Planning	Day 29	Answer Explanations
Day 10	MSE	Day 20	Termination Process and Issues and...	Day 30	Take Your Exam!

Build your own prep plan by visiting:

testprepbooks.com/prep

10

Professional Practice and Ethics

Assessing Competency to Work with Specific Clients

Licensed professional counselors are required to work within the scope of their competence. This means that all counselors must have specialized academic training and receive clinical supervision during their practicum and internship. Counselors can also receive additional training through **Continuing Education Units (CEUs)** or other certifications that qualify them to use certain techniques and methods. For example, a counselor is working with a military veteran suffering from PTSD. The client experiences angry, emotional outbursts with his family, uses substances to cope with the intrusive images he witnessed while in the military, and he has not been able to maintain employment since his discharge. The counselor believes that **Eye Movement Desensitization and Reprocessing (EMDR)** would be the best treatment approach. However, prior to treating a client with EMDR, the counselor must have received specialized training and supervised clinical experience. If the counselor does not have such training, they need to refer the client to a clinician who specializes in EMDR. Otherwise, they could use an alternative treatment method for which they are properly trained.

Statistical Concepts and Methods in Research

Simply defined, **research** means to systematically investigate an experience either to understand what causes it or to develop a theory about how that experience can cause a future event. Systematic investigation can occur through a number of different scientific methods. **Deductive research** focuses on a specific theory and then establishes hypotheses to methodically test the theory in order to support or discredit it. Deductive research often involves setting up experiments, trials, or data collection surveys to collect information related to the theory. **Inductive research** examines information that's already available (such as established datasets like the U.S. Census Report) to highlight data trends and make inferences and/or projections from those patterns. **Research designs** determine how to structure a study based on factors such as variables being tested, the level to which the researcher is manipulating a variable in the study, the types of subjects in the study, what the study is testing or looking for, the frequency and duration of data collection, and whether the data collected is qualitative or quantitative in nature.

Non-Experimental Quantitative Research

Quantitative research utilizes logical, empirical methods of collecting information. This information is called data and is often analyzed using statistics. **Non-experimental quantitative research** includes forms of data collection where the researcher collects data that's already available in some form. They then analyze this dataset to describe the relationship between pre-determined variables. The researcher does not set up a novel system of trials to produce new data, and they can't randomize any data collected. The researcher has no part in manipulating any variables or establishing a separate control group to which they can compare collected data. The lack of a control group, lack of variable manipulation by the researcher, and lack of randomization are often seen as weaknesses in non-experimental quantitative research studies. Some examples of non-experimental quantitative research designs are depicted below:

- **Survey Designs**: These can be conducted through telephone or face-to-face interviews. They can also be conducted through paper or electronic questionnaires (either at an external facility or at

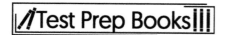

the study participant's home). Survey designs are generally used when research about a particular topic is limited so that more information can be gathered to better shape the research question or topic. Surveys are easy (and usually cost-efficient) to administer, but they can also result in low or biased participant response rates.

- **Correlational Designs**: These analyze the strength of the relationship between two variables in one group. One unique type of correlational design is found in ex post facto studies. The researcher examines two existing groups and analyzes the correlation between the variables of interest. Another unique type of correlational design is found in prediction studies, where the researcher determines a correlation between variables and then uses it to predict other correlations, related events, or future events. The strength and description of the correlation is indicated by the correlation coefficient (r), which falls between -1 and 1. If $r = 0$, it indicates there's no relationship between the two variables, while $r = 1$ indicates a direct, perfect correlation. If r equals a negative value, it indicates an inverse relationship between the two variables. If r equals a positive value, it indicates a direct relationship between the two variables. Regardless of how strong the correlation is between two variables, it doesn't indicate that one causes the other. It simply indicates that these two variables tend to occur (or not occur) together to some degree.

- **Comparative Designs**: These examine data trends to determine a relationship in two groups or datasets that have already been established.

Qualitative Research

Qualitative research is commonly employed in social sciences, including the field of counseling. It typically focuses on the analysis of a group of people (which is sometimes biased) to understand different aspects of human behavior, relationships, and social interactions. The researcher does not manipulate variables when conducting qualitative research. Qualitative research is primarily conducted without rigid structures in place. Data is collected through the following:

- **Case Studies**: These are detailed and documented examples of the topic of interest. They can be real or hypothetical situations. Case studies often record data over a period of time to examine a specific variable of interest. They can examine a situation involving one individual, a family, a larger community of people, or an organization. Case studies frequently look at how people relate to one another and/or to their physical or emotional environment.

- **Focus Groups**: These bring together a relatively small group of individuals. The group can be diverse in nature or have many similar interests. A facilitator guides a discussion within the group to discern information about individual or collective viewpoints about a specific issue.

- **Interviews**: These are typically more personal in nature. Interviews can be conducted in person, over the telephone, or via e-mail or regular mail. The interviewer asks the individual or group a series of meaningful questions related to the research topic. The interview can be structured with the interviewer having pre-set questions to ask, or it can be unstructured with the interviewer asking questions based on the flow of conversation and the answers given by the interviewee(s).

- **Observation**: In an observation, the researcher simply watches the individual or group of interest. However, a number of additional factors usually shapes the development of the

12

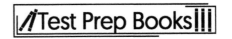

observation study. The researcher can observe the participant(s) in a specific situation or highly controlled context, or the researcher can observe the participant(s) in their day-to-day routine. The participant(s) may or may not know that they are being observed for specific behaviors. The researcher can involve themselves in the context and become part of the observation study. The researcher can also freely write down data from the observations or use a pre-made scale or data sheet to document specific behaviors.

Experimental and Quasi-Experimental Quantitative Research

Experimental quantitative research employs highly controlled processes with the hope of determining a causal relationship between one or more input (independent) variables and one or more outcome (dependent) variables. It uses random sampling and assignment methods to make inferences for larger populations. Typically, it compares a control group (serving as a baseline) to a test group. Ideally, experimental studies or experiments should be able to be replicated numerous times with the same results. The ultimate goal of a well-designed experiment is to declare that a particular variable is responsible for a particular outcome and that, without that variable, the associated outcome wouldn't occur.

Quasi-experimental quantitative research employs many of these same qualities, but it often doesn't use random sampling or assignment in its studies or experiments. Consequently, quasi-experimental research produces results that often don't apply to the population at large. They do, however, often provide meaningful results for certain subgroups of the population.

External Validity

External validity illustrates how well inferences from a sample set can predict similar inferences in a larger population (i.e., can results in a controlled lab setting hold true when replicated in the real world). A sample set with strong external validity allows the researcher to generalize or, in other words, to make strongly supported assumptions about a larger group. For a sample to have strong external validity, it needs to have similar characteristics and context to the larger population about which the researcher is hoping to make inferences. A researcher typically wants to generalize three areas:

- Population: Can inferences from the sample set hold true to a larger group of people beyond the specific people in the sample?

- Environment: Can inferences from the sample set hold true in settings beyond the specific one used in the study?

- Time: Can inferences from the sample set hold true in any season or temporal period?

If results from the sample set can't hold true across these three areas, the external validity of the study is considered threatened or weak. External validity is strengthened by the number of study replications the researcher is able to successfully complete for multiple settings, groups, and contexts. External validity can also be strengthened by ensuring the sample set is as randomized as possible.

Internal Validity

Internal validity illustrates the integrity of the results obtained from a sample set and indicates how reliably a specific study or intervention was conducted. Strong internal validity allows the researcher to confidently link a specific variable or process of the study to the results or outcomes. The strength of a study's internal validity can be threatened by the presence of many independent variables. This can

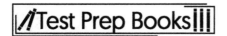

result in confounding, where it's difficult to pinpoint exactly what is causing the changes in the dependent variables. The internal validity can also be threatened by biases (sampling bias, researcher bias, or participant bias) as well as historical, personal, and/or contextual influences outside the researcher's control (natural disasters, political unrest, participant death, or relocation). Internal validity can be strengthened by designing highly controlled study or experiment settings that limit these threats.

Sampling

Sampling is the method of collecting participants for a study. It's a crucial component of the research design and study process. There are a number of different ways to select samples, and each method has pros, cons, and situations where it's the most appropriate one to use.

Simple Random Sampling

For this type of probability sampling, the participants are taken directly from a larger population with the characteristics of interest. Each individual in the larger population has the same chance of being selected for the sample.

- Pros: closely represents the target population, thus allowing for results that are the highest in validity

- Cons: obtaining the sample can be time consuming

- Use When: a highly controlled experiment setting is necessary

Stratified Random Sampling

For this type of probability sampling, the researchers first examine the traits of the larger population, which are often demographic or social traits like age, education status, marital status, and household income. They then divide the population into groups (or strata) based on these traits. Members of the population are only included in one stratum. Researchers then randomly sample across each stratum to create the final sample set for the study.

- Pros: closely represents the target population, which allows for results that are highest in validity. Since the sampling method is so specific, researchers are able to use smaller samples.

- Cons: obtaining the sample can be tedious. Researchers may first need to compile and become acutely knowledgeable about the demographic characteristics of the target population before selecting a representative sample.

- Use When: a highly controlled experiment setting is necessary; demographic, social, and/or economic characteristics of the target population are of special interest in the study; or researchers are studying relationships or interactions between two subsets within the larger population

14

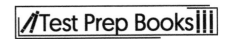

Systematic Random Sampling

For this type of probability sampling, researchers pick a random integer (n), and then select every *n*th person from the target population for the research sample.

- Pros: a simple, cost-effective sampling technique that generally provides a random sample for the researchers. It ensures that sampling occurs evenly throughout an entire target population.

- Cons: researchers need to ensure that their original target population (from which the sample is selected) is randomized and that every individual has an equal probability of being selected. Researchers need to be familiar with the demographics of the target population to ensure that certain trends don't appear across the selected participants and skew the results.

- Use When: a highly controlled experiment setting is necessary; researchers are short on time or funding and need a quick, cost-efficient method to create a random sample

Convenience Sampling

This is a type of non-probability sampling where researchers select participants who are easily accessible due to factors like location, expense, or volunteer recruitment.

- Pros: saves time and is cost-effective since researchers can create their sample based on what permits the easiest and fastest recruiting of participants

- Cons: highly prone to bias. It's difficult to generalize the results for the population at large since the sample selection is not random.

- Use When: conducting initial trials of a new study, when researchers are simply looking for basic information about the larger population (i.e., to create a more detailed hypothesis for future research)

Ad Hoc Sample

For this type of non-probability sampling, researchers must meet a set quota for a certain characteristic and can recruit any participant as long as they have the desired characteristics.

- Pros: allows for greater inclusion of a population that might not otherwise be represented

- Cons: results won't be indicative of the actual population in an area

- Use When: it's necessary that a group within the larger population needs a set level of representation within the study

Purposive Sampling

Another non-probability sampling method used when researchers have a precise purpose or target population in mind.

- Pros: helps increase recruitment numbers in otherwise hard-to-access populations

- Cons: usually unable to generalize the results to larger populations beyond the sample's specific subset

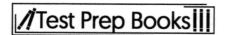

- Use When: researchers have a precise purpose for the study, or a specific group of participants is required that isn't easy to select through probability sampling methods

Levels of Measurement
Levels of measurement describe the type of data collected during a study or experiment.

- **Nominal:** This measurement describes variables that are categories (e.g., gender, dominant hand, height).

- **Ordinal:** This measurement describes variables that can be ranked (e.g., Likert scales, 1 to 10 rating scales).

- **Interval:** This measurement describes variables that use equally spaced intervals (e.g., number of minutes, temperature).

- **Ratio:** This measurement describes anything that has a true "zero" point available (e.g., angles, dollars, cents).

Independent and Dependent Variables and Type I and Type II Errors

A **variable** is one factor in a study or experiment. An **independent variable** is controlled by the researcher and usually influences the **dependent variable** (the factor that's typically measured and recorded by the researcher).

In experiments, the researcher declares a hypothesis that a relationship doesn't exist between two variables, groups, or tangible instances. This hypothesis is referred to as the **null hypothesis**. Errors can be made in accepting or rejecting the null hypothesis based on the outcomes of the experiment. If the researcher rejects the null hypothesis when it's actually true, this is known as a type I error. A **type I error** indicates that a relationship between two variable exists when, in reality, it doesn't. If the researcher fails to reject the null hypothesis when it's actually false, this is known as a type II error. A **type II error** indicates that a relationship between two variables doesn't exist when, in reality, it does. These errors typically result when the experiment or study has weak internal validity.

T-Test

A **t-test** is a statistical testing method used to determine the probability that, when comparing two separate sample sets with different means, the difference in the means is statistically significant. In other words, researchers can infer that the same difference will be found between the same two groups in the target population as opposed to only being found between the two specific sample sets. Usually the t-test is only used when the data sets have normal distributions and low standard deviations. The calculated t-test statistic corresponds to a table of probability values. These values indicate the likelihood that the difference between groups is simply due to chance. Traditionally, if the t-test statistic corresponds with less than a 5 percent probability that the differences between the two data sets are by chance, then researchers can assume that there's a statistically significant difference between the two sample sets.

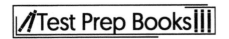

Forms of Hypothesis

A hypothesis typically takes one of two forms:

- **Null Hypothesis**: declares there is no relationship between two variables

- **Alternative Hypothesis**: declares a specific relationship between two variables, or simply states that the null hypothesis is rejected

Analyses of Variance

Variance tests examine the means of two or more sample sets to detect statistically significant differences in the samples. **Analyses of variance tests** (commonly referred to as **ANOVA** tests) are more efficient and accurate than t-tests when there are more than two sample sets. There are multiple types of ANOVA tests. One-way ANOVA tests are used when there's only one factor of influence across the sample sets. Consequently, two- and three-way ANOVA tests exist and are used in the case of additional factors. ANOVA tests can also analyze differences in sample sets where there are multiple dependent and independent variables.

ANOVA tests work by creating ratios of variances between and within the sample sets to determine whether the differences are statistically significant. Calculating these ratios is fairly tedious, and researchers generally use statistical software packages such as SPSS, SAS, or Minitab to input the data sets and run the calculations. SPSS stands for Statistical Package for the Social Science and is one of the most popular packages that performs complex data manipulation with easy instructions. SAS stands for **Statistical Analysis System** and is a software developed for advanced analytics, data management, business intelligence, multivariate analyses, and predictive analytics. **Minitab** is an all-purpose statistical software created for simple interactive use.

Analyses of Covariance

This analysis is a type of ANOVA. This analysis is used to control for potential confounding variables and is commonly referred to as **ANCOVA**. Say a researcher is testing the effect of classical music on elementary students' ability to solve math problems. If the students being tested are in varying grades, then their grade level must be taken into account. This is because math ability generally increases with grade level. ANCOVA provides a way to measure and remove the skewing effects of grade level in order to better understand the correlation that's being tested.

Chi-Square and Bivariate Tabular Analysis

Similar to statistical testing methods like t-tests and ANOVA tests, a **chi-square test** analyzes data between independent groups. However, chi-square tests focus on variables that have categorical data rather than numerical data. They can only be run on data with whole integer tallies or counts, and they're typically used when a researcher has large, normally distributed, and unpaired sample sets.

Bivariate tabular analysis is a basic form of analysis used when the value of an independent variable is known to predict an exact value for the dependent variable. This is most commonly illustrated by a traditional XY plot graph that marks independent variable (X) values across the horizontal axis, and marks dependent variable (Y) values along the vertical axis. Once all of the values are plotted, a relationship (or lack thereof) can be seen between the independent and dependent variables.

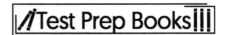

Post Hoc and Nonparametric Tests

Post hoc tests are usually performed after running other tests (e.g., t-tests or ANOVA tests) where it's been determined that statistically significant differences exist between two or more sample sets. At this point, researchers can pick and choose specific groups between which to analyze similarities or differences. Some common post hoc tests are the Least Significant Difference test, Tukey's test, and confidence interval tests, which are often similar to running multiple t-tests. Post hoc tests can be complex and time-consuming to calculate by hand or with simple software, so they often must be completed using sophisticated statistical software packages.

Nonparametric tests are typically used when datasets don't have pre-set parameters, are skewed in distribution, include outliers, or are unconventional in some other way. As a result, nonparametric tests are less likely to be valid in showing strong relationships, similarities, or when differences between groups exist. It's also easier to make a type I error when running nonparametric tests. Some common nonparametric tests include the Mood's Median test, the Kruskal-Wallis test, and the Mann-Whitney test.

Legal and Ethical Counseling

ACA Code of Ethics

Purpose

In general, counselors follow basic ethical guidelines to do no physical or psychological harm to their clients or to society and to provide fair, honest, and compassionate service to their clients and society when making professional decisions. The **ACA Code of Ethics** exists as a resource to provide clear guidelines for counselors to practice by and as a resource for counselors to consult when facing an ethical decision that they're unsure of making. This Code supports the mission of the counseling profession as established by the ACA. The ACA keeps an updated copy of their Code of Ethics, as well as other media and interactive resources relating to ethical practices, on their website at www.counseling.org.

Core Values

The foundation of the ACA Code of Ethics is defined by the following six core values:

- Autonomy: Freedom to govern one's own choices for the future
- Nonmaleficence: Causing the least amount of harm as possible
- Beneficence: Promoting health and wellbeing for the good of the individual and society
- Justice: Treating each individual with fairness and equality
- Fidelity: Displaying trust in professional relationships and maintaining promises
- Veracity: Making sure to provide the truth in all situations and contacts

Ethical Guidelines

The Code of Ethics is comprised of nine sections that cover ethical guidelines to uphold the core values:

- The Counseling Relationship: The counselor-client relationship is one that is built primarily on trust. Counselors have the obligation to make sure the confidentiality and privacy rights of their clients are protected and, therefore, should protect and maintain any documentation recorded during services. Additionally, clients have rights regarding informed consent. Open communication between the client and counselor is essential; in the beginning of the

18

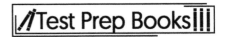

relationship, the counselor must provide the client with information on all services provided, with sensitivity to cultural and developmental diversity. Counselors should also pay special attention to clients who are incapacitated in their abilities to give consent and should seek a balance between the client's own capacities and their capacity to give consent to a more capable individual. Finally, with mandated clients, counselors should seek transparency in areas regarding information they share with other professionals.

- Confidentiality and Privacy: With trust as the cornerstone of the counselor-client relationship, counselors must ensure the confidentiality and privacy of their clients in regards to respecting client rights through multicultural considerations, disclosure of documentation to appropriate professionals, and speaking to their clients about limitations of privacy. Some exceptions to confidentiality include the potential for serious harm to other individuals, end-of-life decisions, information regarding life-threatening diseases, and court-ordered disclosure. Counselors are encouraged to notify clients when disclosing information when possible, with only the minimal amount of information shared.

- Professional Responsibility: Counselors have the obligation to facilitate clear communication when dealing with the public or other professionals. They should practice only within their knowledge of expertise and be careful not to apply or participate in work they are not qualified for. Continuing education is part of the counselor's development as a professional, and the counselor should always be aware of evolving information. It's important for counselors to also monitor their own health and wellness, making sure to refer clients to other competent professionals if they find themselves unable to practice due to health or retirement.

- Relationships with Other Professionals: Developing relationships with other professionals is important for counselors in order to provide their clients with the best possible resources. Being part of interdisciplinary teams is one way for counselors to provide the best, well-rounded services to clients. Counselors should always be respectful to other professionals with different approaches, as long as those approaches are grounded in scientific research. It is important for counselors to develop and maintain relationships with other professionals.

- Evaluation, Assessment, and Interpretation: In order to effectively plan for a client's treatment, general assessments should be made at the beginning of the counselor-client relationship regarding education, mental health, psychology, and career. Clients have a right to know their results and should be informed of the testing and usage of results prior to assessment. Counselors must take into account the cultural background of clients when diagnosing mental disorders, as culture affects the way clients define their problems. Counselors should take care not to perform forensic evaluations on clients they are counseling and vice versa.

- Supervision, Training, and Teaching: It is important for counselors to foster appropriate relationships with their supervisees and students. A client's wellbeing is encouraged not only by counselors but everyone the counselor works with. For counselors who are involved in supervising others, continuing education is important in providing the students or trainees with correct information. Any sexual relationship with current supervisees or students is prohibited, as well as any personal relationship that affects the counselor's ability to be objective. Finally, counselors should be proactive in maintaining a diverse faculty and/or a diverse student body.

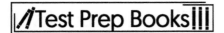

- Research and Publication: When conducting research, counselors must take care to make sure they adhere to federal, state, agency, and institutional policies in dealing with confidentiality. Counselors should keep in mind the rights of their participants and facilitate safe practices during research that do not harm the client's wellbeing. As with any objective research, counselors should take care not to exaggerate or manipulate their findings in any way, even if the outcome is unfavorable. Counselors should take care where the identity of participants is concerned. All parties involved in the research of case examples must be notified prior to publication and give consent after reviewing the publication themselves. It's important for researchers to give credit to all contributors in publication.

- Distance Counseling, Technology, and Social Media: The field of counseling is evolving to include electronic means of helping clients. Counselors should take into consideration the implications of privacy and confidentiality when treating clients online and take precautions in securing these, notifying the clients of any limitations to privacy. It's important to verify the client's identity when using electronic sources throughout the duration of treatment. In distance counseling, counselors must also be aware of the laws in their own state as well as the client's state.

- Resolving Ethical Issues: This section ensures that all counselors act in an ethical and legal manner when dealing with clients and other professionals. It's important for counselors to make known their allegiance to the ACA Code of Ethics and try to resolve ethical issues following this manner. If the conflict cannot be resolved this way, counselors may be obligated to solve the conflict through the appropriate legal and/or government authority.

Ethical Dilemmas

Ethical dilemmas occur when three different conditions are met in a situation. The first is that the counselor must make a decision. If the situation does not require that a decision be made, then there isn't an ethical dilemma. The second is that there are different decisions that could be made or different actions one could take. The third condition is that an ethical ideal will be conceded no matter what decision is made.

One type of ethical dilemma occurs when you have a situation in which two ethical principles are conflicting. This is a pure ethical dilemma because either choice of action involves conceding one of these principles, and there is no way to keep both principles intact. Another type of ethical dilemma occurs when ethical principles conflict with values and/or laws. In these types of situations, a counselor's values may conflict with an ethical principle, and a decision must be made.

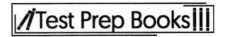
Once you have determined which kind of ethical dilemma you are facing, there are steps to take in order to reach a conclusion and, ultimately, the resolution of the dilemma. The NASW lays out steps that should be taken when attempting to resolve an ethical dilemma.

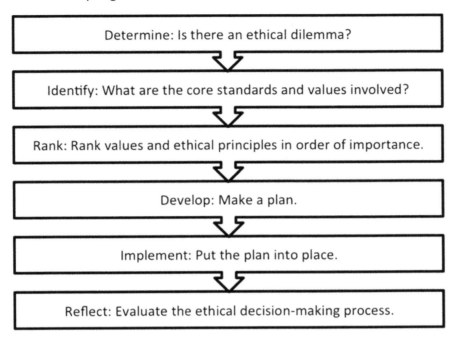

Determine: Is there an ethical dilemma?

Identify: What are the core standards and values involved?

Rank: Rank values and ethical principles in order of importance.

Develop: Make a plan.

Implement: Put the plan into place.

Reflect: Evaluate the ethical decision-making process.

Ethical Issues

Ethical issues can present themselves in any field. In counseling, ethical issues often center on the confidentiality and anonymity of clients, client cases, and data collected about the client (especially in group or family settings). However, counselors are obligated to report any instances of abuse, self-harm that could lead to a fatality, or harm to others that could lead to fatalities. Counselors also need to ensure that clear personal and professional boundaries are maintained between themselves and their client. In all instances of counseling, counselors must exhibit respect and tolerance for individuals of all backgrounds, attitudes, opinions, and beliefs.

Testing

A variety of ethical issues must be considered before, during, and after any test or assessment is administered. To begin, the counselor must be adequately trained and earn any certifications and have the supervision necessary to administer and interpret the test. Tests must be appropriate for the needs of the specific client. Next, the client must provide informed consent, and they must understand the purpose and scope of any test. Test results must remain confidential, which includes access to any virtual information. Finally, tests must be validated for the specific client and be unbiased toward the race, ethnicity, and gender of the client.

Dual Relationships

Dual relationships are clearly outlined in the NBCC Code of Ethics. The Code of Ethics states that counselors should not engage in dual relationships with clients or former clients in which exploitation of the client may occur. The Code of Ethics does recognize that there might be situations where dual

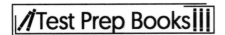
relationships are unavoidable. For example, a counselor might have two jobs, one of which involves providing group therapy to survivors of sexual abuse. It is possible that a member of the aforementioned therapy group could become an employee or client at the counselor's second place of work. In these types of situations, the Code of Ethics suggests that the counselor establish clear boundaries that are sensitive to the client/former client.

Under no circumstances should a counselor ever become involved in a sexual relationship with a client. In addition, the Code of Ethics establishes that counselors must avoid sexual relationships with anyone who is related to or has a close personal relationship with a client or former client. The Code of Ethics also states that counselors should not become involved in sexual relationships with former clients because of the high risk of harm that may occur with such relationships. If, however, a counselor does become involved in a sexual relationship with a former client, the counselor is responsible for demonstrating that the former client entered into the relationship without manipulation or exploitation. The Code of Ethics also specifies that, due to the obvious risk of harm, a counselor should not provide professional services to anyone with whom the counselor has had a previous sexual relationship.

Situations called "**boundary crossings**" are when a counselor does not intend to create a dual relationship but inadvertently does so, as would be the case were a counselor to self-disclose personal information during a therapy session. This is distinguished from a boundary *violation*, which occurs when a dual relationship is established that is inherently coercive or manipulative and therefore harmful to the client. The following are some clues that a boundary crossing is unethical:

- It hinders the counselor's care.
- It prevents the counselor from being impartial.
- It exploits or manipulates the client or another person.
- It harms clients or colleagues.

Dual relationships are sometimes unavoidable in practice, particularly in small communities. However, it is possible to avoid dual relationships that involve boundary violations and ethical violations.

Professional Boundary Issues

Professional boundary issues occur when counselors have multiple types of relationships with a client. This may include a professional, business, or personal relationship. For example, it is permissible to see a client out in public at a restaurant, but not to invite a client to dinner for business or personal reasons. When encountering a client in public, the relationship with the client must be kept confidential. However, if the client chooses to say hello, saying hello in return and quickly ending the encounter would be acceptable.

There are several boundary issues that come with working with clients. These issues are:

- **Intimate contact:** This refers to things such as hugging a client at the end of a working relationship or patting a client on the hand during a crying session. Sexual contact also falls into this category.

- **Personal gain:** This refers to instances in which a counselor engages in activity with a client that results in a monetary (or otherwise valuable) benefit to the counselor. This could involve situations such as referring a client to a business owned by the counselor or a friend/family

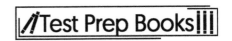

member of the counselor, selling something to a client, or even asking a client for professional suggestions.

- **Emotional and dependency issues**: This refers to instances in which a counselor's own personal issues cause the counselor to have impaired judgment, possibly resulting in other boundary issues, such as a dual relationship with the client.

- **Altruistic instincts**: In some instances, a counselor's own good intentions and concerns for a client can result in boundary violations and confusion about the relationship between the counselor and the client. An example of this would be going to a client's bridal shower or retirement party.

Setting and Maintaining Professional Boundaries

Despite these difficulties, counselors must set and maintain boundaries with their clients and colleagues to ensure an effective practice. Counselors should consistently monitor how their professional boundaries enhance or harm relationships with clients, colleagues, supervisors, and administrators. They must also gauge the impact of their boundaries on the amount of time they devote to work, their ability to cope with stress at work, and the amount of time and energy that they spend on extraneous activities and relationships.

There are several strategies for building and maintaining appropriate professional boundaries and relationships. First, counselors should examine their motivations for giving extra time and attention to a client. If a counselor treats one client differently, this indicates that the boundary may be overextended. Counselors can manage this situation by determining whether the services provided are in line with the client's care plan, the organization's mission, the job description, and scope of practice.

Counselors should also avoid encouraging clients to contact them through personal channels. Clients should use the channels of communication set in place by the organization, such as work email, voicemail, cell phones, pagers, receptionists, on-call staff, and procedures for after-hours referrals to 911, emergency rooms, or mental health crisis centers. Extending the professional boundaries of the counselor role puts colleagues and the organization at risk for failure. It also sets an unfair expectation that other colleagues will extend their professional boundaries. If boundaries are inconsistent between colleagues and within the organization, then clients may become confused and distrust the entire organization.

A third strategy for building appropriate professional boundaries is establishing clear agreements with clients during the initial sessions about the role of a counselor and the dynamics of a client-counselor relationship. When warning signs indicate that healthy boundaries may be in jeopardy, counselors must address the issues with the client clearly, quickly, and sensitively. This involves clarifying the roles and boundaries with the client and asking the client to restate these boundaries to ensure understanding.

A fourth strategy is limiting self-disclosure about the counselor's personal life to information directly related to the client's goals. If there is a dual relationship between the counselor and client, the counselor must preserve the client's confidentiality, physical security, and emotional well-being in social situations.

A fifth strategy is avoiding social media within professional practice. Counselors should not connect with clients on social media. This includes adding clients as friends on Facebook or following clients on

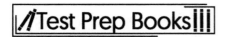

Twitter. Counselors should use discretion and limit the amount of online information that is made available to the public or social network connections to prevent conflicts of interest. Counselors also shouldn't attempt to access online information about clients without prior informed consent. Finally, counselors shouldn't post negative information about colleagues or the organization online.

A sixth strategy is for counselors to foster strong work relationships with their colleagues at the organization. These connections will help counselors cope with stresses, think through questions of ethics and professional relationships, and help maintain a sense of humor. Counselors should be sensitive to signs of bullying in the workplace, as each counselor deserves respect and dignity to ensure social justice for others. It's important that counselors use appropriate channels of supervision and consultation to determine appropriate boundaries in difficult situations. Supervision can also be useful when trying to remedy concerns with existing organization procedures that address or inhibit client needs.

A final strategy for maintaining professional boundaries is ensuring appropriate self-care. This includes taking time for nurturing oneself throughout the workday, maintaining a regular work schedule, and taking time away from the office each day to refocus. Counselors should limit communication when they are away from work to ensure time for rejuvenation, especially during vacations or personal time. They must also be aware of how they handle work stress and monitor how often they take work home. This includes physical work, emotional strain, or hyper-vigilance about work situations. If a counselor consistently struggles to maintain professional relationships and work boundaries, they should seek supervision or outside mental health counseling.

Professional boundaries in counseling are clearly defined limits on the counselor-client relationship that provide a space for the creation of safe connections. Some helpful things to keep in mind include: the line between being friendly and being friends; being with the client versus becoming the client; and understanding the limits and responsibilities of the counselor role.

Mandates and Guidelines

The practice of professional counselors is guided by laws and policies. **Statutory law** is a body of mandates that is created and passed by U.S. Congress and state legislatures. Many of the laws are state-specific and may be more restrictive than federal legislation. Agencies such as schools or mental health facilities can also develop specific guidelines, procedures, and policies. In school systems, the local boards of education can rewrite policies and state regulations to meet the needs of their communities. For example, the ratio of students to counselors differs across the nation. In one state, the mandated ratio can be 1 counselor to 350 students, whereas in another state, the ratio may be 1 to 500. Other mandates may include the requirement of every school to provide comprehensive guidance and counseling programs, such as crisis assessment with referral, dropout prevention, and conflict resolution. Similarly, a large number of state laws require healthcare service plans and insurers to provide some level of coverage for mental health services. Some outliers related to this mandate include copayments, deductibles, and limitations on the number of visits. It is important for a professional counselor to understand the difference between a mandate and a guideline.

A **mandate** is a set of rules and regulations set forth by governing bodies that must be followed when practicing counseling. **Guidelines** are suggestions on how to meet mandates. Ethical standards should guide the professional counselor when conflicting mandates arise. Documentation of the logical course of action is key in legal defense. Mandates that result from federal legislation or court cases will usually cover all counselors. Some of these mandates include child abuse or neglect laws. Counselors who have

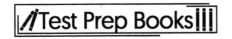
multiple credentials should know the mandates and regulations that apply to their work setting. School counselors rarely require informed consent to meet with students. However, a mental health counselor who works in a school but is employed by an outside agency would have to obtain an informed consent to see these same students.

Sharing Client Information with Third Parties

Because of legal and ethical issues surrounding privacy and informed consent, which are a means of maintaining a client's self-determination and dignity, it is critical that counselors always complete the appropriate forms when information is being shared about the client or decisions are being made on their behalf. Foundational to service provision is to first get written informed consent from the client to participate in services. Clients must fully understand the services being offered and agree to participate before treatment begins. Because it is often valuable for counselors to collaborate with other providers and professionals, it is important to obtain the Consent for Release of Information form before sharing any information with other providers. Clients must also be made fully aware of the reasons for this collaboration and information sharing and be told what information will be shared. Even if the client consents to having information released, the counselor should share only the relevant information with other providers, being careful to still maintain the client's confidentiality and privacy.

Clarifying Counselor/Client Roles

The client system can include not only the client, but those who are in the client's immediate environment, or who have an influential role in the client's life and treatment. A client system may also consist of an organization or community, which may involve many people. It is important to clarify and define the roles of each person involved in the client system, including the counselor, individual client, or the different members of the organization.

Client systems and counselors may initially have differing expectations of their roles in the helping relationship, so it is important that the roles and responsibilities of each are clarified as soon as possible. Although the client may have the expectation that the counselor will have the most active role in treatment, it is important for the client to also be fully engaged and proactive. While the counselor plays a supportive, helpful role, there should be a collaborative effort in which everyone in the client system is working together toward goals that have been set cooperatively. Clients must be actively involved in identifying areas of strengths and weaknesses, setting goals for treatment, choosing providers, and working towards the changes that are needed. In situations where the client system consists of many people, the counselor's role will be to maintain unity and cohesiveness so that goals can be achieved.

Client's Rights and Responsibilities

When providing services, it is important to ensure that clients understand all aspects of the treatment they will receive. In addition to the plan of treatment, it is also necessary to ensure that clients understand the possible risks involved, the costs associated, the length of treatment, and any limitations to confidentiality that might exist due to both mandated reporting laws and third-party payers. Alternatives to the therapeutic plan may also be discussed with clients before beginning treatment. Clients need to be given the opportunity to ask questions and receive answers to ensure they completely comprehend what their therapies will entail. Informed consent should require that the client sign legal documentation stating that they fully understand what will be involved—including all the risks, limitations, and alternatives—prior to beginning treatment. This documentation should become a part of the client's chart.

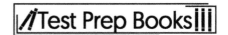

There will be circumstances in which a person may be receiving treatment on an involuntary basis. In these situations, the counselor should fully explain the terms of the treatment as it pertains to the individual's situation, as well as any rights the person does have in regard to refusal. An example of this type of situation would be someone who is court mandated to receive treatment, such as drug and alcohol counseling, anger management, or other therapies.

Sometimes client information needs to be shared with other individuals such as the client's family or other professionals for referrals. In these situations, the client must agree to these disclosures, and consent for disclosure of information must be obtained.

Clients have a right to obtain their records. Counselors are permitted, however, by the Code of Ethics to withhold all or part of the client record from the client if the counselor determines there is a great risk of harm in releasing the information. In these cases, it is important to fully document the request, whether or not the records were released, and the rationale for either releasing or not releasing them.

Limits of Confidentiality and Informing Clients About the Legal Aspects of Counseling

Limits of Confidentiality

Counselors have a duty to protect confidential information of clients. Ethically, client information should not be discussed with anyone other than the client. Legally, a client has a right to keep their medical and therapeutic information confidential. The **Health Insurance Portability and Accountability Act of 1996 (HIPAA)** requires that medical information (including therapeutic and mental health information) be protected and kept confidential. However, there are certain limitations to confidentiality. These generally involve risk of harm to the individual being served, as well as others. Counselors are not as protected as some other professionals when it comes to confidentiality and often find themselves being called to testify in court cases related to their clients. There are also certain situations in which counselors may have to release confidential information to protect the client or satisfy the duty to warn.

Minors

Providing services to minors can be challenging when it comes to confidentiality issues, especially since the legal rules and regulations vary from state to state. At times, there can be a conflict between the counselor's feeling of ethical responsibility to maintain the privacy of the minor and the legal right of parents to be informed of issues discussed. Adolescents in particular may discuss concerns with a counselor that they do not want their parents to be aware of, and it can be a violation of trust if these issues are subsequently revealed to parents. It is imperative that at the start of treatment, the expectations of the counselor's relationship with each person are discussed with the parents and minors, as well as the benefits and limits of confidentiality. Minors should never be promised confidentiality when the counselor cannot keep that promise, but the privacy and individuality of the minor should be maintained as much as possible. In cases where private information about the minor is going to be revealed, counselors should always inform the minor. This holds true regardless as to whether it is with the client's consent, mandated reporting, or due to the parent utilizing their right to information.

Groups

Confidentiality also becomes more complicated when a counselor is working with two or more people, either in a family or group session. All participants must agree that any information shared within the

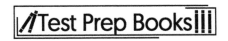

context of treatment will be kept confidential and not shared with others. However, the counselor should stress with clients that they cannot force other members to abide by the confidentiality agreement and that breach of confidentiality is a risk.

Mandated Reporting

It's important to note that counselors are considered mandated reporters in all states. This means there is a legal and ethical obligation to break confidentiality to report any signs and symptoms of child and elder abuse or neglect. In some cases, it will be impossible to know for sure if abuse or neglect is happening. Often the counselor will have only a small amount of information that may raise concerns but must make a report so that an investigation can occur. Any professional who has a suspicion of abuse or neglect of a child or a vulnerable adult must legally make a report to either Child Protective Services or Adult Protective Services, and they cannot be held liable for reports made in good faith.

Self-Harm

Some clients may disclose intent to harm themselves. It is necessary in these situations to fully assess suicidal intent and determine if the client is serious about carrying out a plan for self-harm. It might be sufficient, in cases where a client has considered self-harm but has no clear plan, to complete a safety plan with the client. The safety plan will outline what the client agrees to do should they begin to experience the desire to engage in self-harm. However, if the client has a clear plan of action and access to items necessary to carry out the plan, then confidentiality should be broken to protect the client. This would involve notifying police and having the client committed for observation for their own protection.

Duty to Warn

In addition to protecting clients from themselves, counselors also have a duty to warn third-party individuals if there is threat of harm. **Duty to warn** was established by the 1976 case Tarasoff vs. Regents of the University of California. In this case, a graduate student at the University of California-Berkley had become obsessed with Tatiana Tarasoff. After significant distress, he sought psychological treatment and disclosed to his therapist that he had a plan to kill Tarasoff. Although the psychologist did have the student temporarily committed, he was ultimately released. He eventually stopped seeking treatment and attacked and killed Tarasoff. Tarasoff's family sued the psychologist and various other individuals involved with the university. This case evolved into the duty to warn third parties of potential risk of harm. Satisfying the duty to warn can be done by notifying police or the individual who is the intended victim.

Because ethical dilemmas can involve legal situations, they may also have legal consequences for a counselor or necessitate involving the legal system. For example, a client may disclose that he frequently drinks large amounts of alcohol and then drives his children to school. Ethically, there is an obligation to keep what the client has said in confidence. However, the client's children are being placed in a situation in which they are in great danger of being injured or harmed. Due to laws protecting the welfare of children, the counselor would need to make a report to Child Protective Services. In some states, if someone has a good faith reason to believe that a child is being neglected or abused, and does not report the situation, that person may face a civil lawsuit and even criminal charges.

DETERMINING CLEARLY ESTABLISHED THREATS

One of the difficulties associated with breaking confidentiality to protect a third party is that the threat isn't always clearly established. If a client discloses during treatment that he is going to go home and stab his neighbor, this is clearly a plan of intended harm. However, what about an HIV-positive client who fails to warn sexual partners of her HIV status? What if the client fully understands the risk to her

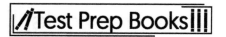

partners and has no intention of disclosing her status? This is a situation which would require thorough documentation, thoughtful debate, and possibly conferencing with colleagues to decide upon the best course of action.

Technology

With technology being utilized extensively by counselors, confidentiality of electronic information is another important issue. Counseling sessions are now being provided by telephone, video chat, and online simulation, and these media open new possibilities for information abuse. If a counselor provides a video therapy session, they should be aware that it is possible for the client to have someone else in the room, off-camera, without informing the counselor or other participants. The same could be true with electronic communication such as texting or email. There is no way to know if a client is forwarding electronic information to third parties without the counselor's knowledge.

Storage of Records

Other issues relating to confidentiality include the storage and maintenance of records and charts. All confidential material should be kept in a secure location and locked at all times. For example, if a counselor takes a clipboard into client rooms to make notes for later documentation, that clipboard should be locked in a drawer when not in use so that no one can turn it over and see confidential information when the counselor is away from their desk. With the use of electronics and computers, there should be policies in place to lock computers when away to avoid anyone seeing notes or other confidential information. Collaboration between colleagues in which clients may be discussed should be done behind closed doors to avoid anyone else hearing the conversation.

Sharing Client Information in Malpractice Lawsuits

There may be instances in which a counselor is sued for malpractice. In these cases, the Code of Ethics states that it is permissible for the counselor to share confidential client information to aid in self-defense, but only so far as is necessary to adequately defend oneself.

Legal and Ethical Issues Regarding Confidentiality

Disclosing Breaks in Confidentiality with Clients

Often when abuse or neglect is suspected, the concern about breaking confidentiality is at the forefront of the mind of the counselor. When disclosing information due to legal requirements, it is always important to discuss the situation with the client. It should be noted that the counselor should evaluate their own safety when discussing disclosure of confidential information with the client. If the counselor believes the situation to be unsafe if/when the client learns of the disclosure, then it is not necessary to alert the client prior to disclosing the confidential information. During informed consent, this requirement to report any signs of abuse or neglect should have been disclosed to the client. This is something that should be discussed in detail with clients during the informed consent process and throughout the relationship.

When such breaks in confidentiality occur, they can damage the relationship. In some cases, it may be necessary or appropriate to disclose to the client that a report is being made. For example, if a new mother has tested positive for cocaine and the infant has tested positive for cocaine while in the hospital, the infant will remain in the Neonatal Intensive Care Unit due to withdrawal. Disclosing to the mother that a report is being made, and why it's being made, could prepare her and create an opportunity to speak further with her about treatment options and other important considerations. It's

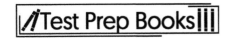
important to note that counselors who fail to report suspected abuse or neglect can be subject to civil penalties and/or prosecution.

Counselor/Agency Policies

Impact of Agency Policy and Function on Service Delivery

Counselors may be employed in a variety of agencies. Some organizations, such as hospitals or government entities, employ diverse professionals. Other types of organizations, such as direct service non-profits or private practice agencies, maintain predominantly social services staff. Agency policies directly and significantly impact the working environment, the services provided, and as a result, the effectiveness of the care clients receive. All agencies should have a mission statement that gives the agency purpose and serves as an umbrella for the agency's smaller goals and objectives. Agency policies must be in the best interest of the client and must support the ethical guidelines to which counselors adhere. They must also be clearly written and available to counselors and clients where appropriate. Counselors and all those providing care to clients should be able to help shape policy development to ensure consistency with client and counselor needs and protection. Policies must address:

- Appropriate confidentiality, consent, and information protection.
- Case management and supervision.
- Cultural competency guidelines.
- Professional development and ongoing trainings.
- Anti-discriminatory/diversity practices.

Payment, Fees, and Insurance Benefits

A topic that must be discussed when obtaining informed consent from clients is payment and fees associated with the counseling services. Fees set by a counselor may be influenced by the standards of living in the local area of practice. A clear outline of the payment policy and fees associated with each counseling session should be provided and explained to the client. One form of payment is termed **sliding fee scale** wherein fees are adjusted depending on the client's income. Professional counselors should consider that a sliding fee scale provides the same service to different clients for varying fees. Counselors who go through credentialing with insurance companies can become network providers.

A fee schedule will be discussed during the contracting phase with an insurance company. After providing counseling services to clients, counselors can bill the insurance. Claims will be reviewed and payment will be made to independent counselors directly. Government insurance options such as Medicare and Medicaid require the professional counselor to be within the network. Clients who do not have insurance or a health savings account can provide payment via private pay with cash or a credit card. The written agreement should include when payment is expected from the client or if the counselor plans to bill the client's insurance. The policy on missed appointments without notice should also be included in the disclosure along with a clear cancellation fee.

Counseling Processes, Procedures, Risks, and Benefits

Counseling Process

Professional relationships with clients develop in six stages. In the first stage, counselors focus their efforts on building rapport and trust with clients. This involves the development of a comfortable and trusting working relationship using listening skills, empathic understanding, cultural sensitivity, and good

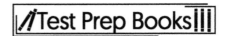

social skills. In the second stage, the counselor identifies the problem(s) that led the client to seek the assistance of a counselor. Together, the counselor and client identify the initial problems that will be addressed, check the understanding of each issue through a conversation, and make appropriate changes as necessary. The third stage involves the counselor using skills that allow him or her to understand the client in deeper ways. The counselor begins to make inferences based on their theoretical orientation about the underlying themes in the client's history. Once these inferences are made, then goals can be established based on these overarching themes.

The fourth stage of professional relationship development involves working on the issues that were identified and agreed upon between the counselor and client. The client takes responsibility for and actively works on the identified issues and themes during and between sessions. As the client successfully works through issues, it becomes increasingly clear that there is little reason for the meetings to continue. Therefore, in stage five, the end of sessions is discussed, and both the client and the counselor work through feelings of loss. The sixth stage occurs after the relationship has ended if clients return with new issues, if they want to revisit old ones, or if they want to delve deeper into their self-understanding. This stage is the post-interview stage and occurs with many—but not all—clients.

Counseling Procedures, Risks, and Benefits

Counseling can provide individuals with the opportunity to learn about themselves with the guidance of a trained professional. It can be a time of self-discovery during which one's strengths and weakness are explored, inventoried, and modified. Counselors are bound by confidentiality, so the counseling environment is a safe one in which clients are free to open up and explore areas of themselves they might not feel comfortable doing otherwise. In addition to working with individuals, counselors are also able to help families and couples create healthier home environments by working on things like conflict resolution, communication skills, and parenting techniques. Individuals can also benefit from group counseling during which they can explore a variety of issues with others who are experiencing the same stressors or problems. Counseling also provides tools that can help to address various mental disorders such as depression, anxiety, bipolar disorder, etc. Counselors are trained to recognize when clients might need medication to help them successfully navigate their emotional issues. They can make referrals to appropriate medical professionals when necessary.

Although there are many benefits to counseling, there are also risks. Counseling can be unsettling for clients since the process explores potentially uncomfortable areas. Old images and memories may surface during and after counseling sessions that may leave clients feeling emotionally dysregulated. Some of the homework assignments may be difficult to complete and may even induce fear (for example, when clients are asked to face frightening situations or objects to overcome phobias). These assignments can be difficult because they challenge the way clients are accustomed to behaving and thinking. For these reasons, all potential clients should be apprised of the risks associated with counseling during the initial assessment and in the informed consent paperwork.

Relationship Phases

At the onset of the process, the counselor and client will progress through the relationship phase, which has four specific phases. These phases may be completed at a varying pace, depending on both parties. Some phases can be completed quickly, while others may take several sessions.

- Phase 1. **Initiation**, or **entry phase**: This is the introduction to the counseling process, which sets the stage for the development of the client/counselor relationship.

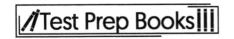

- Phase 2. **Clarification phase**: This phase defines the problem and need for the therapeutic relationship.

- Phase 3. **Structure phase**: The counselor defines the specifics of the relationship, its intended outcomes, and responsibilities of both parties.

- Phase 4. **Relationship phase**: The client and counselor have developed a relationship and will work toward mutually agreed-upon goals.

Advancement of Therapeutic Relationship and Reaching Goals

Once a working relationship is established, the client and counselor will need to develop and maintain positive interactions to ensure the effectiveness of counseling. Positive interactions ensure the therapeutic relationship advances and supports clients in meeting their goals. The counseling relationship has four stages.

- Stage 1. **Exploration of feelings and definition of problem**: Counselors will use rapport-building skills, define the structure of the counseling process and relationship, and work with their clients on goal setting.

- Stage 2. **Consolidation**: This is the process of the clients integrating the information and guidance from the counselor, allowing them to gain additional coping skills and identify alternate ways to solve problems.

- Stage 3. **Planning**: During this phase, clients can begin employing techniques learned in counseling and prepare to manage on their own.

- Stage 4. **Termination**: This is the ending of the therapeutic relationship, when clients feel equipped to manage problems independently and have fully integrated techniques learned in counseling.

Uses and Limits of Social Media

Social media has become a huge part of life for most people, so counselors must be aware of the appropriate uses of social media as well as its limitations. Some counselors may choose to promote their practices through social media. As long as their page is professional, this is a convenient and acceptable tool for marketing. For communication, it is best to provide a phone number and email address on the page rather than allowing messages through the social media page. This helps maintain confidentiality of current or future client information. Counselors may also use social media to connect with other counselors and discuss professional issues. In these instances, it is important that no personal information is shared that could reveal the identities of clients. Aliases should be used to keep specific information about cases that are being discussed from being connected to the counselor or clients. When sharing, commenting, or liking posts on social media, counselors should always be aware that clients might come across anything that is shared publicly. It is crucial to be conscious of whether these interactions and displays on social media could be harmful to clients.

Besides using social media professionally, it is likely that counselors have personal social media accounts. Some clients will want to connect with their counselors through social media, so it is best to address this during the first session. It should be explained that the policy is to never accept friend requests from clients. If this isn't explained up front, the rejection of a friend request could be

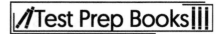

detrimental to the therapeutic relationship and to clients who are emotionally fragile. By establishing and maintaining this policy, boundaries regarding dual relationships remain intact.

Obtaining Informed Consent

The majority of state counseling boards require professional counselors to obtain informed consent from clients prior to providing services. An **informed consent** form is a document signed by both parties agreeing to provide or receive a service. Some of the main topics included on an informed consent form are the qualifications and credentials of the counselor, risks and benefits of receiving the counseling service, goal expectations, and the provider's personal philosophy of counseling. The right to terminate counseling by either party and transfer service to another provider, if applicable, should also be discussed. Confidentiality is a prominent legal aspect of informed consent. The consent form should clearly outline situations in which confidentiality cannot be honored, such as in cases of neglect, intent to harm, and abuse of vulnerable populations. Additionally, informed consent documents should include clear expectations of fees, payment methods, and cancellation policies.

In this day and age, it is common for professionals to use electronic means of communication, such as email or text. It is important that the risks associated with using these avenues are fully disclosed. Depending on the nature of the professional relationship and the needs of the individual, a treatment may necessitate audio taping, videotaping, or observation by a third party. The informed consent of the client should be obtained before any recording takes place. Some counselors will have audio and videotaping as a part of the informed consent documentation when clients begin therapy, and others will have a separate form to be used if and when the need should arise. As long as the client has signed that they understand and give consent, either way will suffice.

Assessing Competency to Provide Informed Consent

In certain instances, a client may have difficulty in fully understanding the information being presented. This could be true especially if there is a language barrier or if the person receiving services either is not fully alert or is disoriented. Appropriate measures should be taken to ensure that the person receiving services fully understands the information provided to satisfy that informed consent has been achieved. This may require utilizing a translator or a third party, such as a durable power of attorney or family member, if the person is not able to make their own decisions. In the event that a client has a conservator or power of attorney acting on their behalf, it is also the role of the counselor to ensure that this person is making decisions that coincide with the wishes of the client.

Confidentiality of Electronic Communication

Counseling is traditionally done in a face-to-face format. With the innovations in technology, virtual counseling is becoming more convenient. Some of the benefits of using technology include the ability to provide services to clients who may live in remote areas, those who do not have access to reliable transportation, and clients who are more comfortable receiving services online versus in person. One of the biggest challenges of using technology is maintaining client confidentiality. Professional counselors should be educated on the use of encryption standards that prevent unauthorized access to counseling sessions. **Encryption** is a safeguard to protect information that is being transferred online. Some common encryption methods include **Transport Layer Security (TLS)** and **OpenPGP encryption.** **OpenPGP encryption** requires a password when accessing an e-mail or data that has been transferred to a recipient.

32

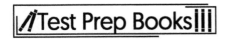
If a data breach occurs, counselors should be prepared to show the efforts taken to safeguard **electronic protected health information (ePHI)**. Counselors may choose to use e-mail services that provide a **Business Associate Agreement (BAA)**, which places the responsibility on the service should a data breach occur. The informed consent should disclose the limitations of providing services via technology. Malfunctioning equipment or connectivity issues may arise and should be discussed with the client prior to providing services. Professional boundaries must also be established, and counselors should be cautious not to display any client information on social media. The **American Counseling Association (ACA)** Code of Ethics states that professional and personal presence in the virtual world should be kept separate.

Establishing Group Rules, Expectations, and Termination Criteria

Group counseling is a method of therapy in which clients with similar needs are grouped together to help share experiences and work toward an individual goal. The counselor's decision to place a client in group therapy is based on several factors, including the client's readiness to change, needs, preferences, and the services required. The decision to place a client in group therapy should be a joint decision between the client and the counselor. Clients should never be forced to participate in group counseling. Before the client can participate in group therapy, rules and expectations should be discussed with the counselor. Counselors will benefit from having a client sign an agreement delineating rules and expectations. Some of the rules group members may be expected to adhere to are confidentiality, privacy, maintaining dignity, abstaining from violence, and regular attendance to the sessions.

Clients should clearly understand that anything said in group counseling should not be shared and no group member is required to answer questions or engage in all activities. A clear expectation of attendance should be explained to the client. Clients are encouraged to remain in group counseling until the group members jointly decide it is time for a member to terminate their group therapy. Counselors acting as group leaders can guide members in determining when a group member is ready to leave. Some of the reasons clients may terminate group counseling include progress toward achieving their goals, a reduction or elimination of their primary symptoms, and the ability to independently cope with their issue. Alternatively, if a client no longer wants to participate in group therapy, their decision to leave should be respected.

Monitoring the Therapeutic Relationship and Building Trust as Needed

Rapport building begins during the initial contact the counselor has with the client, a crucial time for establishing trust and harmony. After building rapport, the client and the counselor can begin working on client issues and continue developing the relationship on deeper levels. The relationship that the client has with the counselor is representative of the relationships the client has in other areas of life; the counselor needs to engage with the client within this framework to effect the greatest change. As the principal conduit for client change and acceptance, the counselor/client relationship is primary to the problem solving and therapy process.

A common occurrence in counseling is **transference**. Without realizing it, the client misdirects feelings about another person onto the counselor. If transference isn't recognized or the counselor doesn't explain the transference to the client, the therapeutic relationship could be damaged if the emotions that the client is feeling are negative. Being mindful of transference and working on these feelings with the client can help to maintain the therapeutic relationship and assist the client in developing appropriate approaches for interactions outside of counseling.

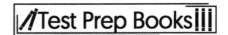

If the counselor cannot develop a positive relationship with the client, the change process is hindered. The counselor/client relationship should be based on trust, empathy, and acceptance by both parties in order to facilitate growth. Some clients may have difficulty building trust with the counselor, and the counselor may need to be patient with the client in order to make treatment goal progress. If the counselor cannot develop an appropriate trusting, empathetic, and accepting relationship with the client, the counselor should seek supervision.

In some cases, the counselor will need to transfer the client because it will be very challenging for the client to make progress if trust does not exist. Counselors should also be alert for countertransference issues in the relationship with the client and address these issues promptly if they occur.

Reviewing Client Records

While the privacy and confidentiality of the client must always be protected, with proper permission it can be beneficial for the counselor to access and view records from others who have played a significant role in the client's life and treatment. This helps to establish a more holistic view of the client and gives a comprehensive perspective of the client's strengths and difficulties. Medical records can provide information about some of the physical and medical reasons behind the client's behaviors, as well as information about the medications the client is taking. Educational and employment records can shed light on how the client functions within the milieus of school and work, providing insight into areas that may need to be addressed with the client. Employment information can also assist the counselor in determining the client's financial eligibility for services. Psychological assessments and psychiatric diagnoses can also help the counselor provide more efficient and knowledgeable treatment. Although the counselor should never depend primarily on secondhand reports, these records can provide a complete picture that may assist in effectively meeting the needs of the client.

When reviewing client records for evaluation, ethical standards must always be upheld. The NBCC Code of Ethics specifically addresses guidelines for using client information for evaluation, including:

- Protecting confidentiality to the fullest extent possible
- Accurately reporting information
- Protecting clients from harm
- Obtaining required client consent for all uses of their information (e.g., supervisory review, reimbursement)
- Making clients aware that the consent can be withdrawn without punishment

Providing Adequate Accommodations for Clients with Disabilities

Enacted by Congress, the **Americans with Disabilities Act of 1990 (ADA)** is a comprehensive civil rights legislation designed to protect individuals with disabilities from discriminatory practices, such as refusal of employment or lack of access to buildings. Disabilities covered under the act include mental and physical impairments that may limit normal activities. An individual considered a viable candidate for employment is one who can perform the necessary activities with reasonable accommodation. Consequently, the ADA requires all workplace and public entities to provide the necessary accommodations and structures for access, unless doing so places an unreasonable burden on the entity. Counselors must abide by all ADA guidelines and provide appropriate accommodations for all clients with disabilities. Additionally, besides meeting the minimum requirements per the ADA,

34

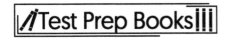

counselors should strive to make any and all additional accommodations for the comfort and ease of clients with disabilities.

Providing Information to Third Parties

Disclosure of client information will be necessary in certain instances. Some clients will require further medical treatment by a mental health provider. In order for a client to attain the best possible outcome, mental health providers will need to be informed of the assessments and interventions performed during the counseling sessions. Counseling services are often paid for by insurance companies. Basic information about the treatment, the client's diagnosis, and the frequency of counseling sessions will be necessary for billing purposes. In addition, clients may share with a counselor that they have a contagious communicable disease. If the disease is life-threatening, a counselor is justified in informing an identifiable third party of the situation. When court ordered, a counselor may reveal limited information about the client's counseling sessions that are relevant to the case. In the case of minors, each state has a minor-consent law that allows clients younger than 18 years of age to seek treatment without parental consent. Counselors should be knowledgeable about their state statutes related to counseling minors without parental knowledge. In any case where an outside agency or individual requests client records, the client must sign an informed consent agreeing to the release of their information.

Developing Reports for External Organizations

Counselors often receive requests to provide reports to the courts and other organizations that may be making decisions regarding the client's life and future. Reports must be written thoughtfully, in a professional and objective manner, and should be drawn from the counselor's notes and observations regarding the client. Reports for external organizations must provide detailed and relevant data and be clear and concise so they can be easily understood. Counselors do not need to provide information beyond what has been requested by a court order, and only in the case of a court order should information be released without the client's prior consent. Even if information must be legally released, the client should be informed of the situation and be aware that the information is being submitted to the external organization. A helpful habit for counselors is to take regular, comprehensive progress notes about visits and interactions with clients. If client records are already available, it is easier to compile a summary report with factual observations and the counselor's professional opinion.

Providing Referral Sources

Counselors frequently encounter clients who need assistance beyond the scope of the agency/counselor from whom they seek help. During assessment or throughout services, a counselor may need to refer a client to another professional for assistance. Counselors should make referrals to those resources in alignment with the best interests of the client. Agencies may also have partnerships with other local organizations that their target population would frequently access. For example, a mental health agency may have an interagency agreement or partnership with a substance abuse provider. It is also essential to discuss with the client why a referral is recommended and ensure the client is comfortable with the decision and understands next steps. When making referrals and sharing information with other providers, counselors must always obtain client consent.

The counselor must be familiar with ethical guidelines surrounding referrals and not refer out simply due to discomfort with or dislike for a client. A counselor who refers out for such personal reasons risks clients feeling abandoned, and the ACA Code of Ethics states that the needs of the clients must be put

35

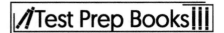

before those of the counselor. In these situations, the counselor should seek supervision and consultation regarding their personal issues. If the counselor is unable to provide appropriate care, then the client should be referred out.

Advocating for Professional and Client Issues

The **philosophy of counseling** includes the belief that counselors should encourage clients to advocate for their own needs. A counselor's duty is to intervene in the early stages of a client's problem to avoid a crisis situation in the future. Counselors may also assist clients with life's challenges, such as finances, job searches, and medical care, by facilitating phone calls or referrals to government assistance programs.

Counselors are often faced with limitations of resources and insufficient representation of the profession. Advocating for their profession involves joining organizations that can make a difference. There are various state and national organizations, such as the American Counseling Association (ACA), that encourage counselors to voice their concerns and advocate for change. Knowledge of public policy allows counselors to participate in committees that can produce changes in legislation.

Supervision

Supervision takes place when a more experienced professional mentors or coaches an emerging professional counselor in fieldwork, practical application, or other service delivery settings. This requires strong interpersonal skills, a sense of respect, and open communication between both parties. The supervisor should be able to provide supportive instruction and guidance without arrogance and condescension; the supervisee should be receptive to instruction and have an honest desire for professional growth and learning. Some commonly used models of supervision in the counseling setting include individual-oriented types of supervision, in which the supervisor may ask the supervisee to reflect upon their interactions with different clients or their personal judgments and biases that may have arisen during a session. The supervisor may also present the supervisee with different forms of research and data and ask the supervisee to utilize the evidence to structure interventions. Finally, the supervisor may provide coaching related to the supervisee's development, by establishing small objectives that lead to larger professional goals.

In peer-oriented and group-oriented approaches, lateral-level colleagues (perhaps with the aid of one or two supervisors) learn from one another by sharing clinical experiences and lessons, new research and literature, or other professional development opportunities. This may take the form of team meetings at the beginning or end of the day, social events where work can be discussed, or conference settings. In some workplaces, individual, peer, and group models may be integrated to provide a more holistic sense of supervision.

Responsibility to Seek Supervision

Sometimes it may be necessary to seek supervision if the counselor experiences burnout, secondary trauma, compassion fatigue, countertransference or the inability to develop a trusting relationship with the client. Although the focus is often on the supervisor's role of ensuring that clients are provided with ethical services by training and evaluating the supervisee, the supervisee's role in supervision is not passive. The counselor should fully engage in the process of supervision and use this relationship to grow and improve. In order to do that, the supervisee must be willing to discuss areas of ethical or legal concern that have arisen in their interactions with clients. They must also be ready to honestly address

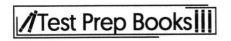

their own struggles and identify their learning needs, and seek the help and advice of the supervisor. This can only happen effectively through genuine self-assessment, which flows from a desire to become a better counselor. The process of self-assessment in supervision can help them see any biases or weaknesses that may be holding them back from fully meeting their clients' needs. If the counselor is defensive or resistant to the supervisory relationship, then they will make little progress.

Factors to consider when receiving feedback during supervision/consultation:

- Counselors can benefit from feedback during supervision or consultation, especially with difficult clients/cases or at significant times in treatment, such as termination.

- When discussing cases, client confidentiality should be protected as much as possible, and client consent to release information should be acquired.

Creating and Maintaining Documentation Throughout the Counseling Process

Purposes of Documentation

Accurate case recording is an integral part of counseling. Keeping accurate client records has many purposes, such as documenting the history and treatment of a client, getting insurance reimbursement, providing counselors a historical account of client sessions, and protecting confidentiality. There are numerous reasons for keeping thorough documentation throughout the counseling process:

- The information contained in a client record can be used to evaluate the effectiveness of services.

- Counseling records serve as a reference for reviewing the client's plan of care and measuring goal achievement. Throughout the course of therapy, counselors may need to refer back to the treatment plan to facilitate interventions. Client records, when combined with other evaluation tools (e.g., client satisfaction surveys, reactions to treatments, accomplishments of goals), can be an effective method of evaluating treatment progress.

- Counselors should record and review any notes pertaining to client behaviors that indicate any chance of clients becoming suicidal or homicidal. These clients will require crisis intervention from other professionals, and their records will need to be reviewed.

- Supervisors may review client records to evaluate the effectiveness of the treatment process, counselor performance, and client progress, or to ensure documentation is being completed accurately and on time.

- Counselors who decide to introduce new techniques, such as group or family counseling, will need to revisit the client's consent and revise the treatment modalities. Clients will need to consent to any amendments indicating a change in therapy techniques.

- Records also provide other counselors with information for continuity of care should the original counselor not be able to continue the sessions.

Litigation and Reimbursement

Accurate case recording is also required to protect the agency from possible legal ramifications and to ensure reimbursement from funders. Counselors must adhere to any state or federal legal requirements

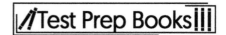
related to storage, disclosure of information, release of client records, and confidential information. Client records should be kept up-to-date, objective, and completed as soon as possible to ensure accuracy of information. Counselors should assume it is always possible that records may be requested as part of legal proceedings. In litigation, the client records will be reviewed by lawyers, and any applicable information will be admitted as evidence during court. Treatment notes should always be clearly written and only include information necessary to the client's treatment to protect confidentiality as much as possible. Because client records are confidential, clients need to sign an informed consent form permitting the access of records by any third party.

Client Reports

Elements of client reports may include developmental history, family history, substance use information, medical history, presenting problem, and recommendations. There are a variety of elements of client reports that may be required by the agency. With the advent of electronic records, client reports are often built into the software that the agency uses. Client reports may also be in **DAP** (data, assessment, plan) format or in the model of **SOAP notes** (subjective, objective, assessment, and plan). Reports are at the agency's discretion, and the counselor should use the format that is required by the agency to develop client reports.

Contracts

As part of the intake process, counselors may wish to develop and agree upon a contract with the client. **Contracts** outline goals and responsibilities of both parties and may help to alleviate potential miscommunication. Important components of a contract include an outline of the service being provided, a description of the counselor's qualifications, and any explanation of the scope of practice. A clause outlining client rights and confidentiality should be included. Lastly, the counselor may wish to include specifics about session time, fees, and consequences of a client being late, missing, or canceling sessions. Contracts can serve to empower clients by clarifying service and allowing clients to take an active role in their therapeutic care. They may also be flexible, allowing either party to modify the contract as needed.

Writing and Maintaining Client Records

Counselors must document their practice with the client. Counselors document sessions with clients as well as client legal mandates, such as visitation with minors in state custody. Documentation may be a combination of narrative and quantitative descriptions, depending on agency requirements. Records should be kept confidential either electronically or in a physical location. New laws require that all records be electronic, and they are called electronic health records. These records must be confidential as stated in the **Health Insurance Portability and Accountability Act of 1996 (HIPAA)**. It is crucial for the counselor to maintain accurate documentation.

Note-Taking Styles

During the assessment and treatment processes, the information from both the subjective and objective data is combined to formulate a concise, yet comprehensive, assessment for the client. In some note-taking practices, the identification of the subjective and objective data along with assessment formation is required. This style of documentation is known as the ***SOAP method***, an acronym that stands for Subjective, Objective, Assessment, and Plan. Another note-taking style that focuses on the subjective and objective data is the BIRP documentation method. ***BIRP*** stands for Behavior, Intervention, Response, and Plan. It is not as commonly used as SOAP.

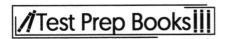

Organization and Storage of Client Information

Organization and storage of client information varies greatly depending on the counselor, the institution, and the requirements of any external funding sources. Information may be stored electronically in online systems or on paper. Important components of information in counseling include: intake forms; personal, medical, and demographic information; assessments and reviews; any diagnoses, intervention, and treatment outlines with measurable goals; and discharge plans or paperwork. Since this is all highly sensitive and confidential information, counselors should be mindful to keep all information updated, accurate, and stored securely.

Awareness and Practice of Self-Care

Due to the highly emotional, interpersonal, and empathic demands of the counseling field, counselors must employ and sustain self-care practices to protect their personal health. Without self-care, counselors are highly susceptible to burnout and compassion fatigue—two risks that occur when working in a field that often provides exposure to disheartening humanitarian situations, abusive intrapersonal relationships, and cases that, for bureaucratic or personal reasons, take a long time to resolve. Unchecked, these experiences can lead the counselor to feel detached from work and hopeless toward cases or to consistently experience the ill effects of chronic stress.

Burnout Symptoms

At times, counselors may experience a sense of disinterest or disengagement from their work, which may signal burnout. Symptoms of burnout can include physical symptoms, such as fatigue, headaches, insomnia, and decreased resistance to illness. Emotional symptoms can include depression, anxiety, boredom, lack of empathy, cynicism, and anger. **Burnout** may be a result of overworking and/or providing service to clients who are not progressing in therapy, thus causing counselors to feel incompetent and ineffective. It is important to know the warning signs of burnout and engage in self-care, which may involve taking a vacation; getting increased supervision or therapy; making changes to one's hours, fees, or practice; or seeking continuing education options.

Self-Care Practices

Self-care practices may include establishing boundaries between one's work and personal life, having a regular meditation practice or other mental exercises that are shown to soothe the nervous system, eating a healthy diet and engaging in regular physical exercise (as these behaviors decrease inflammation in the body and reduce stress hormones), and having a trustworthy support system of friends and colleagues. Introspective exercises, such as daily journaling, can provide the counselor with a better understanding of which activities bring stress to their lives and which activities bring peace. By knowing these, the counselor can bridge the gap to reduce stress in areas they can control, such as setting a clear cut-off time for answering emails or scheduling personal activities that bring them joy. They can adopt healthy coping mechanisms for the areas in which they are unable to control factors that might contribute to their stress, such as an emotional case or external funding issues.

Caseload Management

A **caseload** refers to the number of clients that are assigned to a particular counselor. Managing heavy caseloads can be a challenge for counselors, as it means balancing the needs of many clients with limited time and resources. This may result in poorer quality of services, which directly impacts the client system, and can lead to exhaustion and burnout for the counselor. When possible, a counselor's caseload should be minimized so that more comprehensive services are provided for each client.

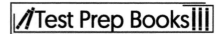

Unfortunately, there are various and complicated reasons that often contribute to higher caseloads in counselor organizations, such as financial restrictions, understaffing, and high numbers of clients. When large caseloads are unavoidable, then counselors must use other strategies to minimize stress and optimize services, including effective time management and more frequent referrals to other providers who can help meet the various needs of the clients. Additionally, it is important for counselors to prioritize client systems according to the complexity of their needs. Balanced and well-managed workloads, although difficult to achieve, can make a significant difference in the level of services provided to client systems and will result in better overall outcomes.

Impairment

Impairment is a professional issue that should be addressed swiftly. Impairment occurs when a counselor's personal problems (e.g., mental health conditions, difficult life circumstances, or alcohol/drug use) have an impact upon their practice. The Code of Ethics states that counselors should seek to rectify their impairment by consulting with colleagues or supervisors, seeking their own treatment, limiting work, and/or terminating client relationships until the impairment has been fully addressed.

Intake, Assessment, and Diagnosis

Biopsychosocial Interview

Interplay of Biological, Psychological, Social, and Spiritual Factors

The **biopsychosocial model** (developed by **George Engle**) incorporates more factors than the traditional biomedical model of illness, which attributed causation only to biological factors, disregarding any other influences. This model posits that health and illness result from the interplay between biological, psychological, and social factors:

- **Biological Factors**: Genetics and other biological factors play a substantial role in human development. Examples of these factors are physical features, such as height, weight, or degree of attractiveness. Is the person healthy or disabled? Can he or she walk, talk, see, and hear? While most believe that others should not be judged by physical appearance, studies show that healthy, attractive, fit persons have certain advantages in life. More people will be attracted to these individuals, which creates an expanded circle of friends and eligible partners. In general, being disabled restricts social, educational, and vocational opportunities.

- **Psychological Factors**: Psychological factors encompass a wide range of symptoms and conditions. These can range from a diagnosis of schizophrenia to mild social anxiety. Many psychological factors can directly impact biological ones and vice versa. Depression may cause insomnia. Anxiety can cause gastrointestinal distress. Anorexia causes restricted food intake to the point of starvation. Chronic pain can cause irritability, anger, depression, and social withdrawal.

- **Social Factors**: Social factors are intimately intertwined with both biological and psychological factors. These are developed in response to the social institutions and influences that one is exposed to. These can include family, school, religious organizations, government, and neighborhoods. The media contributes to people's social context, telling them what is desirable, what is undesirable, and what they need in their lives to be happy. Media influences attitudes about sexuality, violence, consumption of goods, the government, and the way people treat one another. Experiences are based on interpretation, and interpretation is influenced by social context.

In Western culture, particularly in medicine, psychology, and counseling, it is commonly accepted that the interaction of the aforementioned factors determines health outcomes. An individual's health status, their perceptions of and beliefs about health, and their barriers to accessing healthcare exert a combined influence on the likelihood of that individual engaging in healthy behaviors, such as exercising, getting physical exams, or eating well-balanced meals.

For counselors, the biopsychosocial model is helpful in understanding why some individuals are more likely to develop mental health problems. This perspective is also helpful in fighting the stigmatization of mental illness because it promotes the understanding that anyone can develop mental health problems if there is a disruption to the balance of biological, psychological, or social influences. In counseling, this perspective is often expanded and referred to as the **biopsychosocial-spiritual perspective**—the idea that one must also consider the ways in which individuals find meaning in their lives.

41

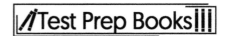

Indicators of Biopsychosocial Stress

Stress can manifest itself in different forms and may result from a threat to the client's functioning, both real and imagined. Some common factors contributing to biopsychosocial stress are natural disasters and disruption of relationships (divorce, death, break-ups, or moving). Other events, such as childhood abuse, bullying, sexual abuse, problems at work, and worries about physical health, may compound or contribute to biopsychosocial stress and manifest in the following symptoms:

- Cognitive
  - Difficulty concentrating
  - Poor memory
  - Anxiousness and worrying
- Emotional
  - Excessive tearfulness
  - Agitation
  - Irritability
  - Feelings of loneliness
  - Depression
  - Unstable moods
  - Feelings of detachment
- Physical
  - Abnormal weight loss or gain
  - Swelling and aches from stiff muscles
  - Digestive problems (nausea, diarrhea, constipation)
  - Insomnia
  - Heart palpitations
  - Chest pain
  - Feelings of being short of breath
  - Breakouts (hives, acne, eczema)
  - Frequent minor illness (colds, headaches)
  - Fatigue
- Behaviors
  - Decreased appetite
  - Withdrawal from preferred activities
  - Nail biting, pacing, pulling of hair, other nervous "tics"
  - Hyperactivity to avoid problems, such as too much exercise
  - Increased aggression

Obtaining Biological, Psychological, Social, and Spiritual Histories

In order for an assessment to be comprehensive, the counselor must gather information and assess the individual holistically, which includes examining systems related to the biological, psychological, and social or sociocultural factors of functioning. In some cases, a spiritual component may be included. This process is based on the **biopsychosocial framework**, which describes the interaction between biological,

42

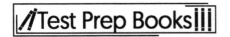
psychological, and social factors. The key components of the biopsychosocial assessment can be broken down into identification, chief complaint, social/environmental issues, history, and mental status exam:

- Identification: Identification consists of the details or demographic information about the client that can be seen with the eye and documented accordingly. Some examples of identification information are age, gender, height, weight, and clothing.

- Chief Complaint: A chief complaint is the client's version of what the overarching problem is. The client's description of the chief complaint may include factors from the past that the client views as an obstacle to optimal functioning. It could also be an issue that was previously resolved but reoccurs, thus requiring the client to develop additional coping skills.

- Social/Environmental Issues: The social and environmental issue component evaluates social development and physical settings. **Social development** is critical to understanding the types of support systems the client has and includes information about the client's primary family group, including parents, siblings, and extended family members. The client's peers and social networks should also be examined. There should be a clear distinction between peers available online (such as through online social networks) and peers the client interacts with face-to-face, as online systems may provide different forms of support than in-person systems. The client's work environment and school or vocational settings should also be noted in this portion of the assessment. The client's current housing situation and view of financial status are also included to determine the type of resources the client has. Legal issues may also be included.

- History: The history component includes events in the client's past. Clients may need to be interviewed several times in order to get a thorough picture of their history. Some information in a client's history, such as events that occurred during the stages of infancy and early childhood, may need to be gathered from collateral sources. Obtaining the client's historical information is usually a multi-stage process and can involve the following methods of data collection:

    o Presenting Problem: Clients should be asked to describe what brings them in for treatment. Although a client may attempt to delve into information that is well in the past, the counselor should redirect the client to emphasize the past week or two. Emphasis is placed on the client's current situation when assessing the presenting problem.

    o Past Personal: When reviewing a client's history, noting biological development may determine whether or not the client hit milestones and the ensuing impact it had on their health. In reviewing biological development, other physical factors should also be assessed for impact on current emotional wellbeing, including those that may no longer persist, like a childhood illness. As much information as possible regarding the client's entire lifespan (birth to present) should be gathered, with attention paid to sexual development.

    o Medical: During the medical component of the assessment process, information should be obtained on the client's previous or current physiological diagnoses. These diagnoses can contribute to the client's current situation. For example, a client with frequent headaches and back pain may be unable to sleep well and therefore may be

43

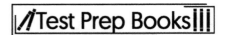

experiencing the physical and psychosocial effects of sleep deprivation. Additional information on other conditions, such as pregnancy, surgeries, or disabilities, should also be explored during this time.

- o Mental Health: Previous mental health diagnoses, symptoms, and/or evaluations should be discussed. If a client discloses prior diagnoses or evaluations, the counselor should determine the following:

    - Whether or not the client has been hospitalized (inpatient)

    - If the client has received supervised treatment in an outpatient setting (to include psychotherapeutic intervention)

    - Whether the client has been prescribed medications

    - If the client has undertaken other treatments related to mental health diagnoses

    - The client's psychological development should also be reviewed. It is important to gather details on how clients view their emotional development, including their general affect.

    - The client's cognitive development, in relation to information previously obtained regarding the biological development, should also be reviewed.

- o Substance Use:

    - Without demonstrating judgment, counselors should encourage clients to disclose whether or not they have used controlled substances. It is important that thorough information is gathered and symptoms related to substance abuse are assessed BEFORE rendering a primary mental health disorder diagnosis.

    - Should a client disclose that they have engaged in the use of substances, information as to the type of substance, frequency of use, and duration of exposure to the lifestyle should be gathered. Additionally, information on what the client perceives as the positive and negative aspects of substance use should be gathered, noting whether or not the client perceives any consequences of substance abuse, such as job loss, decreased contact with family and friends, and effects on physical appearance.

- Mental Status Exam: A mental status exam is a concise, complete evaluation of the client's current mental functioning level regarding **cognitive and behavioral aspects** (rapport-building, mood, thought content, hygiene). There are mini mental status examinations available that allow counselors to provide a snapshot of the client's overall level of functioning with limited resources and time available. Mental status examinations are usually conducted regularly and discreetly through questioning and noting nonverbal indicators (such as appearance) in order for the counselor to best guide the session.

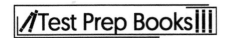

Diagnostic Interview

During the **diagnostic interview** the counselor gathers information in order to make a diagnosis. A combination of data is used, such as the client's developmental and medical histories; results from questionnaires, behavior rating scales, and an **MSE (mental status exam)**; and a list of the client's symptoms. These factors are then used to formulate a diagnosis based on the **DSM-5**. To obtain all of the necessary details from the client, questions can be structured or unstructured. Structured questions will include items from questionnaires and established checklists, such as the HAM-D, used to diagnose mental health disorders. To gain further insight into a client's problem, a more unstructured approach can be used. This could involve discussing the patient's history, asking questions about the client's support system, and inquiring about issues such as sleep habits, concentration, or appetite. The unstructured questions can be open-ended, allowing for more facts to be obtained about the client.

In order to use the client's symptoms to make a diagnosis, the counselor should be familiar with symptoms commonly found in mental and emotional illnesses. Mental and emotional illness can present in a number of ways and vary depending on the illness, the person, and the circumstances. Some symptoms of mental and emotional illness include:

- Chronic feelings of sadness
- Inability to focus
- Extreme mood variation
- Loss of interest in activities one used to enjoy
- Lack of sexual interest or desire
- Intense, and sometimes unexplainable, feelings of guilt, shame, regret, fear, or worry
- Chronic fatigue
- Sleep problems, such as insomnia or sleeping too much
- Feeling overwhelmed by daily routines or tasks
- Substance abuse
- Compulsive or obsessive thoughts or behaviors
- Hallucination
- Thoughts of suicide
- Thoughts of harming oneself or others
- Excessive weight gain or weight loss
- Unexplained anger or irritability
- Detachment from loved ones
- Medically unexplained physical symptoms (psychosomatic) such as headaches, jaw pain, stomach pain, or joint stiffness.

Cultural Formulation Interview

Culture

Cultural context is an essential factor when diagnosing, assessing, or treating individuals with mental illness. **Culture** is defined as the systems of knowledge, concepts, rules, and practices that are learned and passed on throughout generations. Culture is often used as an umbrella-term that encapsulates language, religion/spirituality, family structures, life-cycle stages, ceremonies, customs, and both moral and legal systems. Cultures are considered to be dynamic networks because they change so much over time. Individuals, more often than not, experience different cultures intersecting at once which allows

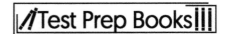

them to gain a more specific understanding of their own identity. This conceptualization of identity then leads to the formation of other beliefs that extend to other areas of life such as relationships, career choices, and education. Due to the importance of culture and how it interacts with our experience as human beings, it is imperative for counselors to evaluate cultural factors when working with people in their practices and not fall into stereotypic or generalizable thinking.

Culture also includes the concepts of race and ethnicity, which are commonly mistaken to be the same thing. Race is a category of identity that differentiates individuals based on physical traits and biological characteristics. Racial categories vary across cultural societies. On a social basis, **race** is a construct that serves as a catalyst for racism, discrimination, and isolation. Existing empirical evidence demonstrates how racism can worsen the effects of mental disorders and racial biases impact diagnostic psychological assessment. Racial minorities are subject to these realities outside of clinical settings, so proper education and cultural competency is required in counselors in order to not emulate these concepts within the therapeutic relationship.

Ethnicity specifies an individual's community or group. They can exist across a common historical, geographical, linguistic, or religious domain. Ethnicity is able to be self-assigned or attributed by other people. In the essence of culture, ethnicities have evolved to intersect and introduce new variations of ethnic identities.

DSM-5 Cultural Formulation Interview
How individuals think about their symptoms or mental illness is greatly influenced by their cultural context. The **Cultural Formulation Interview (CFI)** is designed to evaluate these perspectives in order to gain a comprehensive understanding of the individual's specific experience. It consists of a set of sixteen questions that are typically asked when first meeting a new client during an initial interview. The CFI covers four domains of cultural assessment: cultural definition of the problem; cultural perceptions of cause, context, and support; cultural factors affecting self-coping; and past help seeking.

When obtaining cultural information about the client, counselors should do so in an inviting and welcoming manner. The CFI emulates a person-centered process, meaning that counselors encourage clients to explore their thought processes and experience. By using this approach, the diagnostic assessment becomes more valid and the individual becomes more engaged in the process. Stereotypic thinking is also controlled for as much as possible by this interview because counselors have the ability to understand how the client's particular culture affects their clinical presentation. Other variations of the CFI have been developed in order to assess certain populations such as children and adolescents, the elderly, immigrants, and refugees.

The CFI is such a vital part of diagnostic assessment as it provides extraordinary emphasis on the way mental illness is perceived through a cultural lens. Level of distress, one of the main indicators of psychological illness, can vary in the way it is expressed from culture to culture in how it is communicated (if at all), understood, or felt. A specific psychological experience that is shared among individuals in certain cultural groups, known as a cultural syndrome, may be presented through the CFI. Additionally, cultural idioms of distress and cultural explanations are able to be highlighted and understood through the process of the CFI. Culture will always affect the way in which mental illness presents. By extracting information about the client's experience in this context, counselors can avoid misdiagnosis, obtain useful clinical information, improve rapport and client engagement, guide clinical research, and possibly clarify cultural epidemiology.

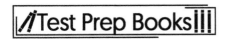

Initial Interview

Interviews are a critical component of counseling wherein clients provide verbal reports, accounts, or narratives that serve as the main source of information and data collected during the assessment process. The basis of the interview is a verbal report that involves introductions between the counselor and client. In some practice settings, the verbal report may be supplemented by an **information sheet** that provides client demographics and a brief overview of the **presenting problem**. Presenting problems are prevailing circumstances, symptoms, or difficulties that the client believes is a problem requiring psychotherapeutic assistance.

Establishing Rapport with the Client

Providing a description of the services provided and what the client can expect during sessions is the counselor's first opportunity to build rapport with the client. Rapport development impacts the thoroughness of the information provided from the client. If the level of rapport is limited, the client may not feel comfortable enough to provide sufficient information. The level of rapport also affects the type of impression the client wishes to make on the counselor. Consequently, it is linked to the client's perception of self-awareness. Some key points to remember are as follows:

- The counselor's own personal characteristics (gender, race, age, etc.) may affect the level of client interaction, based on the client's cultural background.

- Clients may adjust their responses to questions based on how they perceive the counselor's characteristics.

- The counselor's demographics may also have an impact on how the client feels about disclosing sensitive information, such as domestic violence, sexual conduct, or child abuse.

Starting Where the Client is

Once the introductions have been made and an overview of services and interview processes provided, the client should be asked to explain why they came in for treatment. Empowering clients to share their concerns and emphasizing the point of hearing things from their perspective provides the counselor with an opportunity to gauge a client and start "where the client is" in the initial phases of the assessment process. The use of encouraging, neutral phrases will help move the conversation forward and encourage the client to share, e.g., "What brings you in to see me today?" While being encouraging to the client, it is important that counselors are genuine and not phony. Counselors should avoid overly complimentary statements, such as "I'm so glad you came in today!" If the client senses the interest is insincere, they may not wish to share. After engaging the client, they should be allowed to open up, "vent," or speak freely for approximately fifteen minutes.

While the client is delving into any emotions, the counselor should utilize active listening to keep the client engaged. Additionally, it is important to observe the client's **nonverbal cues** (posture, gestures, voice tone and pitch, and facial expressions) that lend to the emotional state. Once the client shares primary concerns, the counselor can focus on what is important to the client. The counselor should observe the client's emotional state, allowing them to feel those emotions freely while providing the account of the problem. Demonstrating empathy is important when responding to the client's emotions. The emotion observed should be acknowledged. For example, if a client is crying, the counselor can state, "You seem saddened about this," to demonstrate empathy. This practice can also hone in on an important area of the client's life that may be addressed later.

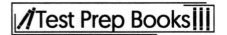
Exploratory Interviewing

Once the client has been allowed to speak freely, the counselor should utilize exploratory interviewing skills to delve into the specifics of topics that seemed particularly troubling for the client during the disclosure of the presenting problem. After the client has revealed the presenting problem and the emotional state has been observed, the client should be asked to delve further into details about current life circumstances. This will provide an opportunity for the counselor to gain additional information related to the context of the client's problem. It also allows the counselor to uncover particularly troubling areas that can be explored later. Moreover, it may reveal certain boundaries for the client who is unwilling or unready to discuss certain details of their life.

Questioning

The counselor should ask questions to provide clarification and deeper insight into the client's problems and level of functioning. Open-ended questions may provide more detail and allow the client to expand into other areas that can be explored later. Closed-ended questions are ideal for fact-finding from a client. Clarification questions should be asked whenever necessary. This may be done through active listening and reflective sharing on the counselor's part, to foster comprehensive communication and further build rapport.

Observation

Observation of client behaviors during the interview may be indicative of how the client behaves or reacts in settings outside of the session. Conversely, clients may act outside of their norm, due to the perceived pressure from the interview process. The aforementioned questions and nonverbal observations are essential to determine factors of the client's personality and the context of presenting issues. Counselors should also be aware that their interactions affect client behaviors and responses during the interview process. For example, the client may mimic rigid body language (folded arms, crossed legs, minimal eye contact) from the counselor and become defensive in speech pattern, pitch, or tone.

Note-Taking of Subjective and Objective Data

Both objective and subjective data are used during the assessment and treatment processes. The client provides their perspective on what happened and the correlated feelings and experiences felt, which is the **subjective data**. Subsequently, the counselor uses the information and may ask finding questions to better understand where the client is emotionally, while teasing out facts related to the client's situation. These facts are **objective data**. If the client has questions as to why notes are taken, the reasoning behind it should be explained, and a copy should be offered to the client to make them feel more comfortable and involved in the interview process.

Determining Diagnosis

Normal vs. Abnormal Behavior

Normal versus abnormal behavior is difficult to distinguish because each person is unique, so creating a standard of normal can be challenging. Though labeling behaviors as normal or abnormal can be problematic, it is important to have some standard by which it is possible to identify those behaviors that are indicative of an underlying psychological condition. Notwithstanding the challenges, it is possible and helpful to have general definitions of normal and abnormal behavior.

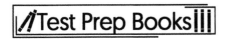

Normal behaviors are those that are common to the majority of the population, as related to emotional functioning, social interactions, and mental capacity. **Abnormal behavior** is considered that which is maladaptive, dysfunctional, and disruptive to life. These behaviors may be an exaggeration of a normal behavior or even an absence of a typical response. They do not conform to the accepted patterns or common behaviors of society. Sadness over the death of a loved one is considered normal but disabling depression that interferes with school and work responsibilities is not. The **DSM-5** is the current standard for determining the diagnostic criteria that distinguishes abnormal behavior from normal.

Four Ds of Abnormality

The **"Four Ds" of Abnormality** assist counselors when trying to identify a psychiatric condition in their clients. Deviance marks a withdrawal from society's concept of appropriate behavior. **Deviant behavior** is a departure from the "norm." The *DSM-5* contains some criteria for diagnosing deviance. The second "D" is dysfunction. **Dysfunction** is behavior that interferes with daily living. Dysfunction is a type of problem that may be serious enough to be considered a disorder. The third "D" is distress. **Distress** is related to a client's dysfunction. That is, to what degree does the dysfunction cause the client distress? A client can experience minor dysfunction and major distress, or major dysfunction and minor distress. The fourth "D" is danger. **Danger** is characterized by danger to self or to others. There are different degrees of danger specific to various types of disorders. **Duration** is sometimes considered a fifth "D," as it may be important to note whether the symptoms of a disorder are fleeting or permanent.

DSM-5

The current **Diagnostic and Statistical Manual of the American Psychiatric Association** (APA) utilized for the classification of mental disorders is the *DSM-5*. It is an update to the APA's previous classification and diagnostic tool from 2013, the **DSM-IV-TR**. The **DSM-5** serves as an authority for psychiatric/mental health diagnosis and functions as a tool for counselors to make treatment recommendations. The *DSM-5* is organized in accordance with the developmental lifespan.

While the *DSM-5* provides classifications and symptoms of mental disorders, causation is not discussed. There are several notable changes to the *DSM-5*:

- The exclusion of Asperger syndrome as a distinct disorder on the autism spectrum

- The loss of some subtype variations for schizophrenia

- The renaming of gender identity disorder to gender dysphoria

- The restructuring of criterion for posttraumatic stress disorder (PTSD) to incorporate application to combat veterans and first responders

- The omission of the bereavement exclusion for depressive disorders

The chapters in the DSM-5 are as follow:

- Neurodevelopmental Disorders
- Schizophrenia Spectrum and other Psychotic Disorders
- Bipolar and Related Disorders
- Depressive Disorders
- Anxiety Disorders

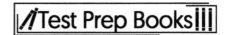
- Obsessive Compulsive and Related Disorders
- Trauma and Stressor Related Disorders
- Dissociative Disorders
- Somatic Symptom Disorders
- Feeding and Eating Disorders
- Elimination Disorders
- Sleep-Wake Disorders
- Sexual Dysfunctions
- Gender Dysphoria
- Disruptive, Impulse Control and Conduct Disorders
- Substance Use and Addictive Disorders
- Neurocognitive Disorders
- Paraphilic Disorders
- Other Disorders

Neurodevelopmental Disorders
Intellectual Disability/Development Disorder
Intellectual disabilities are described in the DSM-5 as neurodevelopmental disorders starting in childhood and are characterized by intellectual difficulties as well as difficulties in several other domains of life, which include conceptual, social, and practical areas. The conceptual domain includes reasoning, memory, knowledge, and language skills. The social domain describes empathy, social judgment, and overall interpersonal skills. The practical domain focuses on areas such as personal self-care, professional responsibilities, and money management skills.

The DSM-5 diagnosis emphasizes the need to meet three criteria:

- Deficits in intellectual functioning that are confirmed by clinical evaluation and standard IQ tests

- Deficits in adaptive functioning that preclude the ability to conform to the standards necessary for independent functioning

- The onset of these deficits in childhood

The fifth edition of the DSM allows for a more comprehensive overview of the individual than the fourth. Intellectual developmental disorder replaces mental retardation in previous editions of the manuals. The substantial changes address the name of the disorder, how it impacts one's overall level of functioning, and improvements to diagnostic criteria to foster more comprehensive patient evaluation. In the DSM-5, all mental disorders will be on a single axis and allotted equal importance.

Communication Disorders
Diagnostic categories in the DSM-5 for **communication disorders** include the following:

- Language disorder
- Speech sound disorder
- Childhood-onset fluency disorder (or stuttering)
- Social (pragmatic) communication disorder
- Unspecified communication disorder

50

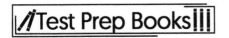

The diagnostic criteria for **language disorder** include an ongoing difficulty and deficit in language acquisition and production, whether written or spoken. Language abilities are also substantially lower than expected for one's age. The diagnostic criteria for **speech sound disorder** include consistent trouble with sound production and a difficulty in verbally communicating coherent, intelligent speech. The diagnostic criteria for **childhood-onset fluency disorder** (or stuttering) are a disruption in fluent and temporal speech patterns and that the interferences are caused by an initial fear of communicating with others. The diagnostic criteria for **social (pragmatic) communication disorder (SCD)** include ongoing troubles with verbal and nonverbal communication such as deficits in interpersonal interactions, a mismatch between a conversation and the context in which it occurs, difficulties in following the rules of interpersonal discussions, and difficulties understanding direct yet abstract use of language. However, autism spectrum disorder is considered exclusionary criterion for this disorder. **Unspecified communication disorder** has no specific description, since symptoms do not meet criteria for any of the other listed disorders; however, this diagnosis is applied when the presence of a communication disorder is suspected.

Autism Spectrum Disorders

Individuals diagnosed with **autism spectrum disorder (ASD)** typically have communication deficits. They are sometimes unable to respond appropriately in conversations, misread nonverbal interactions, have difficulty developing age-appropriate friendships, are extremely dependent upon routines, are unusually sensitive to environmental changes, or are deeply focused on particular items. People previously diagnosed with a well-documented DSM-IV diagnosis of autistic disorder, Asperger's disorder, or pervasive developmental disorder not otherwise specified, should be included under the umbrella diagnosis of autism spectrum disorder. Those who have clear and obvious interpersonal communication deficits, but with symptoms not meeting the criteria for autism spectrum disorder, should be further evaluated for social communication disorder.

Attention-Deficit/Hyperactivity Disorder

Attention-deficit/hyperactivity disorder (ADHD) describes a continual pattern of inattention and hyperactivity that disrupts a person's functioning and overall growth and development. The criteria for ADHD consist of six or more symptoms related to inattention and hyperactivity up until age sixteen, or five or more for those up to age seventeen, that are present for upwards of six months and are inappropriate for one's level of development. The symptoms for inattention consist of not paying close attention to detail, difficulty holding attention for a task, not following through on instructions, trouble organizing, reluctance to putting in mental effort on long-term tasks, losing things often, getting easily distracted, and being forgetful. For impulsivity, the symptoms consist of fidgeting, trouble sitting still, restlessness, struggling to stay quiet, always on the go, excessive talking, answering incomplete questions, difficulty waiting their turn, and often intruding on others. In addition to these criteria, other conditions that must be met include several inattentive and hyperactive symptoms occurring before the age of twelve and in two or more settings. The symptoms interfere with daily functioning and the symptoms aren't better explained by another psychiatric disorder.

The three types of presentations that can occur with ADHD are combined presentation, predominantly inattentive presentation, and predominantly hyperactive-impulsive presentation. **Combined presentation** is provided in the event that enough symptoms related to both inattention and hyperactivity-impulsivity have occurred in the past six months. **Predominantly inattentive presentation** is provided if enough symptoms related to inattention occurred over the past six months, but hyperactivity-impulsivity symptoms were not present. **Predominantly hyperactive-impulsive**

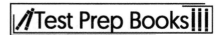

presentation is provided if symptoms of hyperactivity-impulsivity occurred over six months, but symptoms of inattention were not present. A difference between ADHD in the DSM-IV and the DSM-5 is that in the former diagnostic manual, the age of onset was originally at the age of seven, not twelve.

Specific Learning Disorder

A **specific learning disorder (SLD)** is described as a neurodevelopmental disorder that interferes with a person's capacity to learn or use specific skills such as reading, writing, or arithmetic. These skills are regarded as the foundation for academic learning as a whole. SLD isn't synonymous with learning disability as defined by the educational system; however, those with a DSM-5 diagnosis of SLD would be required to also meet the criteria for learning disability set by the educational system.

The DSM-5 diagnostic criteria for SLD include one category of SLD with *specifiers* to illustrate the specific displays of learning difficulties during an evaluation within the three aforementioned major academic domains, and the exclusion of the IQ-achievement discrepancy requirement, which is replaced with four criteria that must be met. **Criterion A** describes that at least one of six symptoms related to learning difficulties have continued for upwards of six months despite receiving additional assistance. **Criterion B** describes the measurement of the affected academic skills being significantly lower than those expected for age five and result in a dysfunction in academic, professional, or daily activities. **Criterion C** describes the age of onset when the problems started occurring, usually during school years or adulthood in some cases, and **Criterion D** specifies which other psychiatric or neurological disorders must be ruled out before a diagnosis of SLD can be substantiated and rendered.

Motor Disorders

In the DSM-5, motor disorders refer to nervous system disorders resulting in abnormal or involuntary movements. These disorders include developmental coordination disorder, stereotypic movement disorder, and tic disorder. **Developmental coordination disorder** (or **dyspraxia**) is a long-term neurological disorder starting in childhood that affects planning of bodily movement and coordination due to brain messages not being accurately transmitted to the body. Impairments in skilled motor movements per a child's chronological age interfere with activities of daily living. The diagnostic criteria for dyspraxia consist of below average coordinated motor skills, persistent interference in daily activities, onset of symptoms in early development, and motor skill deficits that aren't better explained by an intellectual disability. **Stereotypic movement disorder** describes motor behavior that is often repetitive and purposeless, such as hitting, rocking, and shaking oneself. The age of onset is early development. **Tic disorder** describes rapid, sudden, and nonrhythmic movements. The DSM-5 classifies Tourette syndrome and tic disorders as motor disorders under the neurodevelopmental disorder category.

Schizophrenia Spectrum and Other Psychotic Disorders

Schizophrenia is a severe and long-term mental illness typified by symptoms involving disturbances in behavior, perception, and thought that are adversely affecting social or occupational functioning. The DSM-5 outlines five key features of psychotic disorders, which include delusions, hallucinations, disorganized speech, disorganized or catatonic behavior, and negative symptoms. In the DSM-IV, two out of these five symptoms were required to render a diagnosis, though counselors only required one of five symptoms if an individual suffered from bizarre delusions, if hallucinations entailed a running description of their thoughts or behavior, and/or auditory hallucinations involved two or more voices. However, due to poor reliability and in general being too broad, this exception was removed.

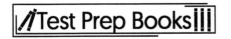

In the current edition of the DSM, diagnosis only requires two of these five symptoms, with at least one symptom being one of the first three criteria. But the most significant change to this diagnostic category is removing subtypes (catatonic, disorganized, paranoid, residual, and undifferentiated). The reasons for doing this have to do with these subtypes not being considered stable conditions, not having any real clinical usefulness, and not having any scientific validity or reliability. However, a catatonic specifier is included and may be used with other psychotic disorders. **Catatonia** can occur across several diagnostic categories without necessarily indicating psychosis. With **schizoaffective disorder**, which creates a connection between mood and psychosis, any mood episode persists throughout the majority of the illness. This change was to help improve the reliability, stability, and validity of the disorder. For **delusional disorder**, the requirement that delusions only be non-bizarre has been eliminated, while a 'bizarre-type' delusion specifier is present. However, shared delusional disorder no longer remains a separate disorder, for it simply exists under the umbrella term of delusional disorder.

Clinician-Rated Dimensions of Psychosis Symptom Severity

Dimensional measures are used by counselors in order to assess the severity and course of mental illness. The clinician-rated dimensions of psychosis are designed to be used in this way, as they measure the main symptoms of psychosis: hallucinations, delusions, disorganized speech, abnormal psychomotor behavior, and negative symptoms of psychosis (e.g., anhedonia and lack of cognitive input). Depending on how the individual responds to these measures, counselors are able to conceptualize the prognosis for their mental illness as well as the treatment methods. The assessment consists of an eight-item measure that allows the counselor to rate the severity of each psychosis symptom of the individual within the past seven days.

Bipolar and Related Disorders

Bipolar and related disorders are distinct categories that include the following:

- Bipolar I
- Bipolar II
- Cyclothymic disorder
- Substance/medication induced bipolar and related disorder
- Bipolar and related disorder due to another medical condition
- Other specified bipolar and related disorder
- Unspecified bipolar and related disorder

For **bipolar I disorder**, criteria include the following:

- Requirement of at least one manic episode
- Psychotic episodes
- The occurrence of mania or a major depressive episode cannot be accounted for by the existence of another psychiatric disorder.

Mania is characterized as an unusually high level of arousal and overall energy, including changes in mood or emotion. For example, someone with bipolar disorder might suddenly leave their job or undertake risky behaviors that bring about momentary feelings of pleasure, such as having sex with multiple partners.

In **bipolar II disorder**, the criteria include the following:

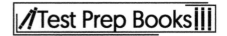

- Occurrence of at least one hypomanic episode
- Occurrence of at least one depressive episode

Hypomania describes a consistent mood elevation with atypical behavior that occurs when depression is absent. For example, someone makes inappropriate sexual advances or spends more money than usual. Also, with bipolar II disorder, the client must never have experienced mania, the symptoms cannot be accounted for by the presence of another psychiatric disorder, and depressive symptoms, as well as those of unpredictable behavior, resulting in a frequent shift between hypomania and depression cause clinically significant distress or functional impairment.

With **cyclothymic disorder**, the criteria include the following:

- Existence of hypomania that does not meet all criteria for hypomanic episodes
- Depression that does not meet all the criteria for depressive episodes for anywhere between one to two years
- Hypomania and depression have each been present for roughly half the time
- The criteria for depression, mania, or hypomania have never been met

Further, symptoms aren't better accounted for by the existence of other psychiatric disorders, aren't the result of substance abuse or another medical condition, and cause clinically significant distress and functional impairment.

For **substance/medication induced bipolar and related disorder**, criteria include the following:

- Ongoing mood disturbance and instances of elevated mood with or without depression
- Anhedonia (lack of pleasure)
- Occurs as a result of exposure to substances or medication
- Symptoms aren't the result of another psychiatric disorder and are causing clinically significant distress, as well as functional impairment.

With **bipolar and related disorder due to another medical condition**, which has been changed from general medical condition, the diagnostic criteria consist of the following:

- Causing clinically significant distress and functional impairment
- Warrants hospitalization
- The presence of psychotic features

By adding both **other specified bipolar and related disorder and unspecified bipolar and related disorder**, the DSM-5 has removed the diagnosis of mood disorder not otherwise specified. Either of these diagnoses are suggested when bipolar symptoms cause clinically significant distress or functional impairment, but do not meet criteria for any of the other diagnostic categories.

Depressive Disorders
Disruptive Mood Dysregulation Disorder
Disruptive mood dysregulation disorder (DMDD) is a relatively recent addition to the DSM. DMDD describes a disorder occurring in early childhood that consists of frequent anger or irritability. Symptoms of DMDD include frequent aggressive outbursts combined with an angry or irritable mood on days without any such aggressive behaviors. These eruptions tend to happen approximately three times per

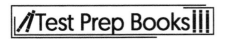

week and at two different settings, such as at school and in the home, and the majority of people in the affected child's life will notice this behavior.

The age of onset for DMDD is prior to age ten, specifically between ages six to eight. The tantrums must be inappropriate to their age of development and persist for at least one year before a diagnosis of DMDD can be rendered. DMDD is common to other disorders such as bipolar disorder and conduct disorder, and comorbidity is fairly common. For instance, children with DMDD tend to also meet criteria for disorders related to attention, behavior, and emotion. Children diagnosed with DMDD are also at an increased risk of developing self-harm and suicidal behaviors. Thus, DMDD is typically common with children already being treated for a psychiatric disorder, although the prevalence is usually lower among the general population.

Major Depressive Disorder

Major depressive disorder (MDD) is characterized by periods of at least two weeks where the individual experiences depressive symptoms subjectively described by the individual as being depressed, sad, or hopeless, along with significant anhedonia (loss of pleasure or interest in activities). To diagnose MDD, at least five of the following nine symptoms must be present for the majority of the time and on most days during the two-week period:

- Depressed mood as subjectively described by the individual or tearful appearance
- Severely diminished interest or pleasure in most activities
- Monthly body weight changes of more than 5% except by dieting, and fluctuating appetite
- Insomnia or hypersomnia
- Observable psychomotor agitation or retardation
- Fatigue
- Feeling worthless or excessively guilty (with or without cause), not normal self-blame or guilt
- Inability to concentrate and indecisiveness
- Recurring thoughts of death, suicidal ideation, or planned or attempted suicide

The presenting symptoms must be causing significant distress and functional impairment and must not be attributed to substance abuse or a different medical condition. Approximately 7% of the US population has at least 1 episode of MDD annually. MDD appears three times more frequently between the ages of 18 to 29 than other age ranges, and 1.5 to 3 times more often in adolescent females than males. Approximately 64% of cases occur with severe impairment. The duration of MDD is a factor in recovery, as long-term MDD may result in several months of recovery—most (4 of 5) recover within a year—though short-term (only a few months) cases may recover quickly.

Premenstrual Dysphoric Disorder

Premenstrual dysphoric disorder (PMDD) is an extreme and debilitating form of premenstrual syndrome. While the symptoms of PMDD can be emotional or physical, mood symptoms must be present in order for a diagnosis of PMDD to be rendered. Anxiety and mood disorders are common in those suffering from PMDD. Criteria for PMDD consists of the following:

- Mood swings
- Irritability
- Depressed mood
- Anxiety

55

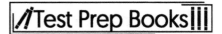

- Decreased interests
- Trouble focusing
- Lethargy
- Changes in appetite
- Sleep difficulties
- Feeling overwhelmed
- Tenderness
- Pain
- Bloating sensation
- Anger
- Feeling hopeless
- Self-deprecating thoughts
- Tension
- Increased social conflicts
- General fatigue

These symptoms must interfere with daily functioning and cause clinically significant distress and are not the result of other preexisting issues such as anxiety, depressive disorders, substance abuse, or a medical condition. When pregnant, women diagnosed with PMDD tend to notice their symptoms disappear; however, after pregnancy, PMDD symptoms can be exacerbated. Suicidal thoughts are also fairly common in women suffering from PMDD. Not unlike premenstrual syndrome, PMDD tends to follow a predictable, cyclical pattern. And while a higher rate of postpartum depression is expected among those with PMDD, research shows that women with PMDD did not have a higher occurrence of it than control groups.

Persistent Depressive Disorder

Formerly known as dysthymic disorder, **persistent depressive disorder (PDD)** describes a depressed mood that occurs most of the time, on more days than not, and has been occurring for upward of two years, as suggested by either one's own personal account or via the observation of others. During this two-year disturbance, the affected individual has never been without symptoms for more than sixty days at a time. Symptoms include the following:

- Poor appetite or overeating
- Poor focus or decision-making abilities
- Feelings of hopelessness
- Low self-esteem
- Low energy or fatigue
- Insomnia or hypersomnia

The depressed client must have two or more of these symptoms before a diagnosis of PDD can be rendered. Also, to be diagnosed with PDD, the client must never have met the criteria for mania, hypomania, a mixed episode, or cyclothymia; and the symptoms are not better accounted for by psychotic disorder and are known to cause clinically significant distress or functional impairment. This disturbance in mood must also not be the direct physiological effects of a substance, medication, or general medical condition. If criteria for major depressive disorder is present for two years, clients can be given comorbid diagnoses of both PDD and major depressive disorder.

56

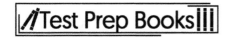
Anxiety Disorders

Specific Phobia

Specific phobia describes a pervasive fear of a certain stimulus and typically occurs in the presence of an object or situation. Common examples of feared stimuli are animals, heights, flying, seeing blood, or receiving an injection. Individuals almost always express a pronounced fear or anxiety in response to the stimuli. Additionally, the fear or anxiety is considered within the context in which it occurs. If the fear does not align with any actual threat caused by the stimuli, then it can be considered a specific phobia. The feared object or stimuli is consistently avoided by the individual or endured with intense discomfort and fear. The anxiety, fear, or avoidance of the stimuli creates significant clinical distress within the individual or severe impairment in areas of functioning.

The fear is persistent, lasting at least six months or more to be considered a clinical diagnosis. In order to diagnose a specific phobia, the anxiety caused by the stimuli cannot be better explained by the symptoms of another disorder such as panic disorder, obsessive-compulsive disorder, post-traumatic stress disorder, separation anxiety disorder, or social anxiety disorder. Specific phobias can be classified by the type of the phobic object: animal, natural environment, blood/injection/injury, situational, or other (for unspecified specific phobias).

Previously, the DSM-IV required that individuals with specific phobia had to be able to recognize the irrationality of the anxiety and it must endure for at least six months if the individual is under the age of eighteen.

Social Anxiety Disorder

Social anxiety disorder (SAD) is characterized as an intense fear or anxiety when in a situation that involves being observed by others. Examples of these situations may include social gatherings, public speaking, or even having a conversation with somebody. For children, the anxiety must also be presented when engaging with peers and not just adults. These social situations do not put the individual at risk in any way other than significant emotional distress. As a result, individuals may consistently avoid these types of instances or endure them with severe anxiety. The fear or anxiety disrupts the individual's daily functioning in a significant way as well as social life. To be confirmed as a diagnosis, the anxiety must last for at least six months, cannot be induced by a substance, and cannot be explained by a symptom of a different mental disorder (panic disorder, agoraphobia, body dysmorphic disorder, etc.). SAD may also be specified as performance only social anxiety disorder, meaning that the anxiety is only present in public interactions.

Separation Anxiety Disorder

Separation anxiety disorder presents itself as excessive fear or anxiety when an individual is separated from their attachment figures (e.g., parents and close relatives). This anxiety is not developmentally appropriate for the individual's age. The anxiety about the separation can manifest in a variety of ways, all of which are representative of impairment in functioning and of clinical significance. People diagnosed with separation anxiety disorder may experience intense distress when anticipating separation from their attachment figures, excessively worry about losing the attachment figures, or even worry about the possibility of an event that would cause the separation. Additionally, individuals with this disorder may avoid leaving their attachment figures and refuse to leave home or go to school. When these individuals are left at home, they may also have excessive fear about being alone. Sleep patterns may also be disrupted in these individuals, as the time spent away from attachment figures can occupy their minds. Nightmares and physical symptoms of illness, like headaches, may occur when

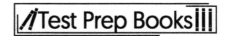

separation occurs or is anticipated. For children, the anxiety needs to persist for at least four weeks for a diagnosis to be rendered. In adults, the anxiety must persist for six months or more.

Selective Mutism

Children diagnosed with **selective mutism** exhibit failure to speak in specific situations. The individual is able to speak in other social interactions and settings, but there is something about being in one environment that prevents the individual from giving auditory information. For example, a child with selective mutism may speak in their home with their nuclear family, but not at all at school or in front of their grandparents. It is vital to understand that selective mutism may greatly impact educational or occupational progression. Teachers may find it extremely difficult in prompting a child to speak and formulate meaningful lesson plans for essential skills, like reading or writing. In addition to the impact on learning, the failure to speak should not be explainable by a lack of knowledge of appropriate linguistics or spoken language needed for oral participation. In order to be classified as a clinical disorder, the disturbance must occur for at least one month.

Selective mutism can only be an accurate diagnosis when the symptoms are not descriptive of a communication disorder and do not occur during the course of autism spectrum disorder, schizophrenia, or any other psychotic disorder.

Obsessive-Compulsive and Related Disorders
Hoarding

Obsessive-compulsive and related disorders cover a variety of mental illnesses that involve obsessions and compulsions, or urges and repetitive behaviors that significantly impair the individual's daily life. In individuals with **hoarding disorder**, there is extreme difficulty parting with possessions, regardless of any actual value attached to them. This results in their living spaces being overly cluttered, often to the point where objects need to be moved in order to get from one room to the next. Hoarding differs from collecting in that the compulsion causes significant distress and impairment for the individual. To diagnose this disorder, the hoarding cannot be due to another medical condition or be better explained by the symptoms of another mental disorder.

Excoriation

The act of **excoriation** involves picking at the skin, often resulting in scars, wounds, or lesions. Excoriation is presented as a compulsion and causes the individual extreme distress in areas of functioning. The compulsion is not due to the physiological effects of a substance, another medical condition, or a symptom of another mental disorder (e.g., tactile hallucinations from a psychotic disorder, attempts to improve a flaw in physical appearance, or a manifestation of non-suicidal self-injury). Individuals with this disorder have made attempts to stop picking their skin, but the compulsion is so strong and ingrained into their reactive tendencies that they manage to engage in this behavior again after a hiatus.

Substance-/Medication-Induced Obsessive-Compulsive and Related Disorder

When there is history of substance or medication use in the individual, combined with obsessions and compulsions, a **substance/medication-induced obsessive-compulsive and related disorder** can be diagnosed. This diagnosis is only applicable when there is evidence that obsessions and compulsions developed after taking a substance and the individual has experienced withdrawal or has been exposed to a medication. The disturbance cannot be better explained by any other obsessive-compulsive

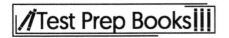

disorder and does not occur within the course of a delirium. Clinically significant distress and impairment in areas of functioning are present within the individual as a result.

Obsessive-Compulsive and Related Disorder Due to Another Medical Condition

This disorder can be taken in the same regard as the previous one. Obsessions and compulsions have the propensity to be symptoms of other medical conditions. For this diagnosis, a pre-existing medical condition is required and serves as the root cause for obsessions and compulsions. There must be evidence from medical records containing information about how the obsessions and compulsions are the result of another medical condition, and it cannot be better explained by any other mental disorder. The disturbance is not present exclusively throughout the course of a delirium and causes significant distress and impairment of functioning.

Trauma- and Stressor-Related Disorders

Reactive Attachment Disorder

While post-traumatic stress disorder is one of the more identifiable trauma- and stressor-related disorders, there are others that are important to consider in order to make an accurate clinical diagnosis. **Reactive attachment disorder (RAD)** describes a consistent pattern of emotionally withdrawn behaviors toward adult caregivers. As the clinical features of this disorder begin to manifest between the ages of nine months and five years, children demonstrate emotionally withdrawn behavior by minimally seeking or responding to comfort when they are distressed. Additionally, a persistent emotional disturbance is presented through minimal responses to others, limited positive affect, or episodes of agitation even in non-threatening situations with adult caregivers.

The child must also have experienced a pattern of developmental intrusions as a result of insufficient care. Social neglect, repeated turnover of caregivers, or being raised in environments where children are not able to form meaningful attachments are all representative of the criteria that identify insufficient care for this disorder. Autism spectrum disorder must be ruled out in order to be diagnosed with reactive attachment disorder.

When confirming a diagnosis of reactive attachment disorder, counselors must understand and be able to differentiate it from autism spectrum disorder (ASD). Many of the symptoms of ASD and RAD are similar; they both involve a lessened positive expression of emotions, cognitive and language impairments, and difficulty with social interactions. What separates these two disorders from each other is that children with RAD must experience the component of severe social neglect, while children with ASD are less likely to have a history with this. Additionally, ASD presents individuals with difficulty in having intentional communication (deliberate, goal-directed language) while RAD still allows children to have social communication levels representative of their intellect.

Disinhibited Social Engagement Disorder

Another trauma- and stressor-related disorder is **disinhibited social engagement disorder (DSED)**. The features of this disorder involve children who are actively interactive with unfamiliar adults, violating social and cultural boundaries. This can be represented by reduced shyness when interacting with strangers, overly familiar physical behavior, lack of attention directed toward actual caregivers, or willingness to accompany an unfamiliar adult with no hesitation. These behaviors are not exclusively due to impulsivity and appear to be socially disinhibited behavior.

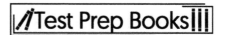

The criteria of this disorder also include that of reactive attachment disorder; a history of social neglect, changing caregivers, or maladaptive attachment environments. In order to be diagnosed as a clinical disorder, the child must at least be nine years of age. This age requirement exists because of the fact that DSED cannot be considered as a diagnosis until a child is mature enough to form selective attachments.

While this disorder has an unknown prevalence rate, research shows that it does appear to have rare occurrences. Of the children that are severely neglected and placed within the foster care system, only about 20% meet the full criteria for DSED. Although it is not a common mental disorder, the impairments of social functioning highlight how impactful an unstable and detached rearing environment can be on a child.

Often, children who have DSED are misdiagnosed with attention-deficit/hyperactivity disorder (ADHD) because of the impulsivity they may present when interacting with strangers. Children with DSED can be distinguished from those with ADHD by not showing difficulties with concentration, attention, or hyperactivity. It is, however, possible for the two disorders to occur concurrently within the same child if they do present issues regarding inattention, hyperactivity, or both combined, as well as the rest of the criteria with ADHD and DSED.

Dissociative Disorders

Dissociative disorders are a classification of mental illness that are centered around identity disturbances, an aberrant construal of consciousness, and interruptions related to memory, emotion, perception, motor control, and behavior. When an individual is diagnosed with a dissociative disorder, all aspects of psychological functioning are severely impacted. The DSM-5 contains dissociative identity disorder, dissociative amnesia, depersonalization/derealization disorder, other specified dissociative disorder, and unspecified dissociative disorder within this section.

Symptoms of dissociation can be experienced as intrusions that alter reality and awareness, causing the individual to have significant difficulty in rationalizing what is real and what is not. Symptoms can also present as an inability to access information that they normally would be able to have access to. For example, if someone is experiencing amnesia manifested by a dissociative disorder, they may not have the ability to recall events that had happened that day.

Frequently, dissociative disorders develop from the result of trauma that has been inflicted upon the individual. Many of the symptoms of dissociation are determined by trauma, such as the tendency to feel embarrassed or confused by the symptoms or even a desire to conceal them from people. For this reason, dissociative disorders are placed right next to the section of trauma- and stressor-related disorders. Many trauma disorders, like post-traumatic stress disorder and acute stress disorder, include dissociative symptoms (e.g., amnesia, flashbacks, numbing, depersonalization/derealization).

Somatic Symptom and Related Disorders

This category of mental disorders, **somatic symptom and related disorders**, is a novel section of the DSM-5. All of these disorders involve physical symptoms that are brought about from mental distress. The diagnoses within this section represent a newly organized version of the somatoform disorders as described in the DSM-IV. The disorders mentioned in this section include somatic symptom disorder, illness anxiety disorder, conversion disorder, factitious disorder, other specified somatic symptom and related disorder and unspecified somatic symptom and related disorder.

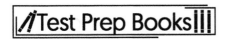

Somatic symptom disorder, the most common diagnosis from this area, focuses on the nuances of discomfort in both physical and emotional measures. While physical pain can cause distress, it is imperative to consider how the individual perceives the pain as well. Individuals with somatic symptom disorder often have extremely high levels of worry. Health concerns may take over the person's life; always seeking treatment and care results in significant impairment in functioning and distress. These individuals think the worst about their health and may describe how it affects other aspects of their lives instead of just their physical discomfort.

It is clear how somatic symptom disorder greatly affects an individual's lifestyle on physical and emotional levels. Cognitive features of this illness include centering their attention on their illness, attributing normal body functions to the illness, interpreting normal body functions as catastrophic or worrisome, and fearing that physical activity may damage their body even further. These individuals may engage in behaviors like constantly checking their bodies for irregularities, constantly seeking medical assistance, and avoiding exercise of any kind. When doctors reassure them that what they are experiencing is mild, people with this disorder will believe that they are not being taken seriously. Due to the physical manifestation of this disorder, people often seek general medical help rather than mental health services. When referred to a mental health service, these individuals may refuse to go in for an initial intake interview with a therapist entirely.

Another disorder within this section is known as **illness anxiety disorder**. This disorder specifically describes clinically significant anxiety about having or possibly contracting a serious illness. These individuals are extremely preoccupied with these thoughts and often seek medical attention. The somatic symptoms that are present, in actuality, are mild or not present at all. The individual is particularly vigilant about their health status, worrying for and caring to any bodily sensation perceived as negative. The preoccupation of the illness must occur for at least six months.

Even after testing negative for serious illness or being reassured by doctors, individuals with illness anxiety disorder still maintain a constant worry or fear related to their health. Illness becomes a prominent feature of their personality and lifestyle. They will often seek out assistance from several medical providers for the same problems that have already been scrutinized by professionals. They examine themselves repeatedly and perform excessive research on medical illnesses they are worried about. The social and family environment becomes extremely at risk for impairment in these individuals as it may prevent them from going to significant events, family gatherings, visiting sick relatives, etc. Environmental stressors may serve as a catalyst for this disorder, considering research suggests that childhood abuse or serious childhood illness may give the individual a predisposition to the development of this disorder as they get older. Illness anxiety disorder is a revised interpretation of hypochondriasis as stated in the DSM-IV.

Feeding and Eating Disorders

Feeding and eating disorders are delineated as a persistent disruption in eating or eating-related behavior. The behavior that results from these disorders involve altering food consumption or digestion that affects individuals on a social, cognitive, and emotional level. The disorders covered in this section are pica, rumination disorder, avoidant/restrictive food intake disorder, anorexia nervosa, bulimia nervosa, and binge-eating disorder.

The diagnostic criteria for rumination disorder, avoidant/restrictive food intake disorder, anorexia nervosa, bulimia nervosa, and binge-eating disorder are mutually exclusive. This describes how an individual can only be diagnosed with one of these disorders based off of what has occurred in their

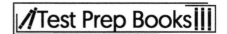

behavior. The explanation for this is despite commonalities that may be depicted in individuals with these disorders, the disorders greatly differ from one another in terms of presentation, clinical prognosis/course, outcome, and types of treatment. The exception is that pica may be diagnosed simultaneously with any other feeding and eating disorder.

Pica describes the act of persistently eating substances that are not food for at least one month. Developmental level is considered for this diagnosis, as young children may often accidentally eat objects other than food, and it is required that the consumption must be disproportionate to an individual's age. The behavior is abnormal when considering the context of the individual's culture. **Rumination disorder** is when an individual repeatedly regurgitates food for over a period of one month. The regurgitation behavior is not attributable to a gastrointestinal issue or any other medical condition. This disturbance does not only occur within the course of anorexia nervosa, bulimia nervosa, binge-eating disorder, or avoidant/restrictive intake disorder.

Avoidant/restrictive food intake disorder is an eating disturbance in which the individual consistently fails to meet nutritional needs. This can be presented as significant weight loss, serious nutritional deficiency, dependence on oral feeding supplements, or severe interference in social and psychological functioning.

Anorexia nervosa, one of the most commonly-known eating disorders, is when the individual restricts their intake of food relative to what their body requires. This leads to a significant low body weight that is less than minimally normal or expected with age, sex, developmental trajectory, and physical health. Individuals have a predominant fear of gaining weight or becoming fat even though they are at an incredibly low weight. Individuals also experience a disturbance in perceiving their body for how it actually looks or denounce the seriousness of the significantly low weight.

Bulimia nervosa is clinically presented as recurrent episodes of binge eating followed by inappropriate compensatory behaviors to prevent weight gain. Some of these behaviors involve self-induced vomiting, misusing laxatives, fasting, or exercising excessively. The binge eating and compensatory behaviors both occur at least once a week for three months. Unlike anorexia nervosa, people with bulimia nervosa often present as average or overweight. It is not uncommon for individuals' behavior to be described as switching off between the two disorders.

Lastly, **binge-eating disorder** is another mental disorder within this section of the DSM-5. This disorder is characterized by recurrent episodes of binge eating and is associated with eating faster than normal, until uncomfortably full, eating large amounts of food when not physically hungry, eating alone due to embarrassment of how much they ate, and feeling disgusted with oneself afterwards. Marked distress occurs from this disorder and the behavior occurs at least once a week for three months.

Elimination Disorders

Unlike other classes of disorders, the **elimination disorders** section in the DSM-5 is particularly succinct. It contains disorders that involve issues with excreting urine and feces from the body. While it is extremely common for young children to have "accidents" when they are young, this problem has the potential to develop into a disorder if it persists past the age of five for more than three months. **Enuresis** describes the repetitive tendency to release urine in places other than a bathroom. The most common type of enuresis that occurs at night is bed-wetting. **Encopresis**, the other type of elimination disorder, involves the process of excreting feces instead of urine. These behaviors may or may not be done on purpose.

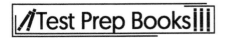

Children with this disorder may experience other symptoms of these disorders such as loss of appetite, abdominal pain, watery bowel movements, lessened interest in physical activity, being withdrawn around friends and family, or even displaying secretive behavior related to bowel movements. The effects caused by an elimination disorder that may impact a child's life can range from mild to severe depending on the symptoms. It is essential for counselors and caregivers to approach children with this disorder with warmth and comfort in order to ease any negative feelings they may have about their symptoms.

Sleep-Wake Disorders

A healthy sleep pattern is a major factor when it comes to psychological functioning. For many, inadequate sleep serves as the root cause of their negative affect. The **sleep-wake disorders** section of the DSM-5 covers all mental disorders that involve issues related to sleep. Insomnia disorder, hypersomnolence disorder, narcolepsy, breathing-related sleep disorders, circadian rhythm sleep-wake disorders, non-rapid eye movement (NREM) sleep arousal disorders, nightmare disorder, rapid eye movement (REM) sleep behavior disorder, restless legs syndrome, and substance/medication-induced sleep disorder are all included within this distinction.

Individuals with sleep-wake disorders mainly present with problems related to inadequate sleep in terms of quality, timing, and amount. All of these areas of sleep will determine how an individual acts in the daytime. Both physical and emotional problems can be attributable to sleep-wake disorders, meaning that counselors must be able to differentiate if the sleep is being affected by symptoms of other mental disorders or a pre-existing medical condition.

The most common sleep-wake disorder is **insomnia disorder**. People with insomnia have a very difficult time falling asleep or staying asleep. While one-third of adults experience insomnia symptoms, only 6–10% meet all of the criteria for insomnia disorder. Symptoms include difficulty falling asleep, staying asleep, or waking up early and having the inability to fall back asleep. The sleep difficulty must persist for three months and occur at least three nights per week in order to fully disrupt functioning on social, academic, or occupational levels.

Sexual Dysfunctions
Sexual Dysfunction Subtypes
Within individuals diagnosed with a sexual disorder, it is imperative to specify the onset of when the difficulty occurred. This is mainly because the timing of when the issue occurs may determine the course of the treatment and the cause for what made the dysfunction apparent in the first place. These specifications are demonstrated through four subtypes within sexual dysfunctions.

The **lifelong subtype** specifies that the sexual problem has been present since the individual's first sexual experiences. If someone who is diagnosed with erectile disorder is placed in the lifelong subtype, then that would specify how the difficulty in obtaining or maintaining an erection has been present ever since the individual became sexually active.

The next subtype is referred to as the **acquired subtype**. This subtype notes that the sexual disturbance has developed after a period of normal sexual functioning. Individuals within this subtype may be more likely to seek treatment because they may be able to recognize the disturbance when it occurs or notice a bodily-related abnormality. Individuals either fall within the lifelong or acquired subtype when specifying the onset of the difficulty.

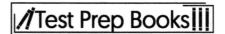

The **generalized subtype** characterizes how the sexual disturbance is not limited to certain types of stimulation, situations, or partners. In contrast, the situational subtype describes how the difficulty is only present within those parameters. If someone is diagnosed with erectile disorder and is placed within the situational subtype, then this offers insight on when the disturbance becomes present. Often, sex therapists work with couples who are experiencing problems related to their sexual relationship. While medical attention may be necessary for some of these disorders, interventions used by therapists to allow open communication of feelings and thoughts about sexual pleasure between partners has the ability to enhance sexual performance as well as satisfaction with their relationship in general.

Genito-Pelvic Pain/Penetration Disorder

For women, penetration during sex has the potential to be painful if not properly operated. However, some individuals with persistent problems related to sexual penetration can be diagnosed with **genito-pelvic pain/penetration disorder**. People with this disorder may experience difficulties with vaginal penetration, intense vulvovaginal or pelvic pain during intercourse, anxiety related to the pain or anticipation of pain, or severe pelvic muscle tension during attempted vaginal intercourse. These symptoms must persist for at least six months and cause great distress to the individual in order for the issue to be classified as a disorder.

Individuals primarily seek treatment for this disorder or just these symptoms in medical settings. The course for this diagnosis is unclear, but there are a few signs that may indicate issues with this disorder that the individual may not be aware of. For example, avoiding the use of tampons persistently has been shown by research to be a common indicator that there may be some issues of discomfort when it comes to vaginal penetration. Additionally, counselors must be able to differentiate this disorder from another medical condition. Lichen sclerosus, endometriosis, pelvic inflammatory disease, and vulvovaginal atrophy are commonly diagnosed in these individuals who actually have genito-pelvic pain/penetration disorder. If a marked fear or anxiety of intercourse is present, then the possibility of this diagnosis must be considered.

Gender Dysphoria

Gender dysphoria encapsulates an entire section within the DSM-5 in addition to being labeled as a mental disorder. When individuals develop an awareness of incongruence in the gender identity that is associated with the sex they were assigned with at birth, they may experience **gender dysphoria**. The incongruence may be accompanied by severe distress in terms of how the individual should not only express themselves physically, but also how they perceive themselves internally with regard to the cultural context. Experiencing gender dysphoria typically manifests in those who identify as transgender, an individual who identifies with a gender or other identity that is different from the sex they were assigned at birth. The diagnostic criteria for gender dysphoria are different for adults, adolescents, and children.

In children, one of the indicators for gender dysphoria is a strong insistence that they are the other gender (male or female) or some alternative identity that is different from the assigned one. Young boys experiencing gender dysphoria may prefer to dress in female attire, whereas young girls may prefer to present as more masculine. Often, young children engage in fantasy play and taking on the role of a different gender during this may also serve as an indication for gender dysphoria. The DSM-5 emphasizes that children strongly prefer the objects, roles, and characteristics of an opposite gender for a period of six months or more.

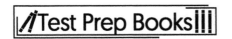

Gender dysphoria is not only presented in children. For many, adolescence and adulthood are when the incongruence becomes more apparent. The course for this disorder will present differently from person to person as everyone's relationship with gender and identity is different. The indicators for adults are essentially the same as they are in children but are more conceptualized as a fully developed awareness. Individuals must have a strong desire to be a different gender, to be treated/referred to as a different gender, and embody the typical feelings and reactions of the gender they truly identify as.

People who experience gender dysphoria are considered sexual minorities as they are often discriminated against on many different scales in a variety of social, occupational, medical, and institutional environments. With this in mind, counselors must be properly educated on the concept of sexual identity as well as develop competency with this population in order to prevent their internal biases from violating proper treatment protocols.

Disruptive, Impulse-Control, and Conduct Disorders

This section of the DSM-5 characterizes issues related to self-control in expressing emotions and behaviors. Specifically, disruptive, impulse-control, and conduct disorders address problematic behaviors that can be directed onto another person (e.g., destruction of property, vandalism, aggression, etc.). What causes these behaviors are issues stemming from emotional reactivity and self-regulating abilities.

The first disorder within this section is **oppositional defiant disorder**. This disorder presents a pattern of angry/irritable moods in addition to defiant behavior. Emotional symptoms include losing temper often, being easily annoyed, or often angry and resentful. Behavioral criteria consist of arguing with authority figures or caregivers, refusing to comply with direction from mentioned figures, annoying others on purpose, or blaming others for their mistakes. A spiteful or vindictive behavioral pattern must occur twice within the past six months. Additionally, these behaviors are directed towards individuals other than immediate family members (parents, siblings, etc.).

Intermittent explosive disorder is the next listing in this section. Verbal aggression, in addition to three instances where the individual damages property or physically assaults another person/animal occurring within a twelve-month period, is what is required for a diagnosis of this disorder. The person must be at least six years of age with the outbursts resulting from anger alone. The situation at hand would normally never elicit an outburst from the average person.

Conduct disorder describes the persistent pattern of violating basic rights and rules of others. This disorder typically develops during the course of childhood and adolescence. This population is highly aggressive and often seen starting physical fights, bullying others, destroying property, conning others, or running away from home. This is the kind of person who will show little to no concern for other people and feel comfortable using them in order to get what they want. Conduct disorder is a necessary prerequisite for children who are later diagnosed with antisocial personality disorder. The other disorders within this section include pyromania, kleptomania, and other specified and unspecified disruptive, impulse-control, and conduct disorders.

Substance-Related and Addictive Disorders

The ten classes of drugs that are covered in this section are alcohol, caffeine, cannabis, hallucinogens, inhalants, opioids, sedatives, hypnotics, stimulants, and tobacco. While these classifications are not fully distinct from one another, each one is still capable of chemically altering the brain's reward pathway. These drugs activate neurotransmitters within the brain to create pleasant feelings or "highs." When

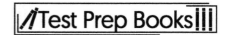
abused, these drugs inhibit the brain from naturally producing these neurotransmitters which can serve as a catalyst for dependency and problems with functioning in all areas of life. This section of the DSM-5 includes gambling disorder, as the behavior associated with gambling is known to activate the reward system in a similar way. Other behavioral addictions such as internet gaming, sex addiction, or shopping addiction are not covered within this section due to the lack of peer-reviewed empirical evidence.

Diagnostic criteria are similar across all of the drug classifications. An individual with a **substance-related addiction** generally displays taking the substance in large amounts or more than was intended, attempting to cut down drug use but consistently failing, spending a great deal of time obtaining substances or recovering from its effects, and a strong craving or desire to use the substance. People with substance abuse disorders may spend the majority of their time interacting with a substance or being in its presence. As a result, significant impairment in functioning, interpersonal issues, and a decrease in responsibilities or recreational activities may occur. Risky use is another factor of substance abuse as it explains how this population may still use the substance in situations that are physically dangerous (e.g., while driving) or even when knowing that the substance is the cause of a current physical or psychological problem.

Tolerance and withdrawal symptoms are also indicators of substance abuse. **Tolerance** is defined as requiring an increased dose of the substance in order to achieve its desired effects. People with substance-use disorders may develop tolerance rather quickly depending on the type of substance and pre-existing brain chemistry. Tolerance needs to be distinguished from the variety of bodily responses that someone taking a substance for the first time might experience. For example, someone who smokes marijuana for the first time may feel little to no effect, while individuals that have the same physical characteristics and ingest the same amount feel the effects at a significant rate. **Withdrawal symptoms** are the body's physical responses to using the drug continuously and then not at all. When heavy drug use is maintained, the blood and tissue concentrations of the body become affected. This can be dangerous and potentially life-threatening to the individual because they may take more of the substance in order to alleviate the withdrawal symptoms. Withdrawal symptoms are specified for each of the drug classes because each substance affects the body differently.

Neurocognitive Disorders

What distinguishes the neurocognitive disorders section from other disorders of the DSM-5 are issues with cognitive functioning that have been acquired instead of developed. Developmental cognitive disorders like ADHD and autism spectrum disorder are instead classified as neurodevelopmental disorders. **Neurocognitive disorders** represent an impairment in functioning that has increased throughout time, and thus the reasoning for the abnormality can be determined. Neurocognitive disorders in the DSM-5 are organized by being major or mild, along with a pre-existing medical condition. Delirium is the only neurocognitive disorder that is not classified this way. Cognitive functioning is measured by six domains: complex attention (selective attention, processing speed), executive functioning (decision-making, planning), learning and memory (short- and long-term), language (processing, expression), perceptual-motor, and social cognition (recognizing emotions, theory of mind).

Delirium can be most simply described as an impairment of attention and awareness. People who experience delirium have extreme difficulty focusing their attention, remembering things, and processing language. Episodes of delirium typically last hours to a few days and may become more or less severe depending on the time of day. Delirium can be caused by substance withdrawal, a side-effect from medication, or another medical condition.

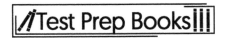

What separates a major neurocognitive disorder from a mild one is the severity of impairment related to cognitive functioning. In major neurocognitive disorders, individuals experience a severe decline in performance of one or more cognitive levels (e.g., language, memory, social cognition). This is based on the level of concern from the individual themselves, an informant, or a clinician. Documentation of cognitive decline or a cognitive assessment is required for the diagnosis as well. This decline in functioning does not exclusively occur during an episode of delirium and at minimum impacts the individual where they cannot live on their own without assistance. On the contrary, a mild neurocognitive disorder does not interfere with the responsibilities of daily living but contains the same criteria for a major neurocognitive disorder. People with mild neurocognitive disorders are able to fully function on their own.

Personality Disorders

When patterns of behavior, emotional responses, and cognition become ingrained within an individual, then it is possible for them to have developed a **personality disorder**. People with personality disorders engage in problematic behaviors and tendencies that are not normally accepted within the cultural context. Past research has shown that personality disorders develop in early childhood and adolescence. For organizational purposes, the DSM-5 separates personality disorders into three clusters: cluster A, odd and eccentric; cluster B, dramatic and erratic; and cluster C, fearful and anxious.

The cluster A personality disorders are paranoid personality disorder, schizoid personality disorder, and schizotypal personality disorder. Individuals with any of these disorders exhibit behavior that is considered odd or eccentric with significant deviation from what is normally accepted. **Paranoid personality disorder** is quite self-explanatory in that this population has extreme difficulty trusting other people and views their motives as evil or harmful. The paranoia is generalizable, leaving these individuals with a very solitary lifestyle. The **schizoid personality disorder** population does not care for social relationships or responsibilities and often have a limited display of emotion. These individuals have no interest in maintaining relationships on any level and do not elicit any warm emotions. People with **schizotypal personality disorder**, on the other hand, are not able to form interpersonal relationships because of their social deficits. These individuals present odd thinking and speech, magical thinking, ideas of reference, and more that prevent them from building relationships with others. These people may physically appear odd through choice of clothing or other stylistic decisions.

Cluster B personality disorders include antisocial personality disorder, borderline personality disorder, histrionic personality disorder, and narcissistic personality disorder. Individuals within this cluster have a difficult time maintaining interpersonal relationships because of their erratic and dramatic emotional reactivity. People with **antisocial personality disorder** have a complete disregard for others and often use other people for their own personal gain. Conduct disorder during childhood is a requirement for a diagnosis of antisocial personality disorders. **Borderline personality disorder** describes those who have unstable personal relationships and intense levels of impulsivity. Common indicators of this disorder include self-harm and black-and-white thinking. These individuals will go to great lengths in order to keep those around them because of their tendency to associate their self-worth with their relationships with other people.

Similarly, **histrionic personality disorder** involves a pattern of attention-seeking behavior. People with histrionic personalities may use their physical appearance to gain attention, have rapid shifts in emotion, and are uncomfortable when they are not the center of attention. Lastly, **narcissistic personality disorder** is diagnosed in those who display a grandiose sense of self, needs constant validation or

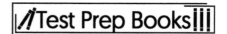

admiration, and has a strong sense of entitlement. The basis for this disorder is that these people thrive off of their feelings about themselves and need reinforcement of their grandiosity from others.

The fearful and anxious personality disorders of cluster C are avoidant personality disorder, dependent personality disorder, and obsessive-compulsive personality disorder. The fear or anxiety within these personality types prevent individuals from forming meaningful relationships, inhibit the development of independence, or become too preoccupied with behavioral tendencies that they cannot live a substantial, healthy lifestyle. When someone is diagnosed with **avoidant personality disorder,** this means that they have an intense fear of interpersonal communication. The fear of rejection or criticism prevents them from taking risks to meet new people and is so ingrained that they believe they are socially incapable of healthily interacting with others.

Dependent personality disorder represents those who have a pervasive need to be taken care of. These people cannot make decisions by themselves, will not create conflict out of worry that their caretaker may leave them, feel extremely uncomfortable being alone, or go to great lengths in order to keep someone around to take care of them. These individuals may feel extreme discomfort or distress when having to move out of their parents' house or going through a breakup with their partner to the point where they do not know what to do with themselves. The last of these disorders, **obsessive-compulsive personality disorder,** emphasizes the pattern of being a perfectionist with no flexibility for mistakes on their own part or those involved in their life. These individuals are unable to complete tasks because they are so caught up in the details. When offered a different perspective on a situation, someone with this personality type would reject it and show stubbornness when working with others. What differentiates this disorder from obsessive-compulsive disorder (OCD) is that the person will not have obsessions and compulsions to the same extent as those with OCD.

Paraphilic Disorders

Patterns of urges, fantasies, or taboo sexual acts that cause distress within an individual are known as **paraphilic disorders** within the DSM-5. These acts may include inanimate objects, children or nonconsenting adults, suffering and humiliation of a sexual partner, or even the person themselves. Paraphilic disorders include voyeuristic disorder, exhibitionistic disorder, frotteuristic disorder, sexual masochism disorder, sexual sadism disorder, pedophilic disorder, fetishistic disorder, and transvestic disorder.

The main idea surrounding these disorders is that despite the pleasure that may be gained from engaging in these acts, individuals with paraphilic disorders still manage to cause severe distress and harm to themselves or other people. Having a paraphilia, an intense sexual interest in something or someone that is not a physically normal, mature, consenting human partner, does not immediately indicate that someone has a paraphilic disorder. A major component of paraphilic disorders is the occurrence of distress as a result from the sexual interest.

MSE

The **MSE (mental status exam)** is a tool used when evaluating a client and is part of the collection of information used to make a diagnosis. The purpose of the MSE is to determine how the client is functioning mentally and emotionally at that specific moment in time, whether it's during the initial interview or any session in the therapy process. The MSE is performed mainly by observation. Counselors can use a variety of checklists, but an MSE should always cover certain items such as the general impression of the client, their emotional state, their thoughts, and their cognitive functioning.

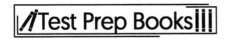

The most obvious will be the overall impression of the client and includes their appearance, attitude, behavior, and motor functioning.

The client's current emotional state should also be noted, observing both their mood and affect. The counselor should observe and note the client's thought content, thought processes, and their self-perception as well as the how they perceive the environment around them. This could include observations of hallucinations or illusions. Additionally, the counselor should pay attention to the client's language and speech patterns. The cognitive portion of the MSE addresses elements such as orientation, memory, concentration, and intelligence. This is the portion of the MSE when observation alone will not be enough. The counselor can utilize various tests and questions to evaluate these areas. It's important that the counselor notes only current observations. Symptoms that the client has reported to be experiencing should not be part of the MSE if they are not observed by the counselor during that interview or session.

Co-Occurring Diagnoses

Co-occurring disorders may also be known as **dual disorders** or **dual diagnoses**. Co-occurring disorders are more prevalent in clients who have substance use history or presently use substances. Substance use is diagnosed when the use of the substance interferes with normal functioning at work, school, home, in relationships, or exacerbates a medical condition. A substance use diagnosis is often made in conjunction with a mood or anxiety related disorder, resulting in a dual diagnosis.

Co-occurring disorders or dual diagnoses may be difficult to diagnose due to the nature of symptom presentation. Some symptoms of addiction or substance abuse may appear to be related to another mental health disorder; conversely, some symptoms of mental health disorder may appear to be related to substance use. On the contrary, there are some signs that a co-occurring disorder is present:

- Mental health symptoms worsening while undergoing treatment: For example, a client suffering from depression may be prescribed anti-depressants to address depressive symptoms. However, if the client is using substances, they may mix other medications with anti-depressants. This can be dangerous in itself but may also create a prolonged false sense of wellbeing while under the influence. Once this feeling fades, it can be confusing for the client to realize whether the prescribed medications are working. Even worse, the client may increase recreational substance use, leading to worse overall mental health symptoms over time.

- Persistent substance use problems with treatment: There are some substance use treatment centers that titrate clients off of one medication and place them on another, such as methadone. This may result in transference of dependence and ongoing substance use while the client is receiving treatment for mental health disorders.

Another scenario is that a client may seek treatment from a substance use treatment center with clinicians that are not equipped to provide adequate mental health treatment for the client. As the mental health problems persist or worsen while undergoing withdrawal, the client may continue to engage in substance use as a coping skill, therefore making the substance use problem appear resistant to treatment.

It is important for co-occurring disorders or dual diagnoses to be treated together because they occur simultaneously. This may be done utilizing a multidisciplinary team approach in an outpatient or

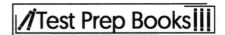

inpatient setting. Treatment of dual diagnoses or co-occurring disorders at the same time in the same setting by the same treatment team is also known as an **integrated treatment** approach.

Determining Level of Care Needed

A client's need for care can fall on a wide spectrum. Some clients may comfortably live in their own residence but attend regularly scheduled meetings with a counselor to receive care. Other clients, after being appropriately assessed, may require institutional care where they can receive medical and therapeutic support as often as is needed. Institutional care may be a long-term or short-term solution for a client. The level of care required for a client is assessed by examining a number of self-sufficiency factors, such as the presence of any formally diagnosed developmental disabilities, physical disabilities, or mental disorders.

Additionally, the client's ability to communicate needs, IQ level, ability to complete self-care tasks (such as dressing, toileting, grooming, etc.) alone or with assistance, and risk of voluntary or involuntary harm to self or others will also be taken into consideration. Based on the client's health and caretaking needs, they may receive outpatient services (such as regular therapeutic appointments), inpatient services (such as a behavioral program that lasts for a predetermined period of time), assisted living in a facility such as a nursing home, or in-home support (such as a home health nurse). Regardless of where a client falls on the care spectrum, services for mental wellness and adjusting to this new context of life will likely be beneficial to care.

Counselors should work with individuals to identify service needs. The methodology for doing so may include:

- Discussion with the individual and/or support system to determine goals for treatment or collaboration to shape goals

- Prioritizing goals and setting clear, measurable objectives

- Determining what a successful outcome of treatment should look like and how this will enrich the individual's quality of life

- Assessing the individual's strengths and available resources and highlighting these throughout treatment rather than focusing on challenges; using these strengths to determine how the individual can be self-sufficient and involved in the process

- Ensuring confidentiality across all interactions and documentation

The level of care an individual requires is an important component of the service delivery plan. The counselor may note the following details:

- Is care medically necessary?

- Can the individual continue to live in their current residence, or is relocation necessary?

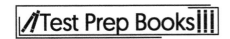

- What level of physical support or assistance does the individual need at this time?

- What level of restriction is needed in care? (For example, more restrictive care would include inpatient treatment, while less restrictive care would include day sessions or community group meetings.)

Determining the Appropriate Modality of Treatment

When utilizing a holistic approach for client assessment and treatment planning, counselors should utilize evidence-based research to support the selected interventions and treatment modalities. The interventions and treatment modalities selected will be based on a number of things, including the client's current level of functioning (based on the biopsychosocial assessment), level of care needed, presenting symptoms, and the counselor's background. Here are some things a counselor will want to consider when constructing interventions or treatment modalities:

- Are the selected interventions evidence-based?

- Do the selected interventions arise from a strengths-based perspective specifically tailored around the client's strengths, interests, and needs?

- Do the associated risks with the selected interventions outweigh the possible positive outcomes?

- Is the selected intervention culturally-sensitive and culturally-appropriate?

- Did the client participate in the construction of the intervention selection and/or consent to it?

- Does the counselor feel comfortable and well-versed in the selected intervention to increase the levels of intensity as needed and provide a continuity of care for the selected modalities?

- Does the selected intervention coincide with the client's financial ability to pay?

Assessing the Presenting Problem and Level of Distress

Use of Objective and Subjective Data

Both objective and subjective data are used during the assessment and treatment processes. The client provides their perspective on what happened and the correlated feelings and experiences felt, which is the **subjective data**. Subsequently, the counselor uses the information and may ask questions to better understand where the client is emotionally, while teasing out facts related to the client's situation. These facts are **objective data**.

Examining the Problem System

The problem system refers to factors that are relevant to the client's presenting problem, which may include other people or environmental elements the client deems relevant to the situation. It is important that questions be asked to determine what the client's perception of the presenting problem is. Additionally, the counselor should determine if there are other legal, medical, or physical issues related to the problem. For a comprehensive assessment, the client should also be asked how long the problem has been present and if there are any triggers they believe contribute to the problem.

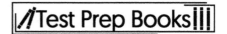

Identification of external supports and access to resources is also key when examining and discussing the problem system.

The presenting problem is generally revealed in the client's statement about why they have come in for treatment. Disclosure of the presenting problem allows the counselor to determine the prevailing concerns deemed important by the client. Counselors can gain a sense of how distressed the client is about the problem or situation and what client expectations are for treatment. The manner in which the client describes the presenting problem can also provide insight as to how emotionally tied the client is to the problem and whether or not the client came in under their own volition.

Discovering Root Causes of the Problem

It is important to determine the true root causes of the presenting problem. Although a client may come in and voice a concern, it may not be the root cause of the issue. Rather, this concern may simply be an item the client feels comfortable discussing. For example, a client who is experiencing sexual issues may initially speak about anxiety before disclosing the actual problem. This may require an investment of time to allow the client to become comfortable trusting the counselor. The history of the problem is important to address because it clarifies any factors contributing to the presenting problem, as well as any deeper underlying issues. Gathering background information on the problem history is also helpful for developing interventions. There are three key areas to address when reviewing the problem history:

- **Onset**: Problem onset addresses when the problem started. It usually includes triggers or events that led up to the start of the problem; these events may also be contributing factors.

- **Progression**: Assessment of the progression of the problem requires determining the frequency of the problem. The counselor should ask questions to determine if the problem is intermittent (how often and for how long), if it is acute or chronic, and if there are multiple problems that may or may not appear in a pattern or recurring cluster.

- **Severity**: Counselors should determine how severe the client feels the problem is, what factors contribute to making the problem more severe, and how the situation impacts the client's adaptive functioning. This may be determined by addressing the following questions:

  o Does the problem affect the client at work?

  o Is there difficulty performing personal care because of the problem?

    ▪ The counselor should ascertain whether or not the client has access to resources that can provide adequate care (running water, shelter, and clothing).

    ▪ The client's living situation should be explored if there are difficulties with personal care activities.

    ▪ The counselor should also ask if there are others for whom the client is responsible, like children or elderly parents/relatives.

  o Has the problem caused the client to withdraw from preferred activities?

  o Has the client used alcohol or other controlled substances to alleviate or escape the problem? If so, for how long and to what degree?

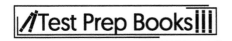

Obtaining and Evaluating Collateral Information

If collateral sources are used, information can also be gathered from one or more of the collateral sources who have insight as to why the client is in need of assistance. **Collateral sources** are persons other than the client, such as family members, police officers, friends, or other medical providers, who can provide information related to the client's levels of functioning, life events, and other potential areas of significance in the client's treatment.

Prior to obtaining collateral information from any source, a signed **release of information (ROI)** form should be obtained from the client (or from a parent/ guardian if the client is a minor). The necessity for an ROI may be waived if there is explicit legal consent granting access to collateral sources. This is most commonly seen during forensic interviews. It is important to explain the purpose behind collecting an ROI to the client. Relatedly, it is also important to make the collateral source aware of the reason behind the request for information on the client.

Information from collateral sources is useful in cases when the client is unable to provide reliable information. The inability to provide reliable information could be due to a number of factors, such as substance abuse issues, severe cognitive impairment, or severe mental illness/disorder. Based on the client's background, there could be a number of collateral sources from which to solicit information. Thus, it is important to filter these sources based on those who have had regular or recent contact with the client.

It is important to select collateral sources that can provide information about significant experiences and events relating to the client's presenting problem. Collateral sources can provide a level of objectivity when discussing the client's situation. Additional examples of collateral sources include physician's reports, police reports, reports from other medical professionals or mental health agencies, school reports, and employment records.

ABCs of a Problem

The **ABCs of a problem** refer to the Antecedent, Behavior, and Consequences linked to a client's perceived problem. The discovery of these items allows the client to define the problem specifically and examine factors affecting emotional wellbeing.

Antecedents to a problem may be prefaced by the involvement of certain individuals in the client's life. It is important to gather understanding on how the client was involved with these individuals and how the client felt affected. Environmental antecedents may also be present.

The client may disclose interactions that lead to problematic **behaviors**, based on the aforementioned information in the evaluation of the antecedent. When addressing the behavior, it is important that counselors gather information on what is said before, during, and after the maladaptive behavior takes place.

The **consequences** to a presenting problem are comprised of both cognitive (internal) and environmental (external) interactions with the behavior. The client and other identified participants linked to the problem will reveal their belief sets and values based on the role played in either sustaining the behavior or attempting to decrease it.

The client's coping skills should be evaluated to determine the type of mechanism they implement when the problem is present and whether or not it is an appropriate coping mechanism for the situation.

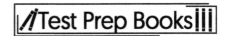

If the client presents with a heightened emotional reaction as a consequence to the problem, it could parlay into another problem and create more complex issues for the client.

At this juncture, the information previously gathered on the client's legal and medical history is beneficial for counselors to incorporate into the assessment process as it may have a significant impact on the factors shaping the client's problem and the resulting consequences.

Evaluating an Individual's Level of Mental Health Functioning

Ideas about what is normal versus what is abnormal with regard to behavior are society-dependent. People tend to equate *normal* with "good" and *abnormal* with "bad," which means that any behavior labeled as abnormal can potentially be stigmatizing. Use of person-centered language is one way to reduce stigma attached to abnormal behavior or behavior health issues (e.g., saying "a person with schizophrenia," rather than "a schizophrenic.")

The "Four Ds" of Abnormality assist health counselors when trying to identify a psychiatric condition in their clients. Deviance marks a withdrawal from society's concept of appropriate behavior. Deviant behavior is a departure from the "norm." The *DSM-5* contains some criteria for diagnosing deviance. The second "D" is dysfunction. Dysfunction is behavior that interferes with daily living. Dysfunction is a type a problem that may be serious enough to be considered a disorder. The third "D" is distress. Distress is related to a client's dysfunction. That is, to what degree does the dysfunction cause the client distress? A client can experience minor dysfunction and major distress, or major dysfunction and minor distress. The fourth "D" is danger. Danger is characterized by danger to self or to others. There are different degrees of danger specific to various types of disorders. Duration is sometimes considered a fifth "D," as it may be important to note whether the symptoms of a disorder are fleeting or permanent.

Screening Clients for Appropriate Services

The treatment plan is dependent on the goals set by the client and counselor. Part of the intake process is obtaining a general overview of why the client is seeking counseling services. Data collection can be performed using various methods. The primary tool used to gather information about the client is an unstructured client interview. Counselors can also observe nonverbal behavior and build rapport during an unstructured interview. Structured interviews are used to ask clients questions that will improve reliability and ensure collection of specific information.

Some tools used to screen clients for appropriate services include questionnaires, checklists, rating scales, and standardized tests. **Standardized testing** is a formal process that produces a score and can be interpreted using a set of guidelines. Examples include personality and aptitude tests, such as the **Minnesota Multiphasic Personality Inventory-2** or the **SAT**. Frequently used projective personality tests include the **Thematic Apperception Test (TAT)** and the **Rorschach Inkblot Test (Rorschach)**. Objective personality tests rely on the client's personal responses and are considered a form of self-reporting. Examples include the **Sixteen Personality Factors Questionnaire (16PF)** and the **Edwards Personal Preference Schedule (EPPS)**. Counselors should choose the screening tool that can best examine the client's presenting problem further.

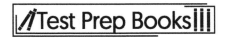

Select, Use, and Interpret Appropriate Assessment Instruments

Administering Tests to Clients

As part of the counseling process, it can be necessary for the counselor to administer tests or assessments to measure and evaluate the client. Tests are a more formalized means to quantify information, guide treatment options, and develop goals. Assessments are more informal. They can include surveys, interviews, and observations. There are a variety of reasons a counselor can choose to administer a test or assessment, such as to:

- help the client gain a better understanding of themselves.
- provide counselors with concrete data.
- ensure a client's needs are within the counselor's scope of practice.
- assist in decision-making and goal-setting for the counseling process.
- provide insight to both the client and the counselor.
- assist in setting clear expectations for clients.
- help the counselor gain a deeper understanding of their client's needs.
- set benchmarks to ensure client and counselor are making progress toward their goals.
- evaluate the effectiveness of counseling interventions.

Psychological and educational tests play a critical role in understanding client backgrounds, belief systems, and perspectives as part of the overall assessment. They also indicate any current or potential psychological, social, or physical needs that the client may have. These pieces of information shape the way counselors develop and tailor interventions for a specific client; they also allow counselors to maintain the highest level of safety for the patient as well as themselves. Psychological testing usually includes an interview component in which the counselor may conduct the initial intake assessment, ask the client personal and family-related questions, and notice body language and other physical behaviors.

Answers to interview questions and body language observations are incorporated into assessments by indicating potential risk or protective factors, individual capacity to accept and receive services, and strengths and challenges that the counselor can incorporate into the client's treatment plan. Clients are also often tested for their communication, comprehension, reasoning, and logic skills in order to determine which methods of intervention will be best received. For example, a client who is unable to communicate verbally may not benefit from simply listening to the counselor providing counseling; a non-verbal, interactive approach will need to be developed for such a client. Clients may also take personality and behavior tests, which allow the counselor to incorporate aspects of the client's beliefs, attitudes, perspectives, and reactions into the assessment.

Major Types of Tests and Inventories

Achievement tests measure knowledge of a specific subject and are primarily used in education. Examples include exit exams for high school diplomas and tests used in the Common Core for educational standards. The General Education Development (GED) and the California Achievement Test are both achievement tests that measure learning.

Aptitude tests measure the capacity for learning and can be used as part of a job application. These tests can measure abstract/conceptual reasoning, verbal reasoning, and/or numerical reasoning. Examples include the Wonderlic Cognitive Ability Test, the Differential Aptitude Test (DAT), the Minnesota Clerical Test, and the Career Ability Placement Survey (CAPS).

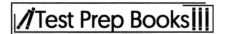

Intelligence tests measure mental capability and potential. One example is the Wechsler Adult Intelligence Scale (WAIS-IV), currently in its fourth edition. The Wechsler Intelligence Scale for Children (WISC-IV), also in its fourth edition, is used for children six years of age to sixteen years eleven months of age and can be completed without reading or writing. There's a separate version of the test for children aged two years six months to seven years seven months, known as the Wechsler Preschool and Primary Scale of Intelligence (WPPSI-III). Examples of other intelligence tests are the Stanford-Binet Intelligence Scale, the Woodcock-Johnson Tests of Cognitive Abilities, and the Kaufman Assessment Battery for Children.

Occupational tests can assess skills, values, or interests as they relate to vocational and occupational choices. Examples include the Strong Interest Inventory, the Self-Directed Search, the O*Net Interest Profiler, the Career Assessment Inventory, and the Kuder Career Interests Assessment.

Personality tests can be objective (rating-scale based) or projective (self-reporting based) and help the counselor and client understand personality traits and underlying beliefs and behaviors. The Myers-Briggs Type Inventory (MBTI) provides a specific psychological type, reflecting the work of Carl Jung. It's often used as part of the career development process. Other rating scale personality tests include the Minnesota Multiphasic Personality Inventory (MMPI-2), the Beck Depression Inventory, and the Tennessee Self-Concept Scale. The Rorschach (inkblot) Test and the Thematic Apperception Test are both projective tests, designed to reveal unconscious thoughts, motives, and views.

Many psychometric instruments exist to assess and diagnose psychological functioning. Some of the most common tests include:

- **Beck Depression Inventory-II (BDI-II):** BDI-II is a twenty-one-question inventory used to measure presence and severity of depression symptoms in individuals aged thirteen years and older.

- **Bricklin Perceptual Scales (BPS):** BPS is a thirty-two-question inventory designed for children who are at least six years old. It examines the perception the child has of each parent or caregiver and is often used in custody cases.

- Millon Instruments:

  - **Millon Clinical Multiaxial Inventory III (MCMI-III):** This 175-question inventory is used to determine indicators of specific psychiatric disorders in adults aged eighteen years and older.

  - **Millon Adolescent Clinical Inventory (MACI):** This 160-question inventory is used to determine indicators of specific psychiatric disorders in adolescents aged thirteen to nineteen years.

  - **Millon Adolescent Personality Inventory (MAPI):** This 150-question inventory is used to determine specific personality indicators in adolescents aged thirteen to eighteen years.

  - **Millon Behavioral Health Inventory (MBHI):** This 165-question inventory is used to determine psychosocial factors that may help or hinder medical intervention in adults aged eighteen years and older.

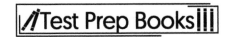

- **Minnesota Multiphasic Personality Inventory (MMPI-2)**: MMPI-2 is a 567-item inventory. It is one of the most widely administered objective personality tests. It is used to determine indicators of psychopathology in adults aged eighteen years and older.

- **Myers-Briggs Type Indicator**: Myers-Briggs is a 93-question inventory widely used to help people aged fourteen years or older determine what personality traits influence their perception of the world and decision-making processes. A preference is identified within each of four different dimensions: extraverted (E) or introverted (I); sensing (S) or intuitive (I); thinking (T) or feeling (F); and judging (J) or perceiving (P).

- **Quality of Life Inventory (QOLI)**: QOLI is a 32-question inventory that determines the perception of personal happiness and satisfaction in individuals aged seventeen years and older.

- **Thematic Apperception Test (TAT)**: TAT is a narrative and visual test that typically requires the individual to create a story and allows the counselor insight into the individual's underlying emotional state, desires, behavioral motives, and needs. It's used for individuals aged five years and older.

- **Rorschach Test**: Rorschach test is a visual test that records an individual's perception and description of various inkblots. It's used to determine underlying personality or thought disorders in individuals aged five years and older.

- **Wechsler Adult Intelligence Scale – Fourth Edition (WAIS-IV)**: WAIS-IV is a series of subtests that assesses cognitive ability in individuals aged sixteen years and older.

Interpreting Test Scores

To begin, any test or assessment should be given under controlled circumstances. The counselor should follow any instructions provided in the test manual. Once completed, the counselor and client can discuss the results. Some best practices for interpreting results are listed below:

- Counselor must thoroughly understand the results

- Counselor should explain results in easily understood terms and be able to provide supporting details and norms as needed

- Counselor should explain and understand average scores and the meanings of results

- Counselor should allow the client to ask questions and review aspects of the test to ensure understanding

- Counselor must explain the ramifications and limitations of any data obtained through testing

Formal and Informal Observations

Qualitative and Quantitative Data

Qualitative data can be collected through interviews, observations, anecdotes, and surveys, and by reviewing literature and other relevant documents. Qualitative data collection methods are often subjective and cannot be generalized to larger samples or populations. Quantitative data can be collected from experiments, recordings of certain events and timed intervals, surveys in which an

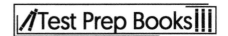

answer choice must be selected for each question, data management systems, and numerical reports. Quantitative data methods are often objective and abstract, and they can be generalized to explain relationships between variables in large populations.

Use of Observation
Basic/Informal Observation
In order to complete a holistic client assessment, it is important that counselors utilize observation to pick up on the nonverbal cues or surrounding environmental aspects. When meeting with a client outside of an office setting, the counselor should observe the condition and location of the client's home and/or work environment when possible.

Additionally, the client's physical characteristics should be observed, which includes some of the aforementioned nonverbal cues of posture, dress, and hygiene, in addition to identifying characteristics such as ethnicity and gender. After meeting with a client, the counselor should take some time to recall the interaction and document identifying information of items observed from the communication.

Observation of Behaviors
It may be necessary for a counselor to observe the client's behaviors rather than solely relying on verbal reports. This is especially true when working with minors who have social and/or behavioral issues as their presenting problem, as well as adults with mental health diagnoses who are unable to contribute competently and verbally to their assessment and report.

A client may be observed in a common setting, such as a school environment or home, to allow the counselor to get a better understanding of how the client functions in a natural environment. The counselor may casually observe how the client functions or may prompt those in the client's personal system to engage in known antecedents. This is done to trigger a particular behavior to gather more information on the client's response. Purposely targeting a behavior to occur in a pre-determined setting (home or office) is known as a **controlled observation**.

In addition to the controlled observation, there are other **formal observation** methods available, wherein specific data is collected on the client in a pre-determined setting. The data must be measurable and is generally used to identify behavioral patterns.

For example, a counselor may note the number of times a self-injurious behavior (like banging of the head) occurs within a setting, while writing down the events that occurred before the behavior (antecedent) and what took place afterwards (consequence). Observing the antecedents, behaviors, and consequences is known as a **functional analysis**.

Observation of Communication Skills
One of the most common means of assessing client's communication skills is through use of verbal dialogue. It is important to note the dialect the client chooses to use, the syncopation of speech, and the length of responses to questions (Are the answers short? Does the client go off on tangents often?) The client's responses are indicators of the presenting problem and an extension of the mental status examination process.

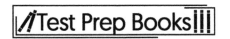

There are numerous areas of communication that can be assessed and addressed, the most common of which are listed here:

- Alertness

    o A common primary indicator of the client's level of consciousness is discernible alertness, commonly assessed with the client's orientation and indicated by a value from one to three.

        ▪ If a client is alert and oriented x1, they are only aware of a person.

        ▪ If a client is alert and oriented x2, then they know the person and place.

        ▪ If a client is alert and oriented x3, then they can state a person, the place, and provide a time period.

    o The client's level of alertness can also be described with adjectives such as lethargic, apathetic, or confused. The counselor can ask questions to determine these elements:

        ▪ "What's your name?"

        ▪ "How old are you?"

        ▪ "Do you know what you're here for?"

        ▪ "What is today's date?"

        ▪ "Who am I?"

- **Speech Patterns**: The rhythm, syncopation, and other behaviors of a client's speech are important in assessing communication. The counselor should document how articulate the client is and note qualities, such as the formation of complete sentences, presence of stuttering, mumbling, curt responses, immature colloquialisms, cursing, and sentence syntax. Additionally, the quality of the client's voice should be assessed for communication patterns. The counselor should observe whether or not the client's tone is appropriate, if the fluctuations are in response to the mood presented, and any persistence of a mechanical tone or rapidity of speech. Moreover, the client's response to the counselor should be noted, gauging the client's degree of cooperation during sessions.

- **Nonverbal Cues**: Not all communication is verbal; nonverbal communication is just as important in client communication. One important nonverbal cue includes the client's facial expressions. Just as it is important to note whether the speech patterns and tone match the flow of conversation, it is equally important to assess whether or not the client's facial expressions are congruent with the present mood and conversation. The counselor should make note of any cues/facial expressions that are in opposition to the words spoken or stated mood (for example, the client stating she is happy, but grimacing or crying). The client's mannerisms should also be observed for communicative deficits or distinctions like fidgeting, flapping, excessive blinking, avoidance of eye contact, rocking, a tense or relaxed posture, and balance. The rate and consciousness of these movements should also be noted. In addition to facial expressions and

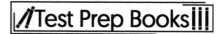

mannerisms, the manner in which a client dresses and the degree of hygiene presented can provide insight to the client's overall functioning.

Assessing for Trauma

In normal circumstances, an individual is typically able to return to a calm state after a stressor passes. Traumatic stress and violence, however, cause long-term effects, and the patient may not be able to recover to a normal state. Indicators of traumatic stress and violence include:

- Unexplained anger or outbursts
- Substance use and abuse
- Uncontrolled behaviors such as binge eating, compulsive shopping, gambling, hoarding, or sex addiction
- Attachment issues
- Chronic and intense feelings of shame, regret, guilt, and/or fear
- Obsessive thoughts or behaviors related to the traumatic event
- Eating disorders
- Self-harm, self-injury, or other self-destructive behaviors
- Sleep problems such as insomnia or sleeping too much
- Intense anxiety, especially in social or crowded situations
- Fear, clinginess, aggression, withdrawal, or regression in developmental behavior in children

Trauma occurs when a client experiences a deeply disturbing experience that yields an intense emotional response. Traumatic events may interfere with a client's baseline level of functioning. It is important for the counselor to have an understanding of the detrimental effects, both visible and invisible, that traumatization can have on a client.

The counselor should have an understanding of the client's baseline level of functioning. This information may be gathered first-hand from the client or through collateral sources if the client is unable or unwilling to provide that information.

The counselor should have an understanding of how to guide the client gently through describing the traumatic experience and the emotions related to it. In doing so, the counselor should have an understanding of the widespread, lasting effects that trauma can have, as well as the multiple recovery and treatment options. This knowledge also helps prevent re-traumatizing the client.

An adult client may present with traumatic stressors due to one or more events that occurred during childhood. Symptoms of anxiety, depression, or other mood disorders that are actually related to the traumatic event(s) may present in session and daily functioning. A counselor should be aware that symptoms of trauma could manifest in places and interactions outside of the client, such as within the family system, with peers, and at work.

Post-Traumatic Stress Disorder (PTSD)

Some people who have experienced trauma or violence will experience an impact significant enough to be diagnosed with PTSD. Symptoms must last for more than one month before the diagnosis of PTSD is considered and must include the following:

- One or more **re-experiencing symptoms** (flashbacks, disturbing dreams, frightening thoughts)

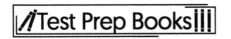

- One or more **avoidance symptoms** (avoiding reminders of the trauma, experiencing emotional "numbing," losing interest in activities that one previously enjoyed)

- Two or more **arousal and reactivity symptoms** (startling easily, experiencing tension, hypervigilance, difficulty falling or staying asleep, eruptions of anger)

- Two or more **cognition and mood symptoms** (difficulty remembering the traumatic event, persistent negative thoughts, excessive feelings of blame or guilt)

Assessing Substance Use

During the intake stage of the counseling process, a counselor may screen clients for substance abuse. The depth of screening will be determined by several factors. Many clients will confess to using substances recreationally or medicinally. The frequency of use, simultaneous use of other substances, and associated medical comorbidities should all be assessed. Counselors should also be aware of the differences between substance abuse and substance dependence. A client who is dependent on a substance is unable to function normally without it. The presence of polydrug use and dependency of substances for social survival should direct the counselor to do an in-depth assessment. Counselors should expect variations in the willingness of clients to respond to substance use questions.

Teenagers will be hesitant to respond honestly for fear of parental involvement. Examples of alcohol and drug screening tools include the **Alcohol Use Disorder Identification Test (AUDIT)** and the **CAGE (cut-annoyed-guilty-eye) questionnaire**. The CAGE questionnaire is a screening tool that determines the likelihood of alcohol problems. The risk is determined by the number of "yes" responses recorded. The **CAGE-Adapted to Include Drugs (AID) questionnaire** is similar to the CAGE tool but includes drug use in its questions. Substance abuse may cause clients to become suicidal or homicidal. Alternatively, chemical dependency may be the result of a suicidal state of mind. It is important to perform a suicide risk assessment concurrently when treating clients with substance abuse. The ultimate goal will be to assist clients in identifying and utilizing alternative coping mechanisms.

Differentiating Substance Use, Intoxication, Withdrawal, and Other Addictions
Substance Use Disorders
The **Diagnostic and Statistical Manual,** generally referred to as the **DSM,** is a comprehensive handbook used by clinicians to determine which mental health diagnosis best fits with presenting symptoms. In older editions of the manual, substance abuse disorders and substance dependence disorders were listed separately, the latter being seen as the more serious of the two. The latest edition, the *DSM-5,* has combined these two disorders into **substance use disorders**. The severity of these disorders is currently broken down by number of presenting symptoms. A client who displays two to three symptoms is considered in the mild range. One displaying four to six symptoms is scored as in the moderate range, and six or more symptoms indicate a severe level of addiction.

The primary distinction between milder and more severe substance use disorders involves the following variables, which are seen in the later stages of addiction:

- **Tolerance:** The need for increased quantities of the substance to achieve desired level of intoxication

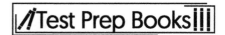

- **Withdrawal:** Onset of undesirable symptoms when the drug or alcohol is not immediately available, which may include tremors, nausea, vomiting, confusion, abnormal heart rhythms, hallucinations, and seizures

- **Cravings:** Increasingly intense urges to consume one's drug or drink of preference

It should be noted that about 50 percent of persons who discontinue use of a substance may experience some form of withdrawal symptoms. Some are mild and do not require medical attention. A small percent experience stroke or seizures that can be life threatening. Clients wishing to attain sobriety by quitting "cold turkey" need careful evaluation and possible medical consultation before entering outpatient treatment for the addiction.

Substance Induced Disorders refer to psychiatric conditions that result from the use of one or more intoxicants. This can occur upon first time use of a substance, such as LSD or synthetic marijuana. More often, the condition is seen following a prolonged and intense use of substances, such as methamphetamines or hallucinogenic drugs. Long term uses of these drugs have, in some cases, caused permanent psychological damage that involves psychosis, depression, paranoia, and other symptoms. The following are the primary substances identified in the *Diagnostic and Statistical Manual*:

- Alcohol
- Inhalants
- Prescription medication
- Sedatives
- Opioids
- Cocaine
- Marijuana
- Hallucinogens

Obtaining Client Self-Reports

One of the ways to obtain data from clients is through self-reporting. **Self-reports** allow clients to disclose their own symptoms, beliefs, attitudes, and behaviors and can be done using a paper survey or electronic test. The Minnesota Multiphasic Personality Inventory (MMPI) is a common tool used to measure personality traits and can help diagnose mental health disorders. **Interest inventories** are a type of affective test that can help clients identify their areas of interest and match these preferences to work contexts. **Symptom checklists** can evaluate the presence and intensity of symptoms that appear with certain disorders and are useful in monitoring symptom reduction after treatment has been established. Examples of symptom checklists include the Beck Depression Inventory, the Connors 3 Rating Scales, and the Child Behavior Checklist. Counselors should be aware of client bias when they report their symptoms. Other factors to consider are the validity and reliability of the chosen test.

Assessment Tools to Identify and Analyze the Presenting Problem

Information can be gathered from the client through a verbal report, or the client can participate by taking assessment tools to assist with identification and analysis of the presenting problem. The counselor may choose from a plethora of worksheets and exercises to engage clients in assessing the various systems in which they are involved. Some of them include the Social Support Network inventory, questionnaires, and perspective worksheets. The more common tools are noted below:

- **Intake Assessment Form**: Clients are asked to complete an assessment form prior to the first session. The counselor may review this form before or after meeting with the client to gain additional insight into the client's needs. The assessment form includes identifying information about the client's household, age, gender, and a brief description of the problem in the client's own words.

- **Genogram**: The counselor can engage the client in creating a genogram, a diagram that depicts the client's family systems, in order to understand significant life events that may indicate familial patterns. Additionally, the genogram can provide insight on the perceived relationship between the client, family, and related support systems.

- **Ecomap**: The ecomap also reviews the client systems, but this diagram extends beyond the family and examines all of the systems in which the client is involved. The client should construct a map of the social relationships in their life, such as work, friendships, church, organizations, and agencies. The social systems are placed in circles. Next, the client should illustrate the connection between the self and relationships with lines. A solid line represents a strong relationship; a dotted or crossed line indicates a fractured relationship. Arrows and other items may be used to add more detail to the relationship status and to help the client and counselor understand the overall function of the relationships.

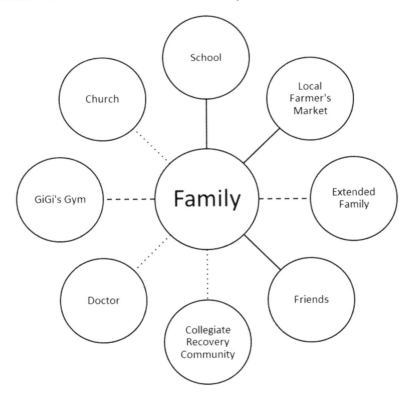

Cross-Cutting Symptom Measures for Adults and Children

Assessing the symptoms of psychiatric illness is one of many central responsibilities psychologists and other mental health professionals engage in. In order to conduct this process in an accurate and organized way, the DSM-5 created the **cross-cutting symptom measures (CCSM)** with separate versions

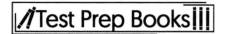

for adults and children. The first level of the CCSM is used to aid psychiatric professionals in determining areas of functioning that may have an impact on treatment and prognosis.

For adults, the measure consists of twenty-three questions that address thirteen psychological areas of functioning. The thirteen domains included within the assessment are depression, anger, mania, anxiety, somatic symptoms, suicidal ideation, psychosis, sleep problems, memory, repetitive thoughts/behaviors, dissociation, personality functioning, and substance use. One to three questions are designated for each domain, measuring how impacted the individual is by the symptom for the last two weeks. For children, the measure is typically completed by a parent or guardian and consists of twenty-five questions that address most of the same domains, with the addition of irritability and inattention domains and excluding personality functioning, dissociation, and memory. For older children and adolescents, ages eleven to seventeen, the counselor may also have the child complete the child-rated version of the measure.

Scoring the CCSM is relatively similar for both the child and adult version. For the adult version, each item is measured on a scale from zero to four, with zero indicating none/not at all, while four indicates severe/nearly every day. A rating of two or more on each item within a domain may signify that the CCSM level two, a more detailed measure, might be necessary in order to gain a better understanding of an individual's symptomology. The child version is also measured on the same five-point scale as the adult version; however, suicidal ideation items are rated on a "yes, no, or don't know" scale. As mentioned before, the CCSM level two provides another way of receiving more information on domains that the individual was highly rated on so the counselor has an even more in-depth comprehension of the patient's clinical formulation.

WHODAS 2.0

The **World Health Organization Disability Assessment Schedule 2.0 (WHODAS 2.0)** is an assessment conducted by clinicians that analyzes any indication of disability in individuals that are eighteen years of age or older. The six domains it covers include understanding/communicating, getting around, self-care, getting along with people, life activities, and participation in society. The WHODAS 2.0 is completed by the individual themself and asks them to rate the difficulty in each specific domain within the last thirty days on a thirty-six-item questionnaire.

There are two versions of the WHODAS 2.0, simple and complex, that counselors use. They differ in their scoring. The simple version allows for the individual to rate the difficulty on a scale from one to five, one being none and five being extreme. These methods are then summed across all of the domains and that determines the degree of impairment in functioning. This version can be scored by hand, making it more preferable for counselors in a busy environment. The complex version, on the other hand, does not use this simple scoring technique. Instead, it uses **item-response-theory- (IRT) based scoring**. IRT-based scoring involves weighing individual items within each domain. This process is completed via computer, and the resulting score is represented on a scale from zero to one hundred, where zero represents no disability and one hundred is full disability.

Interactional Dynamics

Interpersonal relationships refer to interactions (often of a close, friendly, romantic, or intimate nature) between people. They can form due to shared personal, professional, social, charitable, or political interests. Strong interpersonal relationships are built over time as participants are willing to honestly communicate on a regular basis, support one another's well-being, and develop a shared history.

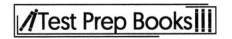

Psychological, evolutionary, and anthropological contexts suggest that humans are an inherently altruistic, community-oriented species that relies on interpersonal relationships to survive and thrive. These types of relationships (when healthy) provide security, a sense of belonging, an exchange of benefits and rewards, and a sense of self-esteem. Healthy interpersonal relationships are characterized by mutual respect, care, and consideration between members. Almost all groups assemble into a power structure of some kind, with natural leaders taking over decision making, resource sharing, and other tasks that affect the group as a whole. **Dysfunctional interpersonal relationships** may be characterized by an extreme power imbalance and dominance by one or more involved members, often leading to submissiveness, learned helplessness, and feelings of low self-esteem in the relationship's less powerful members. Submissive members of a group may find themselves without material resources or respect from the rest of the group.

Ongoing Assessment for At-Risk Behaviors

The counselor conducts risk assessments to determine any influence that could result in harm or increased risk of harm to the individual. Assessing risk can be an ongoing process, as it's important to always have updated, accurate information. Risk-assessment methods will also vary depending on the circumstance (e.g., criminal justice, child abuse or neglect, community care). Some common methodology themes in risk assessment include the following:

- **Universal Risk Screening**: This is a general screening for certain risky behaviors (e.g., violent behavior, substance abuse problems, self-harm) that may result in additional screenings, referral for treatment, or stronger outcomes such as institutionalization (in the instance of high suicide risk, for example). This screening often takes place in initial consultations or as part of the individual's intake forms and may be administered on an ongoing basis (e.g., at every session) to remain current.

- **Unstructured Methods**: These typically include clinical assessments without any specific, prepared structure. While high-level professionals often make judgments during this process, outcomes can sometimes be considered biased and unreliable.

- **Actuarial Methods**: These include highly logical, regimented tests and scales used to predict the likelihood of certain behavior patterns in a specified time frame. While scientific and evaluative in nature, some argue that these methods may place undue blame on individuals or be too inflexible to allow for the likely interplay of many influencing factors in an individual's presenting issue.

- **Structured Professional Judgment**: This combination of the previous two methods is generally the most accepted. It uses structured tools appropriate for the scope of the case but allows for the judgment and flexibility of the counselor to decide what information is useful and to note any external information that may not be caught by standardized assessments.

- **Client's Danger to Self and Others**: Counselors should always be alert to indicators that individuals may pose a threat to themselves or others. These indicators may be obvious or discreet and may include:

  o Substance use and abuse

  o Sudden apathy towards others or society

85

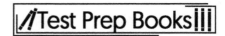

- o Sudden lack of personal care or grooming

- o Isolation

- o Apparent personality change

- o Drastic mood shifts

- o Marked change in mood. Both depressed mood and a positive change in mood can be associated with suicidal thoughts or plans. A sudden positive change may indicate that the individual has made a decision and is no longer experiencing personal turmoil.

- o Verbalization of feelings such as extreme self-loathing, desire to be dead, being a burden to others, or volatility toward others.

Risk Factors for Danger to Self and Others

A client who presents as a danger to self or others should be assessed through a biopsychosocial lens. In addition, tailoring crisis management techniques to the immediate problem can help de-escalate the situation. Open-ended questions should be used to gather as much information from the client as possible. It is also important to consult collateral information from any nearby family members to document other pertinent information about the client.

- The client should be asked if there are plans to harm anyone. If the client states yes, the counselor should determine what the plan entails.

- Any and all threats made should be taken seriously and reported to the proper authorities. Colleagues may be consulted to determine the validity of a threat, if the counselor is unclear on the client's intent.

- Identifying the critical event and antecedent that preceded it is important. The client should be asked to provide as much information on this as they are willing, in order for the counselor to gain a better perspective of the client's point of view.

- Determining whether or not the client has engaged in self-injurious behaviors (SIB) is also important. Here are a few examples of SIB:

- o Excessive use of alcohol or other substances

- o Cutting

- o Banging one's head against a hard object

- o Ignoring necessary medical advice (not taking prescribed pills, leaving a hospital against medical advice)

- The counselor should also evaluate the social and cultural factors that contribute to how the client reacts to stressful situations, including the following:

- o History of violence

- o Stability of relationships (school, work, and home)

    o Social isolation or withdrawal from others

    o Limited access to social resources

- Any recent life stressors that would lead to the client carrying through with a plan to harm self or others

- Assessing the client's current thought process is important. Do they present with confusion, clarity of the situation, or irrational thinking?

- If the client has a clear, concrete plan of action, then the risk for harm to self or others should be considered high.

Risk Factors Related to Suicide

- Previous attempts at committing suicide

- History of cutting

- Multiple hospitalizations related to self-injurious or reckless behavior, such as those noted below:

    o Drug overdose

    o Alcohol poisoning

    o Inhalation of carbon monoxide

- Statement of a plan to commit suicide/suicidal ideations and access to the means to complete it

- Ownership or access to a lethal firearm

- Stated plan to cut one's wrists "the right way"

- Warnings or statements that suicide is planned

- Other factors related to suicide risk

- Age—middle-aged adults present highest suicide risk over other age groups

- Gender—males more likely to commit suicide than females

- Adolescents—high suicide risk, especially those heavily-entrenched in social media groups as a means of support and socialization

- Presence of a mental health disorder

- Life stressors from work or school

- Family history of suicide

- Family discord or other relationship trauma (divorce, break-up, widowed)

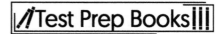

- Excessive drug or alcohol use

- Chronic illness

- Job loss

Pre-Test and Post-Test Measures for Assessing Outcomes

Counselors can employ pre-tests before an intervention to serve as a baseline data set, and they can employ a post-test to measure changes from the baseline. Counselors can also administer surveys, Likert scale questionnaires, or specific intervention evaluation assessments to the client or client system. These tools can measure quantitative results as well as provide an option for anecdotal or testimonial information. Entrance and exit interviews with the client or the client system can also provide a wealth of evaluation information. When evaluating clients face-to-face or through a survey, it's important to create an environment that fosters comfort, open dialogue, and honesty. Clients may feel pressured to provide positive evaluations if they are answering directly to the counselor or if they feel as though a satisfaction survey that they are completing can be traced back to them. This can bias the evaluation process and produce skewed results.

Evaluating Counseling Effectiveness

Evaluation is an important component of any field of study, as it allows counselors to understand which processes are working well and providing results. Evaluation also allows one to identify areas of opportunity and areas for improvement. The process often utilizes data and consumer feedback, and it focuses on processes in place and specific desired outcomes of the practice.

Counselors should continuously evaluate their practice. This evaluation begins with what exactly they would like to evaluate. An evaluation typically focuses on processes (such as clinical intake, client satisfaction, time spent with clients, frequency of sessions, type of intervention) and outcomes (such as were specific goals met for a client, how many clients return after being discharged). Many healthcare organizations provide evaluation tools for counselors, such as benchmark reports that provide client satisfaction responses or practice outcomes.

Methods of practice evaluation are used to measure the effectiveness of treatment. Evaluation is a crucial part of counseling and improves treatment effectiveness, counselor skill, and overall agency management. Evaluation is often required by agency policy and can be a part of supervision. Some level of documentation and evaluation is also typically necessary for reimbursement. Evaluation of policies, programs, and interventions are outlined in the NBCC Code of Ethics. The code recommends the following:

- Counselors should know responsible evaluation procedures, report findings accurately, and use institutional review boards when appropriate.

- Clients must consent to evaluation and be notified of all uses of the information. Counselors need to ensure that clients know participation is voluntary and there are no penalties for refusal or withdrawal of participation.

- Counselors should ensure client confidentiality to the fullest extent possible and only include the information necessary to perform the evaluation.

88

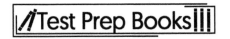

When evaluating practice, the use of several types of evaluation tools are more likely to yield desired results. Also, the use of single-subject designs, surveys, scaling, and other tools can be combined to more effectively evaluate treatment. The following are types of evaluation tools:

- **Goal-Attainment Scaling**: Identified problems are reframed as goals to be addressed. The goals are then given weights or ratings of importance by the client and then the outcomes for each goal are determined using scores.

- **Target Problem Scaling**: Helpful when identified problems are difficult to quantify. The client identifies the severity of each target problem and then rates the changes in the problems as treatment progresses. An overall score is determined to evaluate progress toward all identified problems.

- **Task Achievement Scaling**: Tasks related to an established goal are given ratings when completed to evaluate progress toward goal completion.

- **Surveys**: This tool is used to rate and evaluate a client's feelings about services and may measure satisfaction or the impact of interventions on problems such as depression or anxiety.

Carkhuff's Five-Point Scale

Carl Rogers developed the person-centered, or humanistic, approach to counseling, which stressed the importance of the counseling relationship, as well as the need to evaluate therapy for effectiveness. Rogers believed that three core conditions must exist for therapy to facilitate change: empathy, positive regard, and congruence. Rogers's work was continued by **Robert Carkhuff**, who created a **five-point scale** to measure the core conditions and effectiveness of a counselor. This scale attempts to measure the degree to which the counselor is providing effective levels of empathy, genuineness, concreteness, and respect:

- Level 1. Therapist is contradictory in statements and nonverbal cues and exhibits defensiveness.

- Level 2. Therapist is superficially professional but lacks genuineness.

- Level 3. Therapist does not express defensiveness; there is implied but not overt professionalism.

- Level 4. Therapist is genuine and nondefensive.

- Level 5. Therapist is open and honest and accurately and genuinely reflects ideas and reactions to client.

Areas of Clinical Focus

Adjustment Related to Physical Loss/Injury/Medical Condition

The client's medical history is important information that should be gathered during the intake stage of the counseling process. Medical comorbidities can have an interrelationship with psychiatric illness. Clients who suffer through physical trauma and end up with a disability may have questions related to functionality as members of society, being able to work, and body image changes related to loss of limbs or disfigurement. Pain is a major concern for clients who have chronic injuries and may exacerbate psychological conditions. Clients who receive a diagnosis of terminal diseases such as cancer may go through episodes of hopelessness and despair.

Counselors should be prepared to perform crisis interventions and collaborate with other professionals if needed. Other concerns counselors should be prepared to assess are coping strategies, quality-of-life perception, and the effects of the illness on the client's independence. Clients should be assessed for spiritual or religious beliefs, as they may find comfort in these practices. The client's social support systems, including family and friends, should be established. The degree of social support systems will determine how well a client can handle the treatment and recovery of the illness. Psychological responses to physical illness may lead to anxiety, substance abuse, or depression. Counselors should be prepared to establish a treatment plan that addresses the client's emotional support, coping strategies, and social ties.

Aging/Geriatric Concerns

Aging is an inevitable phase of human development, and the impact is physical, psychological, social, and economic. Self-image is the perception of how one views oneself, but the perception is influenced by societal values. Some cultures revere the elderly and look to them for wisdom and strength. These cultures include the Native Americans, Chinese, Koreans, and Indians. In the United States, there is a different perception of aging. Many elderly Americans feel less valuable or important once they enter retirement. At the same time, they are coping with undesirable body changes and learning to accept that, physically, they can no longer do what they once did. In the U.S., youth and physical attractiveness are highly valued. The elderly are seldom seen as important social figures. They are also less connected with families today, with only 3.7% of homes reporting multigenerational households, per Census Bureau reports. Family support and family contact is less available, currently. For some segments of the population, though, technology has allowed relatives to visit regularly with grandchildren and even participate in family meals or get-togethers.

Geriatric Counseling
Gerontology is the study of biological, cognitive, and psychological features of the aging process. It includes the study of the impact of an aging population on social and economic trends. Gerontologists practice in the fields of medicine, psychology, physical and occupational therapy, as well as counseling. Geriatric counseling practice refers to a range of services provided to the population of those over age 60. Geriatric counselors are found in nursing homes, counseling programs, advocacy centers, and other programs serving seniors. Aging adults must deal with the very real issues of palliative care, hospice, and other end of life issues. The job of counselors is to support them through difficult decision-making processes and to counsel them as they deal with the complicated emotional and spiritual concerns of aging.

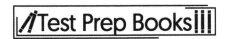

Older Adult Behavior and Development

In gerontology, **aging** is viewed as occurring in four separate processes:

- **Chronological aging**: based on actual years lived

- **Biological aging**: based on physical changes that have an impact on the performance of the body's organs and systems

- **Psychological aging**: based on changes in personality, cognitive ability, adaptive ability, and perception:

  - Basic personality traits appear to be relatively stable through the lifespan, as does an individual's self-image.

  - One aspect that does tend to change, however, is the tendency to become more inwardly focused, which may also result in reduced impulsivity and increased caution.

  - Studies have shown that a pattern of age-related changes in intelligence can typically be observed after age sixty, although changes vary widely across individuals. Furthermore, the somewhat poorer testing results are reflected in **fluid intelligence** (i.e., reasoning, problem-solving, and abstract thinking unrelated to experience or learned information), but not in **crystallized intelligence** (i.e., knowledge based on skills, learning, and experience).

  - Normal age-related changes in memory typically involve acquisition of new information and retrieval of information from memory storage.

  - **Sensory decline** is also a common experience for aging individuals.

- Social aging: based on changes in one's relationships with family, friends, acquaintances, systems, and organizations:

  - Most older persons experience a narrowing of their social networks. However, they are more likely to have more positive interactions within those networks, and they are more likely to experience more positive feelings about family members than younger persons do.

  - **Disengagement theory** states that it is natural and inevitable for older adults to withdraw from their social systems and to reduce interactions with others. This theory has been highly criticized and is incompatible with other well-known psychosocial aging theories.

  - **Activity theory** proposes that social activity serves as a buffer to aging; successful aging occurs among those who maintain their social connections and activity levels.

  - **Continuity theory** proposes that with age, individuals attempt to maintain activities and relationships that were typical for them as younger adults.

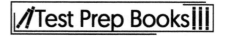

Social Clock Theory (Bernice Neugarten)

Neugarten proposed that every society has a **social clock**: an understood expectation for when certain life events should happen (e.g., getting married, buying a home, having children). When individuals do not adhere to this timeframe, they often experience stress, the sense of disappointing others, or the experience of an internal "clock ticking" and reminding them that time is running out.

Behavioral Problems

Children who struggle with behavioral problems may require counseling services. Professional school counselors often treat students who may require complex counseling services, increased consultations, and collaboration with teachers and administrators. Childhood behavior problems are often the result of anxiety or stress in the home or school setting. In the home setting, one parent may be absent or have extreme or no disciplinary behavior. Children may also be the victims of bullying at school. Behavioral problems are often a way to communicate a lack of social or language skills. Understanding how negative behavior is manifested in children can help create positive change. Counselors should collaborate with teachers and parents to establish a behavior management system. The goal is for children to understand what constitutes acceptable behavior and the consequences of negative behavior. Children with behavioral problems should also feel supported and have a safe place to talk about their feelings. Therapeutic activities, such as sculpting, art, music, and crafts, may help the child project their behavior toward a positive concept. Some of the most common behavioral problems counselors will encounter are abusive language, lying, manipulation, and disrespect.

Bullying

Bullying is widespread among school-aged children and teenagers and may require intervention by a professional school counselor. **Bullying** is defined as intentional, unwanted, and aggressive behavior that is repetitive in relationships in which there is a perceived power differential. There are various types of bullying. **Physical bullying** can be a physical assault or damage to someone's property or belongings. **Verbal bullying** is any type of verbal statements that tease or threaten a person. **Name-calling** is a type of verbal bullying. **Relational bullying** is an attempt to discredit or tarnish another person's reputation by spreading rumors or ignoring the target of bullying. **Cyberbullying**, a growing concern with the influence of social media, is destructive behaviors through e-mail, texting, or social media sites. Those who bully others are more likely to have substance abuse issues later in life and can potentially practice criminal behavior.

Those who are bullied can suffer from emotional distress, suicidal ideation, and a decrease in academic performance. Counselors should be aware of the intervention programs funded by the ACA Foundation. Counselors should also identify advocates who can act as defenders when a bullying incident is occurring. The goal is to empower the person being bullied to speak up and communicate that bullying behavior is not acceptable. Defenders work to involve adults when necessary, support the person being bullied, and encourage empathy in the person doing the bullying. **Workplace bullying**, which can happen to clients of any age, are patterns of behavior that are intended to intimidate, humiliate, offend, or degrade a coworker. Clients affected by workplace bullying can experience a loss of confidence, anxiety, helplessness, and physical symptoms, such as loss of appetite and/or sleep. Clients should be encouraged to review employer violence prevention programs and report the harassment according to the policy.

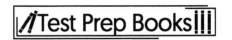

Caregiving Concerns

Impact of Caregiving on Families

There are about 10 million Americans over the age of fifty who are caring for aging parents. In the last fifteen years, thanks to modern medicine, the adult population has begun living longer. As a result, the number of adult children between the ages of fifty and seventy who provide care to aging parents has tripled. This amounts to about 25 percent of adult children who provide either personal or economic assistance.

Research indicates that becoming a personal caregiver to a parent increases the rates of depression, substance abuse, and heart disease. These adult children sometimes take significant financial blows in the form of lost income, earlier than planned retirement, and reduced pension plans, due to leaving the workforce earlier. At the same time, these adult children are assisting their own children as they move towards independence. Those in the youngest generation may still be in college or in the early stages of starting a career and still look to parents for some financial assistance. From a different perspective, the positives of this situation are that children are able to form deeper bonds with grandparents, and the longevity of life in loved ones can have a very positive impact on all involved.

Cultural Adjustments

Impact of Cultural Heritage on Self-Image

Although personal factors play a large role, self-esteem is also based on how closely a person matches the dominant values of his or her culture. For example, Western society tends to value assertiveness, independence, and individuality. Living up to these values is seen as an important accomplishment, and thus, children receive messages about their personal competence and success based on whether or not they are living up to these ideals. Children who are able to exhibit behaviors that are valued within their home and family, as well as those valued by their culture, are more likely to develop a positive self-concept.

One study suggests that across cultures, self-esteem is based on one's control of life and choices, living up to one's "duties," benefiting others or society, and one's achievement. However, the degree to which one's culture values each of those factors has an impact on how the individual derives his or her self-esteem.

A widely cited example of the way that a culture can affect a person's self-image is in the portrayal of women's bodies in the media. In the United States, young women are exposed to underweight models and unrealistically drawn cartoon "heroines," which can lead to the development of unachievable expectations and significant negative perceptions about their bodies.

Impact of Race and Ethnicity on Self-Image

Culture, race, and ethnicity can greatly impact one's self-image, whether one is part of a privileged population or a minority population. One's ethnic and racial background provides a sense of belonging and identity. Depending on a country's treatment of a particular group, self-image can be negatively impacted through racism and discrimination. As mentioned, non-whites are more likely to be arrested than whites and often receive harsher sentences for similar offenses. Racial jokes and racial slurs are common. Stereotypes abound, and some people judge entire racial groups based on the behavior of a few. Such treatment consistently impacts the self-esteem of minority groups. As children become aware of the environment and the culture in which they live, they inevitably notice a lack of prominent

93

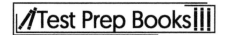

nonwhite politicians, entertainers, CEOs, or multi-millionaires. Non-white Americans who grew up in the fifties or earlier were denied access to restaurants, theaters, high schools, professions, universities, and recreational activities. Even within the last fifty to sixty years, African Americans who had achieved great status in the fields of music, sports, and entertainment were still denied access to certain clubs, hotels, or restaurants.

Every person must explore and come to terms with his or her own culture, ethnicity, and race. Sometimes, this even means rejecting cultural aspects with which he or she disagrees and embracing new and evolving cultural norms. This is a significant part of self-identity development among teenagers and young adults as they are part of a new generation that may be culturally different from their parents. Those that have more exposure to other cultures and backgrounds will have a more open perspective and are better able to evaluate their own culture and ethnicity objectively.

End-of-Life Issues

Death is an inevitable concept. Clients who are nearing end of life may experience emotional distress and functional roadblocks. Poor health, mental health issues, neglect, and depression are common problems experienced by those nearing end of life. Aging is a natural process that can have an effect on purposeful activities of daily living. Clients who lack caregiver involvement and suffer from neglect may require counseling services to address feelings of despair and helplessness. Counselors should be familiar with the various service providers in their communities. These clients may require a referral to a long-term care facility or caregiver services or be enrolled in wellness programs. The overall goal of counseling is to help clients envision a healthy perception of life. Similarly, clients who receive a life-threatening diagnosis may experience anticipatory grief. The client and their family members may require counseling for the expected loss and course of illness. Helping clients acknowledge and express their grief via listening, understanding, and accepting can encourage them to develop coping mechanisms. Counseling for anticipatory grieving can assist with resolving unfinished business before end of life occurs.

In the case of clients who are terminally ill or elderly, counselors play a supportive role in encouraging them to prepare end-of-life forms, such as advanced directives and **Do Not Resuscitate orders (DNRs)**, in conjunction with the appropriate legal and medical authorities. An advance directive is a document that outlines the client's medical treatment wishes in the event that they become unable to make those decisions. Do Not Resuscitate (DNR) is written by the doctor, with the consent of the patient, dictating that if the patient's heart or breathing stop, attempts will not be made to resuscitate. Counselors must empower clients to make decisions that they feel comfortable with and be careful not to impose their own personal biases.

Fear and Panic

Fear is a natural reaction to a specific danger. Fear triggers the flight-or-fight response, which results in physical symptoms such as increased heart rate and respirations. Fear can be a result of phobias, perceived failure, or past experiences, such as violence, war, and aggression. On the other hand, **anxiety** results from the fear of an unspecified danger. The most extreme level of anxiety is known as **panic**. Clients who exhibit panic behavior may experience hallucinations, delusions, the inability to focus, and disorganized thought processes. Some of the screening tools used to detect panic disorders are the five-question **Mental Health Inventory (MHI-5)** and the **Panic Disorder Self-Report Scale (PDSR) questionnaire**.

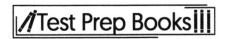

The PDSR contains twenty-four items that are answered in a yes/no format or a five-point Likert scale. Clients experiencing extreme fear and panic have poor situational awareness. Other symptoms include extreme regression and aimless movements. Counselors should speak to clients in firm, simple statements and reinforce reality if a client is experiencing delusions. Clients will benefit from being in quiet settings and minimal environmental stimuli. One of the most effective treatments for clients experiencing panic disorders is **cognitive behavioral therapy (CBT)**. CBT focuses on identifying and modifying thought patterns, which, in turn, can impact emotions and behaviors. Other interventions include exposure therapy and establishing coping mechanisms, such as mindfulness.

Financial Issues

A significant source of stress for many clients is money and financial issues. Financial distress can interfere with personal relationships and family life. The inability to provide for the family, pay debts, or keep up with finances may affect a person's mental and physical health. Clients who experience an unexpected loss of income, bankruptcy, or poverty may seek counseling services to deal with the mental and emotional toll. Mismanagement of money due to lack of financial planning, impulsive purchases, or gambling can also lead to financial issues. Studies have shown that people with financial debt are three times more likely to experience issues with mental health. Other associated risks of financial distress are drug dependency, depression, and contemplation of suicide. Counseling and therapy can help clients identify the emotional need that is met by overspending or impulsive behaviors. The goal is to develop coping tools to suppress the habit. Certified financial therapists focus on the psychological and emotional complications of financial issues and help clients identify the cause of poor financial decisions. Financial therapists can help clients develop money management strategies and productive behaviors.

Poverty is often the foundation of a number of other socioeconomic and health problems faced by individuals, families, and communities. Without resources such as money, transportation, or housing, it becomes difficult to buy healthy food, access medical care, drive to work, have quality childcare, or live in a safe area. For adults in poverty, the extreme level of stress that arises from trying to pay bills, provide basic necessities for themselves and their families, and manage multiple jobs often leads to a number of mental, physical, and emotional problems.

These can include substance abuse, domestic violence, inability to maintain family units and romantic relationships, hopelessness, depression, and desperation. Children who live and grow up in poverty are prone to traumatic and catastrophic health risk factors, such as experiencing or witnessing violence, chronic malnutrition, higher rates of illness, and mood disorders. Experiencing such adverse events in childhood is associated with high levels of stress, impaired functioning, and impaired cognitive ability that can be irreparable. Individuals experiencing poverty are more likely to visit the emergency room for health problems (and often be unable to pay), require government assistance, and commit crimes (often in order to obtain necessary resources). These outcomes create a financial burden on the community and local economy.

Gender Identity Development

Gender identity is the subjective term that describes how people identify their internal sense of self. Regardless of assigned sex at birth, a person may identify as a different gender. Gender identity is usually established by the age of 4 but may happen later or earlier in life. Children can be influenced by social factors, such as gender roles, authority figures, and influential people in their lives. Additionally, children learn language that characterizes males and females and may subconsciously adjust their

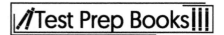

behavior to match gender roles. Societal norms have established ideals of male and female expression, outward appearance, and expected behaviors. Clients who do not conform to a specific gender may often identify themselves as **gender fluid**. Nonexclusive identification of gender is defined **as gender nonbinary**. Clients who identify as neither male nor female, both, or a combination of genders is said to be **gender queer**.

While developing their gender identity, one of the biggest issues clients experience is social isolation. These clients may be discriminated against, stereotyped, or bullied and therefore may experience depression, suicidal ideations, and anxiety. Crisis resources, such as The Trevor Project and the National Suicide Prevention Lifeline, should be provided to clients who express intent to harm themselves. The ACA has endorsed guidelines for counseling clients who are developing their gender identity. Some of the guidelines include using nonsexist language, facilitating client knowledge on the physical and psychological effects of sexism, and increasing their own knowledge on the connection between sexism and other forms of oppression. Joining support groups and community organizations that encourage acceptance of gender identity development can help reduce social isolation. Various organizations, such as Gender Proud, Gender Spectrum, and Gender Diversity, can provide advocacy and help clients feel supported.

Gender Dysphoria

Gender dysphoria encapsulates an entire section within the DSM-5 in addition to being labeled as a mental disorder. When individuals develop an awareness of incongruence in the gender identity that is associated with the sex they were assigned with at birth, they may experience **gender dysphoria**. The incongruence may be accompanied by severe distress in terms of how the individual should not only express themselves physically, but also how they perceive themselves internally with regard to the cultural context. Experiencing gender dysphoria typically manifests in those who identify as transgender, an individual who identifies with a gender or other identity that is different from the sex they were assigned at birth. The diagnostic criteria for gender dysphoria are different for adults, adolescents, and children.

In children, one of the indicators for gender dysphoria is a strong insistence that they are the other gender (male or female) or some alternative identity that is different from the assigned one. Young boys experiencing gender dysphoria may prefer to dress in female attire, whereas young girls may prefer to present as more masculine. Often, young children engage in fantasy play and taking on the role of a different gender during this may also serve as an indication for gender dysphoria. The DSM-5 emphasizes that children strongly prefer the objects, roles, and characteristics of an opposite gender for a period of six months or more.

Gender dysphoria is not only presented in children. For many, adolescence and adulthood are when the incongruence becomes more apparent. The course for this disorder will present differently from person to person as everyone's relationship with gender and identity is different. The indicators for adults are essentially the same as they are in children but are more conceptualized as a fully developed awareness. Individuals must have a strong desire to be a different gender, to be treated/referred to as a different gender, and embody the typical feelings and reactions of the gender they truly identify as.

People who experience gender dysphoria are considered sexual minorities as they are often discriminated against on many different scales in a variety of social, occupational, medical, and institutional environments. With this in mind, counselors must be properly educated on the concept of

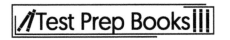

sexual identity as well as develop competency with this population in order to prevent their internal biases from violating proper treatment protocols.

Grief and Loss

The concept of loss is at the root of many depressive episodes. Losses can include anything one holds dearly. Losing a loved one, a pet, a job, housing, or financial or social status can all bring emotional pain. Other losses include the loss of physical or mental health. **Separation** is a form of loss that can occur in many forms, including divorce, military deployment, a job that requires one to move far away, or the loss of custody of a child. Grief is the emotional response to loss. **Grief** includes the main emotion of sadness, but other strong emotions may be present as well. Other feelings include confusion, anger, frustration, anxiety, or guilt.

Although individuals can experience a range of emotions, there are two types of grieving. **Instrumental grieving** is considered more cognitive and focuses on managing emotional reactions and problem solving. It is more *thinking* than *feeling* and is considered a masculine way of dealing with grief. **Intuitive grieving** is more *feeling* than *thinking*. It is thought to be a more feminine way of grieving and focuses on expressing feelings, sharing, and processing emotions.

Elisabeth Kubler-Ross developed the most well-known model for grief in her book *On Death and Dying* in 1969. The five stages model originally pertained to those experiencing the dying process as the result of a terminal illness, but the model has been widely used to understand the grief reactions that people have in response to a number of situations, including loss of a loved one. The five-phase model suggests that individuals pass through at least two of the following stages, and individuals can also cycle back through certain stages:

- **Denial**: This is the first stage. It occurs at the point that the person on some level becomes aware that they have lost someone or something dear, but on another level, they refuse to accept the truth. This stage is generally brief as the person begins to process irrefutable evidence.

- **Anger**: This is a period of venting anger at anyone who the person feels contributed to the loss occurring. It may be towards God, the drunk driver who caused an accident, or the CPS worker who takes a child from the home. In the case of a suicide, there could be anger at the deceased for choosing to leave.

- **Bargaining**: This stage is almost a form of magical thinking. A person may think that if they promise to do better, work harder, or pray harder, the loss process can be reversed. This again is generally a short-lived phase as one realizes that promises made will still not bring back that which has been lost.

- **Depression**: During the fourth stage, a person allows themself to feel the sadness, and they may experience an even deeper emotional pain while learning to accept the loss and move forward. It may be a time of crying, despondency, and anguish. It must be experienced in order to move to the next stage.

- **Acceptance**: The last stage is the point at which the grieving person recognizes that, while the pain is tremendous, they will be able to handle it. Those at this stage understand that time will

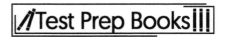
ease some of the suffering. They are learning to make peace with the experience and move forward with their lives.

Counselors can assist clients in dealing with grief by providing support and helping them process emotions and develop skills to adjust to life after a loss. It is important for counselors to understand that individuals experience grief in unique ways and to recognize when grief becomes unmanageable and can lead to more serious concerns, such as depression.

Hopelessness and Depression

Hopelessness is a key characteristic in clients who suffer from depression and suicidal ideations. Clients who experience **hopelessness** believe their current situation will never change. **Depression** is a leading cause of disability and is prevalent in adolescents and more commonly observed in females. In the elderly, symptoms of depression differ from other age groups and often go unnoticed because they commonly occur in combination with other medical illnesses and disabilities. Symptoms of depression in the older adult include confusion, changes in weight or appetite, physical aches and pains, irritability, trouble sleeping, and suicidal thoughts. A caregiver may attribute confusion to a cognitive disorder such as dementia and not address it as possible depression. Hopelessness is considered a cognitive and emotional state and has attributes such as loss of control, negative expectations for the future, and negativism expressed as despair or depression. Counselors can use various screening tools to assess for depression and symptoms of hopelessness.

The **Beck Depression Inventory (BDI)** is used to measure the behavioral manifestations of depression and assess its severity. The BDI is a twenty-one-item self-report inventory that can be used in clients between the ages of 13 and 80. Similarly, the **Beck Hopelessness Scale (BHS)** assesses an individual's negative expectations about their future. The **Hamilton Depression Rating Scale (HAM-D)** is a useful tool that measures depression before, during, and after treatments. This twenty-one-item test is measured on a three-point or five-point scale. The **Children's Depression Inventory (CDI)** is a modified BDI used in children. The CDI can be used in adolescents up until the age of 17 and assesses the severity of depression. Counselors should work with clients to establish a list of worries with possible resolutions. Brainstorming problem-solving solutions and building resilience can assist clients with improving their perception of the future. Other interventions include CBT and interpersonal therapy (IPT) to assist clients with managing negative thoughts and improving their relationships with others.

Loneliness and Attachment

Attachment and Bonding

Understanding attachment and bonding has become more important than ever, especially in relation to changes within the U.S. culture's attitudes about child welfare over the last fifty years. Child Protective Service Teams have become more active in every city. The medical profession, the educational system, and the mental health profession are more informed about children at risk. As a result, more children are being taken from parents, sometimes as early as the day of birth. An older child victim may travel from relative to relative, back to the mother, then into foster or group homes. These children do not have an opportunity to form attachments with their caregivers, nor do caregivers have the opportunity to bond with the children.

Bonding refers to a mother's initial connection to her baby. This occurs within the first hours or days of the birth. Mothers who are able and willing to hold their child close to them shortly after birth generally

98

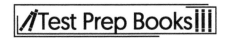
have more positive relationships with the child. When a mother fails to bond, the child is at greater risk for having behavioral problems.

Attachment, on the other hand, refers to a more gradual development of the baby's relationship with their caretaker. A secure attachment naturally grows out of a positive, loving relationship in which there is soothing physical contact, emotional and physical safety, and responsiveness to the child's needs. The baby who has a secure attachment will venture out from their safe base, but immediately seek their mother when fearful or anxious, having learned that mommy will be there to protect them. This type of secure relationship becomes impossible if the child is moved from home to home or has experienced abuse or neglect.

The **attachment theory** is based on the belief that people have the desire to form interpersonal relationships, feel safe, and engage with others. When an interpersonal relationship is disrupted, clients with an **anxious attachment style** can experience distress, grief, and loss. A child whose needs have not been met or who has learned through mistreatment that the world is unfriendly and hostile may develop an avoidant attachment or ambivalent attachment. An **avoidant attachment** is characterized by a detached relationship in which the child does not seek out the caregiver when distressed but acts independently. A child with **ambivalent attachment** shows inconsistency toward the caregiver; sometimes the child clings to them, and at other times, resists their comfort. Establishing a secure, positive attachment with a caregiver is crucial to a child's life-long emotional and social success. The development of attachment disorder is often present in foster children or those adopted later in life and can create much frustration and heartache as the more stable parents step in and attempt to bond with them.

Clients with an **avoidant attachment style** avoid depending on someone else or create distance from others to avoid having anyone depend on them. In times of stress, clients with an avoidant attachment style will withdraw from support systems and experience isolation. The goal of counseling is to make the client understand their attachment needs, communicate them with others, and identify functional coping patterns. Counselors may also use **complimentary interventions** that encourage clients to break old patterns and establish new coping mechanisms. In clients with avoidant attachment styles, practicing empathy and increasing their closeness with others can help decrease loneliness and depression. Counselors can also provide clients with opportunities for social interaction by placing them in group therapy.

Hyper/Hypo Mental Focus

When an individual spends an excessive amount of time thinking about a certain topic or idea or doing a certain activity, it is referred to as hyperfocus. **Hyperfocus** is commonly seen in clients with ADHD or ASD. They have a hard time turning their focus from interesting activities to responsibilities that they don't have much interest in. Often, individuals with ADHD are thought of as having no ability to focus. However, they are capable of focusing their attention continuously for hours on things they enjoy. When the focus can't be switched to important tasks, such as homework or cleaning, it appears that they aren't able to focus. Hyperfocus can become a problem when hours are spent on one thing and duties, or even family and friends, are neglected. Excessive focus can cause individuals to lose awareness of what is going on around them.

They may fail to recognize that they missed a meal or that it is hours past bedtime. Although the intense focus is on something that the individual finds enjoyable, the amount of time spent on the

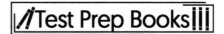

activity and the resulting neglect of other areas of the individual's life can lead to feelings of guilt or anxiety. Since those who tend to hyperfocus do it for the immediate gratification they receive during the activity, one solution for getting them to shift their focus is to create pleasurable feedback in the otherwise boring tasks. Some clients will simply need help diverting their attention to a different task. Creating a schedule with set time-limits for activities (managed with the use of an alarm clock) is a great way to help clients handle issues with hyperfocusing.

On the flip side of hyperfocusing is **hypofocusing**. This is demonstrated by the inability to concentrate. Clients who suffer from PTSD, anxiety, or depressive disorders are often troubled by lack of concentration. There tends to be an emphasis on dismal thoughts that suppresses the ability to focus. Decreased sleep and appetite can also affect the ability to focus; these problems are common with PTSD, anxiety, and depression. Additionally, issues with concentration in clients with depression may be caused by decreased volume of gray-matter in the brain. If a counselor is working with a client who has trouble focusing, the counselor can help the client make a list of necessary but attainable tasks. Being able to reference the list can prevent clients from losing track of what needs to be done. The list should be easily manageable, not daunting. Having a list that can be checked off as tasks are completed can provide the client with a sense of accomplishment that can break the pattern of feeling additional anxiety or depression over being too unfocused to get anything done.

An example of a condition resulting in a hypomental focus state is chronic fatigue. Clients with **chronic fatigue** will verbalize feeling confused, forgetful, anxious, and apprehensive about activities of daily living. Counselors should address the reason for the chronic fatigue. Lifestyle issues that can contribute to fatigue, such as burnout, altered eating habits, and substance abuse, should be addressed and provide a framework for interventions. Clients can benefit from stress reduction skills, recovery programs, or self-care routines, such as yoga and meditation. If a medical condition is suspected, the client should be referred to a medical specialist for treatment.

Intellectual Functioning Issues

Clients with decreased intellectual functioning have diminished learning, problem-solving, and reasoning abilities. Intellectual disabilities usually develop before the age of 18, and these clients exhibit signs of cognitive limitations and lack of adaptive behaviors. Children with decreased intellectual functioning will have issues with abstract thinking, academic learning, and planning. In adults, decreased intellectual functioning results in the inability to follow rules, socially engage with others, or understand important concepts, such as time and financial means. A counselor can use various interventions to treat clients with decreased intellectual functioning, including behavioral therapy, Individualized Education Programs (IEPs), and talk therapy. IEPs are common in schools and require collaboration of school staff to meet the educational needs of the student. Clients with intellectual disabilities require trust, repetition, concrete communication, and simplified language. Counselors should be aware that up to 40 percent of clients with an intellectual disability will have mental health challenges, such as anxiety and depression, and should be addressed accordingly.

Insomnia and Sleep Issues

Sleep deprivation occurs when a person does not get the optimal amount of sleep on a daily basis. Lack of sleep or trouble sleeping can lead to issues such as unstable mood, chronic fatigue, and medical comorbidities. Chronic sleep deprivation may result in delusions and hallucinations. **Insomnia** is the most common sleep disorder reported and can be associated with anxiety, depression, and

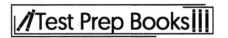

posttraumatic stress disorder (PTSD). Counselors should explore the root cause of sleep disorders and develop interventions related to the source of the problem.

Counseling should primarily focus on having the client change behaviors, develop relaxation skills, and establish sleep goals. There are various methods a counselor can use to address sleep disorders, such as keeping a sleep diary, improving sleep hygiene, and discussing dark therapy. **Sleep diaries** can help determine any causative triggers that disturb sleep patterns. **Sleep hygiene** is a personalized plan in which the client develops a list of activities to perform and/or avoid before bedtime. **Dark therapy** involves restricting light sources, which can delay the circadian clock. Clients should be encouraged to limit exposure to blue light that is found in screens, such as cellphones and televisions, before bedtime. CBT is commonly used in clients with insomnia and aims to change sleep schedules and habits that can contribute to sleep disturbances.

Maladaptive Eating Behaviors

An **eating disorder** is a persistent disturbance in eating behaviors that leads to poor health. Maladaptive eating patterns can lead to psychological, physical, and emotional disturbances. Some of the most common eating disorders are anorexia nervosa, bulimia nervosa, and binge-eating disorder. Clients who practice extreme forms of dieting can also be classified as having an eating disorder. Extreme dieting can lead to sleep disturbances, decreased energy, mood swings, irritability, and social isolation. Additionally, clients who experience high levels of emotional or mental stress can use food to suppress their negative thoughts. This type of maladaptive eating behavior can be attributed to atypical depression. **Atypical depression** results from chronic stress and a sustained level of increased cortisol in the body. Cortisol is a stress hormone that increases appetite.

Stress eating satisfies the client's emotional needs as opposed to their physical hunger. Clients who experience these maladaptive eating behaviors may also experience low self-esteem and anxiety. Adolescents are the population most commonly affected by eating disorders and may develop maladaptive behaviors because of bullying, body shaming, or peer pressure. Screening tools, such as the **SCOFF questionnaire** (Sick, Control, One, Fat, Food), the **Body Attitudes Questionnaire**, and the **Eating Disorder Inventory**, are useful in assessing the presence of an eating disorder. Behavioral therapy is an important part of recovery and aims to help clients build good eating habits, stop harmful behaviors, and develop healthy coping skills. Clients may be placed in group therapy to obtain support from others who experience the same condition. Counselors should encourage clients to develop healthy coping skills to deal with emotional distress and ultimately be comfortable in their own body.

Remarriage/Recommitment

After separating from a partner or divorcing a spouse, people experience a sense of loss and may go through stages of grief. There are multiple **stages of grief**, including denial, anger, bargaining, depression, and acceptance. The final stage is **rebuilding**. During this stage, acceptance of the situation increases and a plan for the future emerges. Clients may seek counseling to process their emotions, learn to establish healthy boundaries with their former partners, and attempt to rebuild their lives. Counseling can help clients identify unhealthy behaviors that ended the relationship. It is important to include the client's new partner in the counseling so they can establish a sense of vulnerability and increase effective communication. Some of the problems to address include jealousy, lack of closure in previous relationships, resentment, and lack of trust. Counselors who specialize in couples counseling

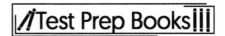

should focus on helping partners communicate their needs and develop healthy solutions to their conflicts.

Developmental Processes, Tasks, and Issues

Client needs in counseling vary depending on their developmental stage. Counselors should be aware of the challenges their clients face as they progress through their lifespan. In every psychosocial stage, there are two concepts all clients will face. For example, children from the age of 3 to 6 years will experience **initiative versus guilt**; through imaginative play, children begin to experiment with who they are. If they do not feel supported by their parental figures, they may feel guilty about not following a set of rules. In middle adulthood (approximately ages 40 to 65), **generativity versus stagnation** challenges a person to contribute something meaningful to new generations.

Failure to do so will lead to stagnation without a meaningful sense of accomplishment. Knowledge of the different developmental stages can help the counselor guide the client through anticipated challenges and put their problems into perspective. A client's culture and diversity factors may also influence how they meet their developmental tasks. Clients who have low socioeconomic status or are victims of racism, prejudice, or oppression may have limited opportunities to reach their developmental goals. Interventions include individual, family, and group counseling. Classroom guidance can facilitate younger clients' understanding of the emotional, cognitive, physical, and social aspects of self-development.

Obsessive Thoughts and Behaviors

Obsessions are impulsive thoughts that are persistent and recurring in the mind. Obsessions and compulsions often exist together. **Compulsive behaviors** are ritualistic and aim to decrease the severe anxiety that is caused by not performing them. Clients with an **obsessive-compulsive personality** have an overwhelming need to follow a strict set of rules, moral codes, and fixed routines. On the other hand, clients diagnosed with **obsessive-compulsive disorder (OCD)** have a pattern of unwanted thoughts followed by a repetitive compulsion, and an intense need to carry out compulsive behaviors. Examples of obsessive themes include violence, sexual ideation, contamination, and doubt. For example, a client who believes that every surface is contaminated may avoid touching all objects and will repeatedly wash their hands if forced to touch a surface.

Other clients may return to their home to check the door lock many times a day to satisfy the intrusive thought of doubt. There are a couple of interventions counselors can use during therapy to decrease the compulsion that follows the obsessive thought. **Exposure and response prevention (ERP)** aims to control the anxiety of not reacting to a particular obsession. The goal is to have the client confront the obsession and refrain from performing the usual compulsive action. CBT can help clients place their obsessions into perspective. The goal is to recognize unrealistic thoughts and become desensitized to the obsession. Clients should also be encouraged to develop coping skills to deal with the anxiety caused by not reacting to an obsessive thought. When counseling children with OCD, parents should be educated on supportive strategies. Praising the child when they resist compulsions, allowing uncertainty, and avoiding criticism can reassure control of the issue.

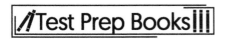

Occupation and Career Development

One of the most important aspects of an adult's life is their career choice. Career counseling can help clients choose, change, or leave a particular occupation by providing resources, interpreting aptitude assessments, or discussing the development of career choices. Counselors should assist clients in identifying their strengths, personality type, and skills set. The **Myers-Briggs Type Indicator (MBTI)** is a tool used to determine personality type based on self-reporting. Choosing a career based on personality type can decrease the probability that an individual will experience burnout in their occupation. Some of the topics to discuss with clients during career counseling are financial goals, educational capacity, advancement opportunities, and work environments. Demanding occupations may lead to job stress, and clients may present with psychological issues, such as depression, anxiety, and substance abuse, or physical symptoms, such as decreased appetite, difficulty sleeping, and headaches. Counselors can help clients identify patterns that contribute to stress and develop relaxation techniques, such as meditation, yoga, and deep breathing, to decrease the effects of burnout.

Considerations When Providing Counseling Services

Adults with Disabilities

Individuals with disabilities have additional challenges in the career planning process. Disabilities include physical limitations, learning disabilities, cognitive impairment, mental health issues, as well as veterans in the Wounded Warrior class. Fortunately, there are many resources available, including the **Americans with Disabilities Act**, **the Job Accommodation Network (JAN)**, the **Department of Labor Disability Employment Policy (ODEP)**, and many other national and community programs. Counselors can help clients to understand their legal rights and to learn how to educate employers about options during the application and interview process. Many employers can (and are required by law to) offer accommodations to assist with employment opportunities. In addition, most areas have service organizations that assist with career planning and can even offer on-the-job coaching.

Sexual Orientation

In recent years, there's been increased awareness and sensitivity to lesbian, gay, bisexual, and transgender (LGBT) individuals. However, like any minority group, they can be subject to discrimination and bias. For counselors, it's essential to be aware of LGBT issues in career development. Discrimination can occur in the interview process and on the job, and many states and countries don't provide legal protection to LGBT employees. An increasing number of employers value diversity in their workforce, and an April 2013 study shows that 88% of Fortune 500 companies enforce non-discrimination policies. Counselors working with LGBT individuals can utilize several strategies to increase the effectiveness of counseling. Making clients feel safe by demonstrating an understanding of LGBT culture is important, as well as avoiding stereotyping. Counselors should consult with other professionals as needed, use current resources on LGBT society, and refer out when necessary. Lastly, counselors should engage in open discussions about LGBT issues and help each client develop career goals unique to their personal situation.

Physical Issues Related to Anxiety

Anxiety is defined as having a sense of dread, uncertainty, or uneasiness. Although anxiety usually disturbs thought processes, it can also manifest through physical symptoms. Some of the most common physical signs of anxiety are elevated heart rate, sweating, dizziness, tense muscles, and headaches. Physical symptoms that are more severe, such as difficulty breathing, can signal a panic attack.

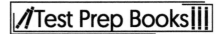

Counselors should be able to recognize that anxiety will affect each client differently. Based on the level of anxiety, counselors can develop interventions to help the client develop healthy coping skills. The most common type of therapy to treat the symptoms of anxiety is CBT. **CBT** works by retraining how clients think via exposure. For example, if a client struggles with being out in public for long periods of time, progressive exposure to social situations in time increments may ease the anxiety. **Biofeedback** is another form of therapy that helps clients understand the physical reaction to anxiety and become aware of how their bodies respond to triggers. Introducing self-care habits, such as exercise, meditation, yoga, and journaling, can help clients reduce their anxiety and, consequently, their physical symptoms.

Physical Issues Related to Depression

Depression is usually characterized by feelings of hopelessness, anger, sadness, and suicidal ideation. However, depression can also cause physical manifestations. Eating disorders are common, and clients may experience decreased appetite and weight loss or increased cravings that lead to binge behaviors. Depression can lead to slow body movements, slouched posture, back pain, and headaches. In children and teenagers, oversleeping and overeating are common manifestations. In the older adult, fatigue and non-medical impotence are physical signs that are often overlooked and may delay a depression diagnosis. Goal setting during an initial counseling session can help clients determine what priorities to address. Counselors can help clients recognize their strengths and use them to change behaviors and develop healthy coping mechanisms. Common goals of overcoming depression include improving physical well-being, building meaningful relationships, and performing productive activities of daily living. Counselors should also encourage clients to develop healthy lifestyle habits, such as exercise, which releases endorphins; eating foods that are rich in omega-3 fatty acids, which increases serotonin; and meditation, which can increase dopamine levels.

Physical and Emotional Issues Related to Trauma

Trauma affects everyone differently. The reaction depends on the person's emotional resiliency, history of past trauma, and other factors. Some trauma survivors exhibit symptoms that clearly meet the criteria for PTSD, while others exhibit smaller clusters of symptoms, such as anxiety or depression. Others show little or no symptoms. Below is an overview of common responses:

- **Foreshortened future**: This refers to the sense that one's life is shortened or forever altered and that a normal life may never be experienced again.

- **Emotional responses**: These may be fear, sadness, shame, anger, guilt, and/or anxiety.

- **Physical reactions**: Survivors of trauma often have multiple somatic issues, including gastrointestinal complaints, neurological problems, poor sleep, and muscle pain.

- **Hyperarousal**: Trauma survivors often become hypervigilant. They are frightened by neutral stimuli, such as a dog barking or a child screaming. They may experience a continual feeling that something terrible is going to happen.

- **Intrusive thoughts**: Survivors can become flooded with unwanted thoughts and memories about the trauma.

- **Trigger/flashbacks**: Triggers are stimuli that set off memories and provide a sensory reminder of the traumatic event.

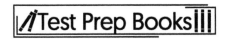

- **Dissociation**: This coping mechanism allows the person to "check out" temporarily. This process severs connections to the painful memories.

- **Self-harm**: Some survivors use self-harm as a means of distraction from emotional pain. This could transition into more serious self-harm and can result in suicidal behaviors if not treated.

- **Substance abuse**: Many survivors use substances to medicate unpleasant emotions, such as fear or shame.

Common Effects of Stress, Trauma, and Violence

Many people equate stress with an emotional experience, but stress can actually have a profound effect on the body, cognition, and behavior as well.

Common Effects of Stress		
Body	**Mood**	**Behavior**
Headache	Anxiety	Overeating or under eating
Muscle tension or pain	Restlessness	Angry outbursts
Chest pain	Lack of motivation or focus	Drug or alcohol abuse
Fatigue	Irritability or anger	Tobacco use
Change in sex drive	Sadness or depression	Social withdrawal
Stomach upset		
Sleep problems		

Although everyone experiences some degree of stress, stress becomes trauma when the intensity of the stress causes a person to feel helpless and seriously threatened, either physically or psychologically. Unfortunately, trauma and violence are common experiences for both adults and children, and the risk for traumatic and/or violent events is particularly high for individuals suffering from mental illness. Some people will experience a trauma with little to no lasting impact, while others may struggle with the aftermath of the trauma for the rest of their lives.

Many variables can either exacerbate or ameliorate the impact of trauma:

- Whether the event occurred once or was ongoing
- Whether the event occurred during childhood or adulthood
- Intensity of the traumatic event
- Personal experience vs. observation
- Ability to access supportive resources
- The way in which people and systems respond to the individual who has been traumatized

Potential effects of trauma and violence:

- Substance use and abuse
- Mental health problems
- Risk-taking behavior
- Self-injurious behavior
- Increased likelihood or exacerbation of chronic illnesses, including cardiovascular disease
- Difficulties with daily functioning, including navigating careers and relationships

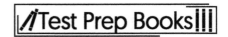

Process Addictions

Behavioral process addictions are compulsive activities performed to satisfy an impulse. Clients with process addictions perform activities despite the possible consequences. Addictions are particularly problematic when they interfere with the ability to function academically, socially, and professionally. Clients who develop habitual behaviors that result in guilt, distress, or shame can benefit from counseling to decrease the anxiety caused by abstaining from the addiction. Common process addictions include chronic gambling, sex urges, hoarding, excessive exercising, and unrestrained shopping. Clients with a **gambling addiction** may lie about the extent of their gambling, ignore family and work responsibilities, progressively increase the amount that is gambled, and use gambling as a means to escape life problems.

Compulsive spending is classified by investing an excessive amount of time and resources to shop. The Bergen Shopping Addiction Scale is a screening tool that measures the severity of a shopping addiction. The scale consists of twenty-eight statements that rate each item in a five-point continuum of agreement. Behaviors that increase the likelihood of a shopping addiction include consistent and obsessive thoughts about shopping, using shopping as a mood stabilizer, inability to decrease the amount of shopping, and guilt if the activity is not performed. Process addictions require discovering the underlying emotional need that necessitates the compulsive behaviors. Counselors should work with clients to establish adaptive skills and impulse control. CBT, support groups, and twelve-step programs can help clients overcome process addictions. The development of new hobbies, avoiding places that encourage the behavioral addiction, and strengthening supportive relationships can facilitate recovery.

Indicators of Addictions to Gambling, Sex, Food, and Media

Addictions and compulsive behaviors can damage health, finances, social status, and relationships. Even some behaviors—such as exercise and work—are recognized as positive behaviors, but when taken to extremes, unpleasant consequences develop. For example, exercise addiction, in its least damaging form, may create anxiety when physical or weather conditions prevent participation. In more extreme cases, certain athletes will continue to train in spite of illness or injury, exacerbating the physical problem and sometimes causing permanent disabilities.

Those addicted to pornography find that having close and intimate contact with their long-term partner is less exciting than viewing stimulating films or pictures. This creates intimacy problems and difficulty in one's primary relationship. The Internet has made it easier for people to access these materials, sometimes at no cost, creating a greater number of persons who view it addictively.

Some people who struggle with shopping addictions—sometimes called "**shopaholics**"—may become hoarders or financially destroy themselves and their family. They may make foolish purchases when more basic needs of the family are not being fulfilled. For example, many people who struggle with addiction have closets full of clothes never worn or may own fifteen pairs of sunglasses.

Like exercise, overworking—sometimes referred to as "**workaholism**"—may also be viewed as positive by some standards. In the end, however, those working many hours of overtime may result in a life out of balance. They may also be using work as a means to avoid other responsibilities, such as family life. It can create stress and low energy, and it can lead to physical and emotional problems.

Overeating, based upon the number of obese and overweight persons in our culture, is on the rise. Some people use food much in the same way that others use alcohol or drugs—to feel a sense of

106

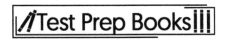
pleasure or to numb feelings of depression or anxiety. The consequences of obesity are numerous from a social and physical standpoint, with the most severe of these being the high risk for heart disease or stroke.

Some individuals are addicted to self-harm in the form of cutting, scratching, or mutilating themselves. This is often described as a means to bring relief from emotional pain as one focuses on the physical sensation of pain to distract from the emotional sensation. It may also be a type of self-punishment. Some people have horrendous scars from this compulsion. Others may contract infections. It is theorized that persons who self-mutilate are at higher risk of suicide than those who do not, making it a possible precursor to suicidal ideations.

Racism, Discrimination, and Oppression

Discrimination is the unfair or unequal treatment of a person or group, based upon a characteristic, such as race, ethnicity, religion, age, sex, or sexual orientation. There are several forms of discrimination that minorities experience.

Direct discrimination refers to unfair treatment based on someone's characteristics. An example would be refusing to hire someone because of their ethnicity.

Indirect discrimination refers to situations in which a policy applies the same to everyone, but a person or group of people are negatively impacted due to certain characteristics. For example, a company might require that everyone help unload shipments that come to the office. The policy is the same for everyone, but it's discriminatory towards any disabled employees. In a workplace environment, indirect discrimination can sometimes be allowed if there's a compelling reason for the requirement. For example, firefighters have to meet certain physical criteria due to the nature of their work.

Another form of discrimination is *harassment*. This involves unwanted bullying or humiliation intentionally directed to a person of minority status. *Secondary victimization* refers to the unfair treatment received when a person reports discrimination and is not supported by authorities.

Effects of discrimination on the individual may include depression, anxiety, other mental health issues, and medical/health-related problems caused by lack of access to health resources. Effects of discrimination on society include diminished resources (e.g., employment, educational opportunities, healthcare) and a culture characterized by fear, anger, or apathy.

Religious Values Conflict

Religion and spirituality are two distinguishable terms that can cause distress in an individual if not followed according to their ideals. **Spirituality** is a sense of connection to the universe, nature, or a higher power that may not be directly identified. Individuals who share a common faith and practice a particular set of beliefs may identify themselves with a formalized **religion**. Religion can influence a person's life and may be helpful in coping with hardship. When religions operate under principles that deviate from their doctrine, an individual may question their faith, which can lead to unstable emotional and mental well-being. Clients who are questioning their faith may experience anxiety and can potentially self-harm, experience suicidal ideation, and have substance abuse issues. Clients who experience religious discrimination and are potential victims of physical violence may have PTSD, depression, and mental distress. Counseling should focus on guidance as opposed to supporting or rejecting a person's beliefs. Clients should be encouraged to reconcile the areas of conflict between

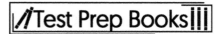

their life and religion and uncover areas of concern. Helping the client align their emotional needs with their fundamental beliefs can help them develop a greater understanding of mental and spiritual well-being.

Retirement Concerns

Planning for retirement usually includes financial stability and affordability of living. However, retirement can also lead to emotional and mental instability. Work provides a social structure and sense of community. Careers often fulfill a sense of purpose and passion. Retirement can cause emotional distress and lead to feelings of uselessness, loneliness, boredom, and disillusionment. Retirement can cause an identity crisis, and clients will be seeking counseling to establish a new sense of productivity. There are several interventions counselors can implement to help clients adjust to retirement. Setting small goals and establishing milestones can give clients a sense of purpose. Clients should be encouraged to become involved within the community and build friendships to avoid the isolation that follows retirement. Setting up a schedule for the day's activities allows for structure and can help clients feel a sense of normalcy to their routine. Volunteering, developing new hobbies, and expanding social ties can decrease the mental and emotional effects of retirement.

Ruminating and/or Intrusive Thoughts

Persistently focusing on a situation or thought process is known as **rumination**. Ruminating thoughts are concerns with possible loss, failure, or hopelessness. People who experience rumination focus on negative thoughts, feelings, and past experiences. As intrusive thoughts persist, the result can be in anger, sadness, and agitation. Rumination is a maladaptive form of self-reflection and focuses on psychological distress. Clients who have ruminating thoughts are more likely to become depressed and develop unhealthy coping mechanisms, such as alcohol abuse and binge-eating habits. **The Ruminative Response Scale (RRS)** is a twenty-two-item questionnaire that measures the intensity of ruminating thoughts when feeling sad. CBT for ruminating thoughts focuses on developing new ways of thinking and targets the issues that are causing the intrusive thoughts. **Functional analysis** is a component of CBT that aims to identify problematic thinking and change behaviors that exacerbate habitual thought processes. During behavioral activation and cognitive restructuring, clients take action, reward healthy behaviors, and learn reality-based thinking. The goal of counseling for rumination is to encourage mindfulness and defuse negative thoughts.

Separation from Primary Caregivers

Throughout their development, children form attachments to their primary caregivers. **Secure attachment** is a healthy bond between a child and a caregiver. Some of the behaviors that define secure attachment include eye contact, verbal and nonverbal display of emotions, and recognition of familiar caregivers. Other forms of attachment include the anxious-resistant insecure, anxious-avoidant insecure, and the disorganized/disoriented style. These attachment styles typically indicate that the child's needs are not consistently met by the caregiver. A weak attachment bond can result from early separation from caregivers and lead to social and emotional developmental issues. Signs that children have insecure attachments include rejection of emotional connections, frequent crying, avoidance of eye contact, and lack of interest in interactive play.

To determine the effect of detachment from a child and their caregiver, the **Strange Situation test** can be performed prior to initiating counseling. The test consists of eight episodes lasting a couple of

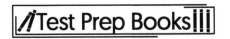

minutes in which the caregiver, child, and a stranger are introduced, separated, and later reunited. In a secure attachment style, separation anxiety is marked when the caregiver leaves the child. In the resistant attachment style, the child will display intense distress when the caregiver leaves. In the avoidant attachment style, children show no sign of distress when left alone. Counseling can help children understand healthy relationships, develop coping skills for separation anxiety, and form constructive bonds with caregivers. Interventions include behavioral therapy, such as systematic desensitization and flooding. Gradual exposure to anxiety-producing situations can diminish the fear that is initially experienced.

Sexual Functioning Concerns

Sexual dysfunction is characterized as any problem that prevents an individual from obtaining satisfaction from sexual activity. More than 40 percent of women and 30 percent of men report issues with sexual functioning. There are four categories of sexual dysfunction: a lack of sexual desire, inability to become sexually aroused during intercourse, delayed or absent climax, and pain during intercourse. Sexual dysfunction has both physical and psychological causes. Physical causes include heart disease, diabetes, high blood pressure, hormonal imbalances, among many others. Psychological causes include stress, anxiety, depression, body image issues, and past sexual trauma. Counseling should focus on the underlying cause of sexual dysfunction. For example, clients who have a history of sexual assault may benefit from **depth therapy**, which focuses on unconscious feelings and aims to change unhealthy coping behaviors. After recovering from sexual trauma, sex therapy can address intimacy concerns. Sex counseling can help individual clients and couples reflect on their internal conflicts and concerns. The goal of counseling is to remove mental and emotional barriers that prevent clients from achieving sexual satisfaction.

Sleeping Habits

A disturbance in sleep patterns is known as a **sleep-wake disorder**. Sleep-wake disorders can affect mental, emotional, and physical health. Several psychological factors that affect the sleep cycle include depression, anxiety, trauma, and stress. Sleeping less than the recommended hours can lead to sleep deprivation. Sleep deprivation can cause fatigue, impaired judgment, and trouble focusing. Alternatively, consistently sleeping more than the recommended hours can lead to headaches, back pain, lack of productivity, and depression. Poor sleep habits, such as late or early bedtimes, remaining in bed for prolonged periods of time, and excessive daytime napping, can cause sleep-wake disorders. It is important to recognize if poor mental health is affecting sleep or if sleep disorders are causing disruptions in mental health. Counselors should focus on the behaviors or emotional disturbances causing the disruption in sleeping habits. Interventions include helping clients set a consistent sleep schedule, create bedtime rituals, and eliminate stimuli before bedtime.

Spiritual and Existential Concerns

Spirituality is a sense of connection to the universe, nature, or a higher power that may not be directly identified. An individual may continuously be searching for an ultimate meaning of life or personal growth. Spirituality can also connect people to one another and is expressed via various rituals, such as meditation, yoga, and dance. Spiritual beliefs may also provide social and emotional support, offer comfort in times of grief, and provide ethical guidelines for a way of life. When an individual questions their spirituality and is faced with a life challenge, such as the loss of a loved one or diagnosis of a

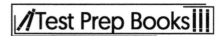
chronic health condition, they may struggle to find meaning in life. Similarly, clients who experience doubts about their place in life and develop an internal conflict may experience an **existential crisis**.

Some of the reasons an individual may experience an existential crisis include unresolved emotional challenges, unfulfilled social lives, inability to overcome guilt, and overall dissatisfaction with their path in life. The sense of hopelessness can lead to depression and anxiety. Clients seeking counseling for spiritual or existential concerns may struggle with self-compassion or a lack of belonging or may be unconcerned with life. **Pastoral counseling** is a realm of practice with education on theology and can help clients discover their own spirituality. Being empathetic and incorporating a twelve-step program can guide clients toward resolving their spiritual concerns. Encouraging clients to replace pessimism with positive thoughts, reflect on reasons for being grateful, and identify positive qualities in oneself can help to resolve an existential crisis.

Stress Management

Types of Stress
Crisis situations and stress have a variety of causes. **External stress** exists outside of a person's control and can include natural disasters, loss, illness of self or a family member, crime, poverty, or job change. Internal distress is the reaction to external stress but may be chronic and exist at all times due to an individual's coping skills and personal choices. Positive events, such as marriage, childbirth, a new job, or relocation, can cause eustress, which is considered positive stress. Major life changes can cause transitional stress, which may be short term but still requires strategies for managing. Stress management techniques include maintaining one's physical health, adequate sleep, relaxation techniques, and engaging in enjoyable activities or hobbies.

Stress Management
Counselors will often encounter clients with stress related problems and should be well versed in stress management techniques to offer clients suggestions for this issue. Counselors may engage clients to practice relaxation techniques in order to manage stressors. Clients may engage in physical exercise at their physician's discretion to relieve stress. Deep breathing exercises are also beneficial in relieving stress. Clients may work to change fallacious thinking patterns and distorted perceptions to reduce stress through treatment such as cognitive behavior therapy or rational emotive therapy. Clients may be stressed concerning basic living needs and counselors can link clients to services in the community to assist them with these issues. If clients are at the safety and physical stages of the hierarchy of needs, these stressors should be addressed before other issues are included in the therapeutic process.

Substance Use/Addiction Issues

Addiction is a complex process involving biological, social, cultural, and genetic factors. There is some disagreement in the addiction treatment community about the causes and best treatments for substance abuse disorders. There are several models of addiction.

The earliest theory of addiction is called the **_Moral Model_**. This model implies that the person abuses substances because they are morally weak. The **addict** is viewed as a sinner or criminal and one who does not have the intestinal fortitude to change negative behaviors, therefore choosing to wallow in the misery of their sins.

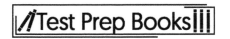

The **disease model or medical model of addiction**, upon which the twelve-step program of **Alcoholics Anonymous (AA)** is based, specifies that the addict suffers from an illness that will never be cured and is progressive in its development. Even if the individual ceases alcohol intake, the disease remains. AA literature indicates that when one relapses, even after years of sobriety, the addict picks up, not where he left off, but where the disease would have taken him if the drinking had continued. It is seen as a medical disorder and, at times, referred to in the Big Book of AA as having an allergy, with alcohol as the identified allergen. This theory is accepted and understood by many successful AA participants who have maintained sobriety throughout this program for years and who have shared their experience of strength and hope to help others struggling with addiction.

The **bio-psychosocial model of addiction** focuses on the role of the environment. Cultural and social factors influence one's beliefs and attitudes about substance use. In certain religions, it is unacceptable to use alcohol. In others, it may be encouraged—such as the huge sale and consumption of beer at Catholic picnics and fish fries. An addict's observation of others and their patterns of alcohol ingestion influences their attraction to drug or alcohol use as a means for tension relief or a form of celebration. Exposure to family or community members who use large quantities of intoxicants may serve to normalize dysfunctional patterns of use. Some youth observing parents consuming a quart of vodka each night may believe their family members are just normal drinkers, whereas other youth are raised in environments where alcohol is unacceptable or served only on rare occasions.

The **learning theory of addiction** is based on concepts related to positive reinforcement. The assumption underpinning this model is that addiction is a learned behavior through operant conditioning, classical conditioning, and social learning. Social learning takes place through observation. Learning theory posits that the interplay between these three factors contribute to the initiation, maintenance, and relapse of addictive behaviors. The intoxicant serves as an immediate reinforcement in the form of increased euphoria or relaxation. In some cases, it also deters withdrawal symptoms. Both of these forms of reinforcement increase the likelihood that the behavior will be repeated in an effort to recreate the sensation of feeling better.

Genetic theory of addiction is based on research indicating that biological children of parents who struggle with addiction or alcoholics are more prone to addiction than children of non-alcoholics. According to genetic therapy, this genetic predisposition towards addiction accounts for about half of one's susceptibility to becoming an addict. Theorists of this model agree that other factors, such as social experiences, have an impact upon the formation of an addiction.

The repercussions of the addict's behavior can affect many significant aspects of life. The impact of addictions is felt not only by the addict, but everyone in that person's family and circle of social support. Those most powerfully affected are the immediate family members—particularly those who live under the same roof as the addict. Friends, extended family, co-workers, and employers also experience fallout from the addict's behaviors.

The spouses or partners of people who struggle with addiction often feel depressed, anxious, and angry. Persons in the throes of addiction often lie and steal to maintain their habit. It is not uncommon for people who struggle with addiction to steal from friends, family, or employers. Families must deal with the anxiety of not knowing when their loved one will come home or what mood or condition the person may demonstrate upon arriving home. Some families must deal with the shame of seeing their loved one arrested or knowing that this person harmed others while under the influence. Others simply

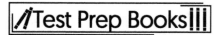

become embarrassed by behaviors that loved ones exhibit in public or their failure to show up for an important event, such as a graduation.

Children of parents who struggle with addiction experience embarrassment, fear, anxiety, and sadness. They are more likely to be abused or neglected, especially in single parent homes. Children may suffer when money intended for basic needs is spent on drugs or alcohol instead. When abuse and/or neglect are reported to CPS, these children may be taken from parents and placed in a series of group or foster homes. In some cases, custody is completely severed. Such experiences may lead to deep psychological scars for those closest to the addict.

Effects of Substance Use

The following lists the effects of substance use. These include physical problems, mental health problems, social problems, and financial problems:

- Physical Problems: Common physical problems include organ damage, gastrointestinal issues, birth defects in children exposed to drugs or alcohol during pregnancy, and increased exposure to HIV and hepatitis. In addition, there is a risk of death by overdose.

- Mental Health Problems: Persons addicted to drugs or alcohol are prone to mental health disorders, such as depression, anxiety, memory loss, aggression, mood swings, paranoia, and psychosis. Some of these issues persist long after the person has stopped using the addictive substance.

- Social Problems: As mentioned, the people closest to the addict suffer much emotional pain. Family and friends cannot rely on the person to follow through with important responsibilities. The addict may be involved in illegal activities leading to arrest, loss of income, and loss of custody of children. Others begin to distance themselves from the person for self-protection. Some families may disown or shun the addict and set up legal barriers to prevent contact. The addict may begin a series of revolving door stays at jails, hospitals, and halfway houses.

- Financial Problems: Addicts and alcoholics may experience dire financial consequences. They have trouble keeping steady employment. They may destroy their credit status, deplete savings accounts, or fail to do their share to meet financial needs of the family and household. Medical and social problems, such as arrest, can impact financial stability. Prolonged unemployment causes loss of vehicles, homes, and other assets, and may eventually lead to homelessness.

Effects of Intoxication

Intoxication effects can vary considerably depending on what drug or combined drugs have been consumed. Depressants, such as alcohol, opioids, or some prescription drugs have some of the following components:

- Sense of euphoria
- Decreased coordination
- Staggering or unsteady gait
- Speech impairment
- Judgment impairment
- Memory impairment

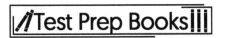
- Disinhibited behavior
- Mental confusion

The following effects may be seen in those abusing cocaine or amphetamines:

- Increased energy/hyperactivity
- Sense of euphoria
- Increased heart rate
- Decreased need for sleep or rest
- Agitation
- Anxiety
- Paranoia
- Psychosis

Those persons abusing hallucinogens may experience the following:

- Sense of euphoria, wellbeing, or relaxation
- Hallucinations
- Distorted perceptions of self, body, time, or space
- Increased heart rate and blood pressure
- Numbness
- Anxiety, sometimes leading to sense of panic

Effects of Withdrawal

Withdrawal symptoms vary from individual to individual, and the process is impacted by the type of drug consumed, the length of time the drug was used, and the current health status of the addict. Some withdrawal symptoms are psychological and do not involve physiological changes. There may still be a sense of anxiety, sadness, or irritability as one stops using the substance.

Withdrawal, in its more serious forms, can be life-threatening. There may be seizures, strokes, or heart attacks. Some withdrawal symptoms, such as those seen with methamphetamine, mimic mental illness. In areas where this drug is widely used, emergency rooms must use drug testing to determine if this is an onset of paranoid schizophrenia or the effect of amphetamine withdrawal. Those showing psychotic symptoms generally become asymptomatic after three or four days. Some people withdrawing from alcohol or other substances experience tactile hallucinations. They may see and feel insects on their skin or in their environment, causing them to aggressively scratch at their skin.

Withdrawal causes much physical discomfort that may include vomiting, diarrhea, stomach pain, profuse sweating, tremors, headaches, and spikes in heart rate or blood pressure. Persons with severe withdrawal symptoms or those with frail health should be monitored by a physician or placed in a hospital for observation. Withdrawal symptoms or the fear of experiencing them often propel the addict to seek more of the drug of preference in order to avoid these unpleasant and life-threatening experiences.

Suicidal Thoughts and Behaviors

Suicidal ideation is an emergent thought process that should be addressed promptly. Suicidal thoughts or behaviors can occur as a result of experiencing severe anxiety, depression, hopelessness, or panic

113

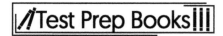

attacks. When clients express suicidal ideation, counselors should promptly perform a suicide risk assessment. There are various tools used to assess for suicide risk, such as the **Columbia-Suicide Severity Rating Scale (C-SSRS)**, the **Beck Scale for Suicide Ideation**, and the **Suicide Assessment Checklist**. In general, these tools assess the suicidal intent of the client. Counselors should also observe for warning signs, such as direct or indirect suicidal statements, depressive symptoms, emotional disturbances, negative behavioral thoughts, and situational challenges. Some of these signs include long-term depression, preoccupation with death, suicide notes, and lack of interest in life. Specific information should be obtained if the client verbalizes that they have a suicide plan. Clients should be questioned on the frequency of suicidal thoughts and if the means to carry out the specific plan are available. Crisis interventions, such as emergency hotlines, hospitalization, and notification of social support systems, may be warranted.

Terminal Illness Issues

A medical diagnosis of a terminal illness is impactful. Examples of terminal diagnoses include cancer, acquired immunodeficiency syndrome (AIDS), and Lou Gehrig's disease (ALS). End of life is expected within a short time frame, and a person may feel intense grief, sadness, and despair. Support systems may also be emotionally affected by the individual's diagnosis. Clients and their loved ones often seek counseling to come to terms with the diagnosis and find resolution of their feelings. Clients trying to cope with their diagnosis may experience guilt, regret, fear, frustration, and uncertainty about their life. Loved ones who take on the role of a caregiver can develop anxiety, depression, resentment, and burnout. Counseling interventions will commonly address feelings during the stages of grief (denial, anger, bargaining, depression, acceptance, and rebuilding). Clients may be encouraged to join support groups for the terminally ill and seek companionship from those going through the same situation. The goal of counseling is to have the client and their loved ones process their feelings, communicate their needs, and find emotional relief.

Visual and Auditory Hallucinations

Hallucinations are false perceptions of reality. The most common types of hallucinations are visual and auditory. A person may see and/or hear someone or something that does not exist. Hallucinations occur as a result of multiple conditions, including schizophrenia, psychosis, extreme emotional or mental stress, and as a side effect of medications. Substance abuse can also cause hallucinations, which are more prominent during withdrawals. Auditory hallucinations can sometimes direct a person to perform a harmful action. Clients experiencing auditory hallucinations should be questioned regarding suicidal or homicidal intent. Counseling interventions for clients experiencing hallucinations include assessing and acknowledging the client's feelings about the hallucinations, being objective about reality, and developing coping strategies to manage the hallucinations. CBT can help clients restructure delusional beliefs and distinguish what is real and what is not. Counselors should explore when hallucinations are more likely to occur and encourage clients to perform distracting activities, such as singing, reading, or talking to a friend, when experiencing the issue.

Worry and Anxiety

Worrying, defined as dwelling over actual or possible problems, is a symptom of many mental health diagnoses, such as generalized anxiety, psychosis, OCD, and PTSD. It is important for counselors to assess other underlying factors, such as toxic relationships, financial concerns, and workplace issues, and develop interventions that address those circumstances. Excessive worry can prevent clients from

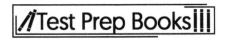

finding enjoyment in everyday activities. Individuals who obsess over potential scenarios can experience distress, insomnia, and panic attacks. CBT can help clients identify when the worry happens and break the cycle of negative thinking by identifying fears and putting them into perspective. Clients can also be encouraged to make a list of specific stressors, identify behavior patterns, and develop strategies that will minimize the time spent worrying. Activities such as exercising, socializing with friends, and listening to music can minimize the negative thoughts that occur with worry and anxiety.

Adoption Issues

Many children who go through the adoption process do not have a positive outcome. Issues with the foster care system, neglectful adoptive parents, or issues with placement can lead to emotional stress and trauma. Children may also experience anxiety and anger from not knowing their background. The rate of teens who develop behavior disorders is almost double for those who are adopted. While in foster homes, up to 45 percent of children leave the system and can experience homelessness, unemployment, and imprisonment. Other problems adopted children face include attachment issues, developmental delays, and decreased trust. Counseling interventions to help clients cope with adoption issues include family therapy, play therapy, and support groups. **Family therapy** can help caregivers and children learn to relate to one another and establish empathy. **Play therapy** allows children to verbalize their thoughts and emotions through self-expression and can help counselors develop strategies to support the child. **Support groups** may help clients find people who share similar thoughts, encourage each other, and discuss problem-solving techniques for emotional challenges.

Blended Family Issues

A high percentage of children live in a **blended family** with a biological parent, a stepparent, and possible stepsiblings. Children who are part of a blended family may experience stress from conflict between separated parents or siblings, differing parenting styles, and opposite family routines. Children who become part of a blended family may resent the new parent, be bullied by stepsiblings, or express their frustration through behavioral outbursts. Alternatively, adults who become stepparents can experience tension in the family due to ongoing communication with their partner's ex or trying to gain acceptance from the child. Counseling can provide blended families with an opportunity to establish roles, boundaries, and parenting goals. Family therapy can help children express their concerns and allow the caregivers to show their affection. Couples counseling can help partners adjust to their new blended family life and provide open communication about challenges and compromises.

Child Abuse–Related Concerns

Children develop attachment early in life. The bond that is created between a child and their parental figure is determined by the amount of nurturing and how well the child's emotional and physiological needs are meet. Children who develop a sense of trust that is later broken will develop emotional disorders. Child abuse is reported frequently and can be in the form of neglect, exploitation, abandonment, physical, or sexual. Teachers are often the first to notice signs of child abuse. A child may present with physical signs, such as unexplained cuts or bruises. The child's behavior may also be erratic, and interacting with others may be troubling. Children who are abused by their parents or an older authority figure will struggle with anxiety, fear, and severe emotional distress. The mental and emotional effects of abuse can also linger into adulthood and interfere with academic performance, social interactions, and independence.

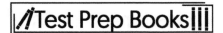

Counselors who treat young clients who experience abuse can intervene with psychodynamic techniques such as play therapy. Play therapy allows the child to imitate or re-create the experience, enabling the counselor to discuss right from wrong with the child and help them develop healthy coping skills to begin the healing process. Talk therapy is a goal-oriented technique that aims to remedy unhealthy behaviors that result from trauma. Talk therapy is geared toward clients who understand the concept of abuse. The overall goal of counseling is to provide the child with a safe environment to express their emotions and begin the healing process.

Child Development

The term **child development** refers to the process of human growth from birth until the end of adolescence. It encompasses physical, emotional, and psychological changes that take place during those years. Child development examines the process of growth and life transitions during the first eighteen years of life as the infant moves from complete dependency to increasing autonomy. It is recognized that there are certain sequential milestones, but each individual is unique in terms of developmental advancement. Child development is influenced by social, economic, and cultural factors. Because the way in which children develop today impacts how society will function in the future, it is essential that parents, educators, child care providers, and those in the medical field have a clear grasp of what elements are crucial in terms of successfully transitioning a child into the role of an independent adult.

Social skills and emotional intelligence are developed as children age. To understand the needs and behavior changes throughout life, **Erikson's Stages of Psychosocial Development** serves as a reference for the different stages of growth. There are eight stages in life, and four of them happen throughout childhood. It is important to meet the needs in every stage because lack of fulfillment can lead to issues such as abandonment, academic challenges, neglect, and intellectual disabilities. During **infancy**, the need for a safe environment is established when parental figures meet their infants' needs and provide trusting behavior. If the emotional and physiological needs are not met, infants are faced with mistrust.

During the **toddler** stage, children begin to develop their own independence and autonomy. Defiance and stubbornness are common during this stage. If autonomy is not established, they are left with a sense of shame and doubt. Initiative versus guilt occurs during the **preschool years** and focuses on developing social roles and emotions through imaginative play. During **school age**, relationships and academic performance are important. Children who struggle with bullying or inferiority may experience mental health problems such as depression and anxiety. Other events that may interfere with positive development include child abuse, domestic violence between parents, parental divorce, homelessness, and death of a loved one. Counseling can help young clients process emotions and experiences through play therapy, art therapy, or family therapy. For instance, family therapy can strengthen relationships and help family members understand and meet each other's developmental needs.

Adolescence

Adolescence is the sometimes-rocky path from the end of childhood to the onset of adulthood. It is a time of tremendous change, experimentation, and learning lessons. The changes are far-reaching, with the most apparent being changes in physical appearance and the emergence of sexuality. At the same time, adolescents are changing cognitively and emotionally and learning to view the world through new eyes. Adolescent development is usually categorized into three stages. These are early adolescence (ages ten to fourteen), middle adolescence (ages fifteen to sixteen), and late adolescence (ages seventeen to twenty-one).

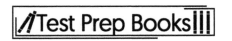

During **early adolescence**, the child's sense of identity is beginning to emerge. They are less interested in time spent with parents and more interested in being with peers. Close friendships may be forged during this time. In this stage, the child may be moody, sometimes rude, and occasionally oppositional. Limit testing is common, as is experimentation with drugs, alcohol, or cigarettes. Girls are more likely to exhibit early signs of sexual maturity than boys at this point. It is a period of exploration of the body and becoming more aware of new sensations. This leads to concerns about being physically attractive.

In **middle adolescence**, the child continues to move toward eventual independence. The peer group becomes more central, and parents are viewed as less likable than before, due to a new awareness of parental flaws. There is a greater preoccupation with body image, personal style, and intellectual interests. The child can now experience insight and may spend time analyzing inner experiences or relationships. Sexual orientation and identity are becoming more clearly defined, but it is still in a formative stage.

In **late adolescence**, there is greater movement towards independence as demonstrated by a stronger ability to feel compassion, expressing ideas through words, expanding interests in career paths, self-reliance, and a concern for the future. Sexuality is expressed in more mature and more stable relationships. The child can now set goals and follow through with them successfully. Some sadness may be present due to the inevitable separation from parents and their changing social relationships.

Knowledge of adolescent development is a standard for the practice of counseling with adolescents. Adolescents who mature early may also be at increased risk for early sexual activity, teenage pregnancy, and STDs. For boys, late maturation appears to be more problematic than early maturation; late maturing boys are at increased risk for bullying, parental conflict, academic problems, and depression.

Identity Development

Identity includes **self-concept** and **self-esteem**. Self-concept is the beliefs one holds about oneself. Self-esteem is how one feels about one's self-concept.

The physical changes of adolescence can have a strong influence on an adolescent's self-esteem. Adolescents also incorporate comments from others, particularly parents and friends, into their identity. Counselors can help with adolescent identity development simply by asking questions and being available to listen, while suspending judgment.

Adolescents also undergo important emotional development and begin to hone the skills that are necessary for stress management and effective relationships with others. Some of the skills necessary for stress management are recognizing and managing one's own emotions, developing empathy for others, learning appropriate and constructive methods of managing conflict, and learning to work cooperatively rather than competitively.

A normal part of adolescence is a yearning for independence. Counselors can help parents understand that the desire for independence is healthy and age-appropriate. They can educate both parents and adolescents about the importance of positive peer relationships during this time. Peer groups help adolescents learn about the world outside of their families and identify how they differ from their parents. Adolescents who are accepted by their peers and who have positive peer relationships may have better psychosocial outcomes in both adolescence and adulthood.

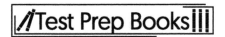

An increase in conflict with parents is normal during adolescence and seems to be most prevalent between girls and mothers. Parents may need reassurance that this conflict does not represent rejection, but rather a normal striving for independence.

Some theories seek to explain the prevalence of risk-taking behaviors among adolescents. One theory of risk-taking behavior explains that the need for excitement and sensation seeking outweighs any potential dangers that may come from sensation seeking. Another theory says that risk-taking often occurs within groups as a way to gain status and acceptance among peers. Additionally, adolescents who engage in risk-taking behavior may be modeling adult behavior that has been romanticized.

There are many ways in which counselors and parents can provide guidance to young people with regard to their risk-taking behavior. They should become comfortable discussing uncomfortable topics, so that adolescents can safely talk about their decision-making and peer pressure. Additionally, it is wise to steer adolescents toward healthy outlets that channel their talents or get them involved in positive activities.

Adolescent resilience and positive outcomes are associated with these factors:

- Having a stable and positive relationship with at least one involved and caring adult (e.g., parent, coach, teacher, family member, community member)

- Developing a sense of self-meaning, often through a church or spiritual outlet

- Attending a school that has high, but realistic, expectations and supports its students

- Living in a warm and nurturing home

- Having adequate ability to manage stress

Atypical Sexual Growth and Development

While not everyone develops sexually on exactly the same timeline, there are certain expectations that define healthy and unhealthy sexual development. It is important to understand red flags that may be signs of unhealthy sexual development. These may be brought on by abuse or by exposure to sexually explicit scenes. Children who are preoccupied with sexuality at an early age and whose behaviors differ from peers their own age may be at risk. Other indicators include attempting adult-like sexual interactions. These behaviors may include oral to genital contact or some form of penetration of another person's body.

These issues should raise concerns:

- A child overly pre-occupied with sexual thoughts, language, or behaviors, rather than in more age-appropriate play

- Child engaging in sex play with children who are much older or much younger

- Child using sexual behavior to harm others

- Child involved in sexual play with animals

- Child uses explicit sexual language that is not age appropriate

118

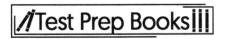

A **sexually-reactive child** refers to one who is exposed to sexual stimuli prior to being sexually mature enough to understand the implications. The child becomes overly preoccupied with sexual matters and often acts out what they witnessed or experienced.

Dating and Relationship Problems

Relationships typically go through three phases. During the **romance or rejection phase**, a couple begins to learn about each another and build intimacy. Idealization occurs during this phase, and partners may ignore each other's flaws for fear of conflict or rejection. During the **trust or disillusionment phase**, partners will encounter more disagreements regarding activities of daily life. Couples who have positive conflict resolution strategies will establish trust and learn to rely on one another during challenging times. Couples who are unable to overcome their differences may constantly argue and grow apart. The final phase is **adjustment or separation**. Couples who are able to respect differences in opinion and trust each other will adjust and stay together. Those who are unable to compromise will separate emotionally and end the relationship. Unhealthy relationships have similar characteristics and include jealousy, insecurity, unsuccessful resolution of disagreements, lack of romance, and imbalanced responsibilities. The **Gottman Method** is an intervention that helps partners identify each other's aspirations and worries and teaches conflict management. Couples counseling can help partners address concerns, identify areas of differences, develop conflict resolution techniques, and improve communication.

Divorce

Separation of marriage can occur for several reasons, including lack of commitment, disproportionate responsibilities, poor communication skills, an affair, and abuse. After divorce, partners may experience anger, guilt, grief, and anxiety. Additionally, divorced couples with children may experience intense stress. Individuals who experience a divorce may be unable to cope with adjustments, such as finances, social relationships, and single lifestyles. The goal of counseling is to help clients navigate through the divorce or recover emotionally and mentally after a divorce. Couples therapy can facilitate a healthy divorce and establish guidelines regarding financial obligations, living arrangements, and parenting. Individual therapy helps clients gain a new perspective on life and develop coping skills to deal with depression, anxiety, or stress caused by the divorce. Clients should be encouraged to perform stress-reducing activities, such as self-care, meditation, exercise, and contacting friends for support.

Family Abuse and Violence

People may experience abuse at the hands of strangers, caretakers, or close friends and family. The effects of abuse are traumatic, pervasive, and long lasting. Beyond affecting the abused parties, abuse often impacts those who are close to the victims. Physical, sexual, and psychological child abuse can lead to impaired intellect, learning disabilities, deficits in trust and language skills, and long-term inappropriate behaviors or lack of coping mechanisms. As abused children grow, they may be unable to make healthy friendships or desire or maintain intimate relationships. They may have failed marriages, or they may perpetuate the cycle of abuse when they become parents. They may often feel unworthy or that they did something to cause the abuse. This often has an impact on their attachment styles and how they relate to others.

In adults, abuse may cause permanent or temporary physical damage, low self-esteem, shame, despair, or feelings of helplessness. Victims of abuse as an adult may experience mental health disorders such

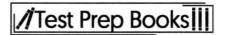
anxiety and depression. If children witness their loved ones experiencing abuse, it may be traumatic for them, or they may normalize the behavior and perpetuate abuse themselves. Elder abuse, especially in nursing homes, often goes undetected as victims may be weak or losing mental faculties. Elders are especially vulnerable to physical and financial abuse. Effects may include rapid physical or mental deterioration, submissiveness, bedsores, increased rate of illness, or premature death. In traumatic cases, both children and adults may become severely depressed or anxious. They may abuse substances or commit suicide.

Victims of abuse and neglect are most often children, the elderly, or someone suffering from a physical or mental disability. Because of their vulnerability, these populations are most at risk of mistreatment. One of the most challenging aspects of dealing with abuse or neglect is that victims are often hesitant to report abuse. This may be due to fear of the perpetrator or a conflicted sense of loyalty toward that person, who may be a close relative or friend. It is often communicated to victims that they are the cause of the abuse, and they mistakenly take on the responsibility for the bad things happening to them. The effects of abuse vary depending on many factors, including the severity level of the abuse, the response of other adults or caregivers when the abuse is reported, and the age of the victim at the time of abuse.

Physically, there may be injuries, wounds, or even sexually transmitted diseases in the case of sexual abuse. Oftentimes, these physical symptoms are what is observed by outsiders and can be the first sign of potential abuse. Evidence of neglect may also show up physically—e.g., if a person loses weight, is not wearing adequate clothes, or is not taken for necessary medical attention. A child inexplicably missing school for multiple days may also be an indication of a problem. Psychologically, abuse impacts a person in many ways. Their whole view of self may revolve around the abuse suffered, resulting in low self-esteem and feelings of worthlessness and loneliness.

Additionally, mental illnesses, such as anxiety or depression, may arise, and victims may even engage in self-harm or attempt suicide. Behavioral changes may also occur, and a child may begin acting out at home or school. When a person endures sexual abuse, they may later begin acting out sexually or become either sexually promiscuous or sexually withdrawn. There is a higher level of drug and alcohol abuse among victims of abuse, as well as criminal activity. The wounds from abuse are varied and extensive, but with a strong social support and appropriate counseling, victims of abuse can be extremely resilient and even go on to help other survivors of abuse.

Physical Abuse

Physical abuse is the intentional act of physical force that may result in pain, injury, or impairment to a child or other dependent. Physical abuse is typically thought of as violent acts such as hitting, kicking, burning, etc., but it may also include extreme physical discipline, force-feeding, and some uses of drugs or restraints. **Physical indicators of physical abuse** are multiple physical injuries in various stages of healing; physical injuries that are inconsistent with an individual's account of how the injuries occurred; multiple injuries, accidents, or unexplained illnesses occurring over a period of time; and injuries reflecting the object used to inflict the injury (e.g., cigarette burns, tooth marks, bruising in the shape of finger/hand marks). **Behavioral indicators of physical abuse** are flinching; offering inconsistent explanations of injuries or being unable to remember how injuries occurred; exhibiting wariness around adults or authority figures; aggression or abusive behavior toward others; and withdrawn, sad, depressed, or even suicidal behavior.

The following are indicators of physical abuse that may be seen in children:

120

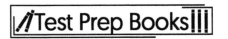

- Presence of bruises or marks
- Mistrust of others, evidenced by cringing or shying away
- Fear of going home
- Increased aggressive behavior, bullying of others
- History of acting-out, suicidal behaviors, and/or school problems
- Frequent vomiting
- Parent or caregiver appears unconcerned about the child's physical condition, no explanations offered for injuries

Sexual Abuse

Sexual abuse is forced or coerced sexual contact or exposure, usually by someone older or in a position of authority over the victim. Sexual abuse can also include forcing someone to watch sexual acts or receive messages involving unwanted sexual content. The impact of sexual abuse is complex, and the emotional and psychological response to the trauma may evolve as the victim gets older and understands more fully what happened to them. Children who suffer sexual abuse may struggle from confusion about the abuse, especially if they are told by the perpetrator that it is right and good and if that person is someone with whom they have a relationship of trust. They may be blamed by the perpetrator for the abuse, which leads to further feelings of confusion and guilt. If they report the abuse to someone who does not believe it, the long-term effects of the abuse may be even greater, as well as the guilt, self-doubt, and shame. A history of sexual abuse will normally impact a person's relationships with others throughout life, and there may be issues of trust as well as confused feelings toward sex.

The following are indicators of sexual abuse in a child:

- The statement that one has been sexually assaulted
- Mistrust or fear of those who bear resemblance to the abuser, potentially due to gender or size (children may be mistrustful of all adults)
- Changes in behavior
- Depression
- Anxiety with presenting symptoms (hair loss, fluctuations in weight)
- Increased fearfulness (possible night terrors and enuresis/bed wetting from children)
- Withdrawal from preferred activities/social isolation
- Compulsive masturbation
- Substance abuse
- Overly-sexualized behavior

The following are indicators of sexual abuse that may be seen in the parent or caregiver:

- Demonstrating inappropriate behaviors
- Role confusion, distortion of child's role in the family
- Jealousness or over-protection of the victim
- Excessive, abnormal alone time with the child
- Lack of appropriate social and emotional contacts outside the home
- Substance and/or alcohol abuse
- Parent or caregiver reports being sexually abused previously (possible normalization or continuation of the cyclic behavior)

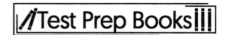

Psychological Abuse and Neglect

The following are indicators of neglect in children:

- Reports of no one around to provide care
- Appearance of being malnourished, always hungry
- Excessive sleepiness
- Untreated medical problems
- Parent or caregiver demonstrates lack of interest
- Parent or caregiver chronically ill (physically or mentally)
- Parent or caregiver history of neglect from their parent or caregiver
- Description of or visibly-unsafe home environment

The following are indicators of psychological abuse and neglect:

- Extreme fluctuations between aggression and passiveness
- Manifestation of emotional stress through nail biting, hair loss, rocking, bed-wetting
- Presence of low self-esteem with self-defeating statements. for example, *no one likes me, no one cares about me, I can't do anything right*
- Excessive desire to be a people pleaser
- Developmental delays or presentation being younger or slower (speech or movement) than age-appropriate
- Caregiver or parent belittles the child
- Client is treated lesser than other individuals in the family

Interpersonal Partner Violence Concerns

Partner violence takes place in an intimate relationship where one of the partners is physically, verbally, or sexually aggressive towards the other. **Physical abuse** includes hitting, choking, or biting that may result in bodily injury. **Emotional abuse** and **psychological abuse** can include threats, verbal statements that diminish self-worth, and actions that prevent socialization. **Sexual abuse** is any sex act that is forced, coerced, or demeaning to an individual. There is also typically a high level of social and financial control, as well as psychological manipulation or belittling. The most obvious indicators of partner violence are physical injuries such as bruises, broken bones, or black eyes. Emotional symptoms—such as excessive crying or fear—may also be observed, in addition to controlling or obsessive behavior on the part of the abusive partner. However, indicators of partner violence may also take the form of more subtle symptoms, such as depression, anxiety, or distrust of people. Drug or alcohol abuse is often associated with partner violence, and there is a higher risk of violence when drugs or alcohol are involved.

Intimate partner violence occurs when one of the partners seeks to exercise control over the other. While the majority of perpetrators of violence are men, this is not always the case, and domestic violence can be perpetrated by both men and women in either heterosexual or homosexual relationships. Overt physical acts of aggression are often intermittent and may be precipitated by an increase in anger on the part of the abusive partner. Other forms of control, manipulation, and psychological or verbal abuse are more continual, creating an atmosphere of fear and helplessness. In spite of the aggression and control of the abusive partner, the victimized partner of violence often hesitates to reveal the abuse to anyone and will choose to stay with the abusive partner. This dynamic

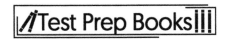

results from the conflicted sense of loyalty the partner feels, especially in cases where they may have had children together.

In situations of intimate partner violence, the abusive partner often alternates abusive behavior with kindness and affection and may apologize and promise to change. This causes the victim to justify or minimize the periods of violence and emphasize the more positive aspects of the relationship. An abusive partner may use the acts of kindness as a constant form of guilt and manipulation, causing the other partner to feel ungrateful if they reveal the abuse to anyone. Additionally, fear of the abuser or a misplaced sense of shame may prevent the victim from telling anyone of the abuse. Only when the costs of leaving the relationship are outweighed by the benefits, will the victimized partner take steps to get out of the abusive situation. In such cases, counselors must provide a safe relationship of trust for the abused individual.

The impact of intimate partner violence is pervasive and profound. The abused partner not only bears physical scars, but also emotional and psychological wounds such as distorted self-image, insecurity, shame, and guilt. These can lead to depression, anxiety, self-harm behaviors, or suicide. In addition to the partner, children who are exposed to domestic violence are also deeply impacted and may struggle in school, at home, and in present and future relationships. There is also a high correlation between intimate partner violence and the perpetration of child abuse.

Individuals who stay in an abusive relationship for a long period of time can develop physical and psychological problems. Some psychological effects of domestic violence include anxiety, depression, trust issues, fear of intimacy, suicidal thoughts, and emotional distancing. Counseling can help treat the lasting effects of domestic violence. Domestic violence survivors require counseling that helps build upon their individual strengths and improve their self-esteem. Individual therapy can help identify the pattern of violence and establish a plan to keep the client safe. Group therapy allows clients to normalize their feelings by sharing experiences with others who have gone through the same situation. Providing a creative outlet, such as music or art, can also help clients express their emotions.

Marital or Partner Communication Problems

Troubled relationships can often be attributed to poor communication. Many individuals find it hard to talk about their troubles as a result of negative childhood experiences or past failed relationships that affected them emotionally and psychologically. There are four different styles of communication. The **assertive communication style** is characterized by clear, honest, and direct statements that positively express feelings and thoughts. An **aggressive style of communication** focuses on expressing feelings with a clear disregard of the other's feelings. Partners with an aggressive communication style may make the other person feel like their opinions are not valued. **Passive communicators** rarely voice their feelings or opinions and may become overwhelmed by their partner's decisions. **Passive-aggressive communication** is characterized by unclear or confusing statements and may lead to internal frustration and resentment. Counselors should take communication styles into consideration when developing interventions between partners that help improve the quality and frequency of communication. The goal is to encourage partners to have open lines of communication, voice their emotions, practice active listening, and respect each other's opinions.

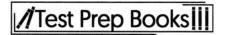

Parenting/Co-Parenting Conflicts

Good parenting practices are essential for raising emotionally healthy children. When parents, either married or divorced, have conflicting parenting styles, both the children and the marriage can be negatively affected. Through counseling, parents can discover their parenting styles and work together to provide their children with consistent parenting. Child psychologists vary on what types of parenting styles are most effective, but there are four generally recognized styles of parenting:

- **Authoritarian parenting style:** This style of parenting reinforces the role of parent as controller and decision maker. Children are rarely given input into decisions impacting their lives, and the parent takes on a dictatorial role. Children raised by this kind of parent are often obedient and tend to be proficient. The drawback is that they do not rank high on the happiness scale.

- **Authoritative parenting style:** This style of parenting allows for a greater sense of democracy in which children are given some degree of input into issues that impact their lives. There is a healthy balance between firmness and affection. Children raised in this environment tend to be capable, successful, and happy individuals.

- **Permissive parenting style:** This type of parenting allows children to be more expressive and freer with both feelings and actions; they are allowed to behave in whatever manner they please. There are very few rules, and no consequences will be given, even if a rule is violated. These children are more likely to experience problems in school and relationships with others. In the long run, they are often unhappy with their lives.

- **Uninvolved parenting style:** This form of parenting often occurs in dysfunctional families in which parents are emotionally or physically unavailable. They may be remiss in setting clear expectations, yet they may overreact when the child misbehaves or fails to understand what is expected. This is often seen in families where poverty is extreme or addictions or mental illnesses are present.

The authoritative style of parenting is considered to be the most effective form of parenting, yet much depends on the individual child or parent and the economic situation or cultural setting. One rule of thumb is that whatever style one chooses, it is helpful to remain consistent. A parent who is permissive one day and authoritarian the next sends mixed and confusing messages to the child. It is also important that the child is completely aware of rules, expectations, and what consequences may follow if the rules are broken. Communicating a sense that children are loved, wanted, and accepted is one of the most important parts of parenting.

Emotional Dysregulation

Emotional dysregulation is a mood disorder that makes it difficult to regulate emotional responses and behaviors. Individuals with emotional dysregulation may be seen as aggressive, controlling, entitled, or problematic. Emotional dysregulation may be caused by an abusive childhood, brain injuries, or a disruptive home environment. Those who experience emotional dysregulation have a difficult time maintaining personal and professional relationships due to their conflicting and misunderstood behavior. One of the most common interventions to treat emotional dysregulation is **dialectical behavior therapy (DBT)**, which incorporates CBT and methods that help create mindfulness, such as meditation, music, and yoga. The goal of DBT is to help clients establish skills for confronting their

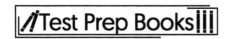

emotions and regulating the behavioral response. Other interventions include anger management to identify stressors and Schema Therapy, which helps to identify and change unhealthy ways of thinking.

Treatment Planning

Collaborating with Clients to Establish Treatment Goals and Objectives

Counselors should always treat the individual as the expert on the individual's life, and while counselors should gather relevant external and collateral information, they should make all efforts not to allow these sources to supersede information provided by the individual. Counselors should involve the individual as much as possible in problem identification and resolution planning by asking about details about the individual's life, any presenting issues and what might be causing them, what kinds of changes the individual would like to make, how these changes might enrich quality of life, and real and perceived fears. All of these details should be acknowledged, respected, valued, and referred to when planning and implementing interventions. Counselors should also tailor interventions to highlight and utilize established strengths and resources of the individual.

Collaboration should begin at the intake process. This is a period in which the counselor can make assessments, but they can also get information directly from clients about why they are in the session and what they hope to achieve. The counselor can also ask clients the steps they believe they need to take to reach their desired outcomes. While clients may or may not provide useful or feasible answers, this process still sets the tone that allows clients to feel acknowledged and involved in their own care.

In the intake session or in the sessions that immediately follow, the counselor can invite the client to develop objectives to reach their goals. This may also include establishing accountability tools, documenting plans of action to address potential barriers and how to overcome them, and any other support protocols that clients may need for their individual situations. Inviting the client to take a collaborative perspective in designing interventions, establishing objectives, and developing program goals allows the client to feel empowered and engaged as an active member of the problem-solving process. These factors are associated with higher incidences of positive outcomes, as they encourage clients to feel accountable for their behaviors, actions, and personal changes.

Goal setting should occur in collaboration with a client's treatment plan. Intervention strategies, tasks, and timeframes should correspond with the desired goal and objectives. The primary goal should be to assist clients in returning to pre-crisis functioning. However, there will likely be additional and related goals and tasks as the plan of action is implemented.

Goals can take the form of **SMART goals**, which are specific, measurable, achievable, relevant, and time-bound. **Specific** means detailing why you want to accomplish the goal, what specifically there is to accomplish, who is involved, the setting for the goal, and what kind of resources are involved. **Measurable** means designating a system of tracking your goals in order to stay motivated. **Achievable** is making sure that the goal is realistic, such as looking at financial factors or other limitations. **Relevant** means making sure it's the right time for the goal, if it matches your needs, or if the goal seems worthwhile to pursue. Finally, **time-bound** is developing a target date so that there is a clear deadline to focus on.

126

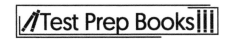

In family or couples counseling, goals may be reciprocal or shared:

- **Reciprocal goals**: Complimentary goals agreed upon by members of a system related to the same target problem (e.g., a father's goal is to offer more compliments to his son, while son agrees to increase verbal acknowledgement to father's positive feedback).

- **Shared goals**: When members of a system choose the same goal that addresses an identified problem (e.g., spouses each agree to communicate needs more frequently).

Depending on the client's specific case, this process may take one session or may take much longer. Counselors should continuously show patience, compassion, and a welcoming desire to engage the client in the process.

Establishing Short- and Long-Term Counseling Goals Consistent with Clients' Diagnoses

Interventions matched to client problems are based on the biopsychosocial assessment information, empirical data, and research collected by the counselor during sessions and during counselor education. The components of the biopsychosocial assessment gather client factors that help guide the counselor in applying a theoretical model that will work best in designing an intervention to treat the client's presenting issue effectively.

Setting goals is an important aspect of the therapeutic process. Talk therapy may seem unstructured or capable of lasting for long periods of time; however, both the client and the counselor are responsible for setting and working toward measurable change. Goals of counseling can include the desire for physical change, such as getting into shape or losing weight, and career aspirations and/or social goals, such as gaining increased support or modifying relationships. Other types of goals can be emotional, spiritual, and intellectual. Goals can be immediate, short term, or long term, and clients may want to achieve several goals at different paces.

Identifying Barriers and Strengths Regarding Goal Attainment

Assessing the Ability and Motivation to Engage in Intervention

Counselors must be able to identify indicators of motivation and resistance in order to determine how to engage the client and progress through treatment effectively. If a client is motivated, then they are likely to be more participative in treatment and positively respond to interventions.

Indicators of motivation are transparent and include a client voluntarily coming in for treatment and expressing a willingness to be actively involved in treatment. As time progresses, the client's level of engagement with the counselor is an indicator of motivation as well. It is important for counselors to determine whether the client feels empowered with the interventions to remedy the problem or if the client is dependent upon the counselor to provide the solution.

Resistance is likely to be more present in clients who are involuntarily seeking treatment, such as through a court order. Resistance may take the form of clients minimizing the effects of their behaviors, rationalizing their behaviors, or believing there is no problem to address. A client may also appear disengaged during sessions or directly state that they will not take the recommended steps toward resolution. Resistant clients may frequently arrive late, cancel, or fail to show up for sessions.

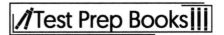
Indicators of Client's Strengths and Challenges

Noticing a client's different characteristics can indicate particular strengths. Strengths are biological, physical, mental, social, spiritual, or emotional abilities that help them to solve problems and keep the mind, body, and spirit in a stable state. The counselor might also notice areas requiring intervention or treatment plans for the individual's overall growth. Focus is on the following indicators:

- Intelligence quotient (IQ) and cognitive ability
- Willingness to learn
- Willingness to understand oneself without judgment
- Ability to accept both positive feedback and constructive criticism
- Desire for personal growth
- Willingness to change
- Ability and desire to learn new concepts
- Temperament
- Optimistic or pessimistic thought patterns
- Reaction patterns to stressors (both initially and over time)
- Self-esteem
- Self-efficacy
- Self-worth
- Accountability for one's actions
- Emotional quotient (EQ), also called emotional intelligence (EI)
- Status and complexity of close relationships and friendships
- Ability to trust and depend on others
- Ability to be trustworthy and dependable
- Ability to empathize and sympathize
- Perspective on society at large
- Self-awareness
- Moods and what external events or internal thought processes affect them
- Involvement in social institutions (e.g., religious groups, social clubs)
- State of physical health
- State of finances
- Socioeconomic status

Assessment of Client's Strengths, Resources, and Challenges

Once the client has identified the existing problem and systems, the client's **internal support systems** should be assessed, which includes examining the client's strengths and coping abilities. As with other facets of the assessment process, the client can provide a verbal report answering an open-ended question about what they view as current strengths and weaknesses.

Additionally, the counselor can ask the client to provide a narrative related to a recent experience (it does not necessarily have to be linked to the presenting problem), in order to showcase strengths and weaknesses. Using finding questions can guide the client to describe their reaction to events comprehensively, to identify what favorable actions were taken, and to research what alternative actions could be taken. The counselor may then summarize back to the client the strengths they heard in the narrative. This ensures that the client feels heard and understood.

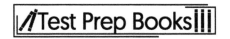

The counselor may also use scales to assess the client's strengths and weaknesses. A **dual perspective worksheet** may be utilized to identify the supports and obstacles perceived by the client in current social interactions. The worksheet helps create a visual map of the areas of strength the client can rely on as a means of improving areas of functioning, while simultaneously allowing the client to see areas that could use additional improvement. The counselor can create a treatment plan with the client to develop or enhance coping skills, focusing on strengthening weaker areas and utilizing stronger ones.

Ego Strength

Ego strength is the ability of the individual to be resilient in the face of stressors. Generally, individuals with high ego strength will be able to return to a normal emotional state after experiencing crisis. They will be able to appropriately process it and cope with the demand of doing so. Positive or high ego strength is marked by:

- the ability to acknowledge mood shifts without getting overwhelmed
- the ability to cope positively with loss and setbacks
- realizing painful or sad feelings will decrease in intensity over time
- taking personal responsibility for actions and reactions
- self-discipline in the face of temptation or addictive urges
- setting and respecting firm limits and boundaries
- avoiding people who are negative influences
- learning from mistakes rather than blaming oneself or someone else

Consequently, the absence of these indicators may reveal areas around which to tailor intervention or treatment. These indicators may be determined through verbal discussion or standardized assessments.

Factors in Successful Intervention/Treatment

Assessing the client's support systems and strengths can be utilized to hypothesize how the client will respond to treatment. Some of the factors that determine a client's success are listed here:

- Cognitive Skills
  - rationalization
  - intellectual capacity and abilities
  - creativity and innovation
  - drive and initiative
- Internal Supports/Interpersonal Skills
  - problem solving
  - ability to empathize
  - confidence/sense of self
  - relationship sustainability
  - sense of purpose
- Coping Skills
  - ability to multi-task
  - self-regulation
  - ability to navigate uncertainty
  - optimism
  - temperament
- Other Factors

129

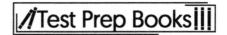

- o income, associated socioeconomic status
- o physical health
- o community involvement
- o external supports (church, family, and friends)

Client Resistance

Resistance to counseling, at some point, may be unavoidable. The process of change is difficult, and clients may become overtly or unconsciously oppositional when faced with the need to adjust thoughts or behaviors. In psychoanalytic terms, clients are resistant in an attempt to avoid anxiety brought up through the counseling process. Resistance can be very obvious, such as canceling or delaying appointments, not following through, or not fully engaging in the process. Resistance can also be subtler; clients can display resistance through disinterest or noncompliance. The counselor can contribute to client resistance through inadequate therapeutic interventions, such as having an agenda that does not meet clients' needs. Although resistance can interfere with the process, it can also be very powerful when dealt with effectively. Counselors need to pay close attention to resistance, understand its origins, and work to help clients recognize and work through blockages.

Responding to Resistant Behaviors

Clients may show resistance to treatment or to the counselor for a variety of reasons, including personality, misdirected anger, confusion, self-protection, fear, or anxiety. Clients often show resistance when they have been required by a court or social services to cooperate with a counselor or have been pressurized in some other way to participate in services. Before making judgments about a client's resistance, it is important for the counselor to first try to understand them through active and empathetic listening. Before clients will listen to counselors, they need to be reassured that they have been fully heard.

Counselors should acknowledge and validate the client's concerns. A relationship of trust needs to be built, which can be a slower process when clients begin with resistant behaviors, but this is the only way to ultimately overcome that resistance. No matter how skilled a counselor is, if there is resistance and a lack of trust in the relationship, then progress will be limited. Client engagement in services is vital, and it is only when the counselor helps empower the client to identify and work toward their own solutions that there will be real success. The goal is for the client and counselor to be on the same team, collaborating together to work towards the client's desired goals.

Referring Clients for Different Levels of Treatment

When planning a client's treatment, the counselor will need to decide which type of therapeutic environment will coincide best with the client's needs. The most extreme level of treatment is inpatient. **Inpatient treatment** provides professional supervision and monitoring along with daily counseling sessions. Clients who require inpatient treatment will be diagnosed with more problematic and complicated mental health issues or issues that are chronic or unusual. Inpatient treatment will provide an orderly routine, allowing focus to be on therapy, and it will eliminate environmental factors that aggravate the client's issue. This level of treatment is best for clients who can commit to weeks or months in a treatment facility. Inpatient treatment should be chosen for clients who are in danger of harming themselves or others and/or if their condition is interfering with day-to-day functioning. In cases of substance use, if the client has attempted treatment in the past and relapsed, inpatient treatment is a viable option.

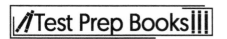

The next level under inpatient treatment is **residential**. This type of treatment environment is more like a home. Clients are monitored but not to the same degree as they would be in inpatient treatment. Inpatient treatment is preferable for problems such as eating disorders or substance abuse. The daily focus will be on treatment. Counselors should refer clients to residential treatment if they don't need constant supervision but still need to get out of an environment that encourages or provokes the problem. In residential treatment, clients benefit from the group environment where others who are going through the same problems support and push each other to reach their goals.

The most flexible option for treatment is outpatient as it allows clients to continue working or going to school while going through therapy. Clients who only need to meet for sessions once a week or once a month should receive outpatient treatment. **Outpatient treatment** allows clients to retain privacy regarding treatment while learning how to cope in their usual environment. The options for outpatient treatment include short- and long-term counseling and individual, group, or family therapy. Typically, clients who are referred to outpatient treatment show more motivation to change and will show signs of being able to commit to this level of treatment. Outpatient treatment is acceptable for clients who suffer from disorders such as depression or anxiety. Occasionally, after inpatient treatment, patients will need to maintain treatment in an outpatient setting.

Referring to Others for Concurrent Treatment

Counselors sometimes work concurrently with other providers of mental health services. One of the most common examples is when counselors work with psychiatrists. If a counselor believes that their client is not making sufficient improvement or their symptoms are worsening, they can refer the client to a psychiatrist for medication evaluation while continuing to counsel the client.

Counselors can also refer their clients to another counselor if the client desires another type of therapy (e.g., marriage counseling). In such cases, individual counselors may maintain communication with the other counselor, but they are not required to do so. The level of collaboration with other mental health providers should always be done with the client's best interests in mind.

Guiding Treatment Planning

Formulating a Treatment Plan

While formulating the treatment plan, the counselor should assess the level of care needed for a client with the whole person in mind and a desire for continuity of care. As the counselor starts where the client is, the treatment plan process should reflect levels of care that are in line with the client's needs, adjusting the intensity up or down based on the level of need as reflected in ongoing assessments and review processes.

To develop an intervention plan, the counselor and individual may collaborate. If that isn't possible, the counselor may want to involve the individual in order to have an informed, engaged, and receptive participant. The methodology may include:

- Clear discussion and a written definition of the presenting issue, including supporting anecdotal evidence, observations, and (possibly) statistical data.

- Discussion of what may contribute to or cause the problem and how it affects other aspects of the individual's daily life.

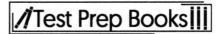

- Discussion of possible resolutions to the presenting issue.

- Discussion of components of the individual's life that support resolution and what may be obstacles.

- Development of objectives for success that are specific, measurable, achievable, relevant, and time-specific (known as SMART).

- Establishment of a method to evaluate progress.

Creating SMART objectives allows for data-driven and measurable intervention plans. When creating objectives, counselors should be able to measure the following:

- The desired behavior that is exhibited

- The number of times the desired behavior is exhibited over a period of time

- The conditions in which the desired behavior must be exhibited

- Progress from the undesired behavior to the desired behavior through baseline evaluation and evaluation at pre-determined intervals

Contracts

Once goals are determined, a contract is the next step to engage the client in services. Contracts can be formal or informal, and written or verbal depending on the policies of the agency and the nature of treatment. A **contract** between client and counselor provides a set of expectations and guidelines for treatment. Clients should be made aware the contract is a commitment by both parties, but not a legal document. Components of the contract include goals, assignments of tasks, timeframes, frequency of sessions, methods for determining progress, and how updates or revisions of the contract can occur. Other items that can be included are lengths of sessions, financial arrangements, procedures for cancelling appointments, etc.

Termination Process and Issues and Follow-Up After Discharge

Ethical Issues Regarding Termination

Termination of the relationship occurs when the client and the counselor have reached treatment goals. Even though the relationship is terminated, the client may feel warmly toward the counselor, and congruence and empathy may still be part of the relationship. Some clients may require maintenance sessions to continue stability, but when termination is the next clear stage in the relationship, psychotherapy sessions should end.

In the case of a client choosing to prematurely terminate services, the counselor should clearly explain the risks to the client and also carefully document all meetings and interactions to protect against legal ramifications. **Abandonment**, which refers to the counselor terminating services prematurely without adequate reason or in an improper manner, is considered malpractice and can lead to lawsuits. When the counselor decides to end the working relationship, they must ensure that the client is adequately prepared and warned about the end of services and that the client is emotionally equipped to deal with the termination. Counselors can refer clients to other types of providers, who can continue working with the client after their own services have ceased. If a counselor needs to terminate services early, such as

132

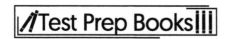

in the case of leaving a job, they should connect the client to a new counselor who can continue to provide the same level of services.

Discharge Planning

An important part of treatment planning is **discharge planning**. There are numerous reasons that services for a client may end. Clients may feel that they no longer need the services, that they are not compatible with the counselor providing the services, that an increased level of care is needed that is beyond the scope of the counselor, or they may have successfully met goals for treatment.

Discharge planning should begin with the onset of the initial assessment for the client. The counselor should not delay discharge planning, as discharge may occur at any time. Making the client aware of the choices for discharge and the discharge planning process empowers the client during treatment. It also provides continuity of care for the client.

The main purpose of discharge planning is to develop a plan of care that goes beyond the current treatment sessions to promote success once services have concluded. In the event the client is going to a higher level of care or to a different professional, effective discharge planning is useful in disseminating pertinent information about the client to assist in continuity of care and effective treatment. In this sense, the current counselor should prepare to become a collateral source linked to the client's level of care for the next professional.

In addition to benefitting the other counselors the client may meet with, effective discharge planning is a benefit to the client as well. If services have been completed successfully and the client has met the stated goals, then discharge planning ensures the client has a plan to sustain a stable level of function and maintain the successes achieved. This is particularly useful with clients who suffer from substance use or other addictive behaviors, as effective discharge planning can prevent relapse.

Upon the conclusion of the client discharging from services, a discharge summary should be created and placed in the client's file. The ***discharge summary*** should include the following information:

- Reason for discharge
- Description of treatment goals and the degree to which they were met
- Client's response to the interventions
- Description of the client's levels of functioning
- Baseline
- Progress during treatment
- Functioning at discharge
- Recommendations for follow-up care
- Links to community resources
- Appointment dates for other providers (if available)
- Provision of additional contacts, client supports
- Description of potential risks post-discharge
- Contact information for post-discharge support and crisis intervention

Indicators of Client Readiness for Termination

When clients have made significant progress on the treatment plan, goals, and objectives, the counselor can begin planning for termination. Depending on the identified goals and objectives, a standardized assessment can be used to determine how much progress has been made. Counselor practices vary

133

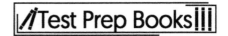
depending on what level of goal attainment should be completed before termination (i.e., some, most, all). Other options can be offered to the client for continued work and learning such as groups, workshops, and reading materials. In many instances, services are terminated due to limitations by insurance or other funding sources. It is extremely important in these circumstances that the counselor assists the client in locating additional resources that can be used following service termination. When preparing clients for termination, counselors should discuss the following topics with the client:

- Initial reasons for requesting help
- What skills the client initially lacked that led to initiating services
- Skills developed as a result of treatment and how those new skills will help the client with future challenges
- Ways the client will continue to build on new skills development
- counselor and client feelings about termination

Follow-Up After Discharge

At the final session, the counselor and client can schedule a follow-up session at a predetermined time to evaluate the client's continued progress after termination. Another option is to propose a time to meet and alert the client that the counselor will contact the client to schedule a follow up. The **follow-up session** enables the counselor the opportunity to determine how well the client has progressed and to determine the effectiveness of the intervention(s) used during sessions.

Transitions in Group Membership

There are two kinds of groups in counseling: open and closed. A **closed group** has a specific starting date, and only the clients who begin on that date are admitted to the group. Once the group starts, no other clients are permitted to join. In an **open group**, clients can begin and end treatment at any time during the life of the group. Prior to the beginning of either type of group, counselors should interview all potential members individually to determine their suitability for the group. Once new members are admitted, the counselor should go over the group's rules and describe the limits of confidentiality.

When a group is coming to end, counselors should prepare their clients in advance. This can be done by addressing issues such as the sadness some members may experience because they have come to rely upon the group for support or they have formed bonds within the group. Counselors can facilitate this process by having open conversations and encouraging clients to express their feelings. In preparation for termination, counselors should also talk about the progress made by the group members. Additionally, counselors can provide referrals to individual counselors if clients need or desire further treatment. Helping clients transition out of group therapy is an important stage of the process.

Using Assessment Instrument Results to Facilitate Client Decision-Making

Psychometric assessment tools can provide valuable pieces of information. Many assessment tools are available for free, while others must be purchased. Assessment tools often come with rating scales that indicate the level of training needed to interpret the results. **Assessment instruments** can be used at the beginning of treatment to help counselors make diagnostic decisions. Counselors can also have clients take personality assessments, which can provide them with information about the best ways to work with their clients. Some counselors use a battery of tests that provide them with multifaceted views of their clients' disorders and personality structures. Assessment tools can also be used throughout counseling to give counselors feedback on the effectiveness of their treatment methods. If the testing

134

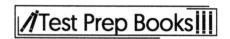
devices indicate that a client's symptoms are remaining the same or worsening, then counselors might consider changing their treatment plans.

Reviewing and Revising the Treatment Plan

Treatment evaluation is a necessary part of direct practice. Counselors should strive to exercise best practice techniques by using evidence-based practice evaluation. It is beneficial for clients to see the progress they have made, while simultaneously providing information to funders and insurance companies that typically require documentation and outcome measures for reimbursement of services. Other benefits include providing indicators that interventions should be modified or that treatment is complete and termination is warranted. Several factors are important in the evaluation of a client's progress, including identifying specific issues to be addressed; creating appropriate goals, objectives, and tasks; using effective and relevant techniques and tools to measure success; and routinely documenting progress.

Client progress may be measured using a quantitative or qualitative approach used in research. **Quantitative measures** relate to the rate of occurrence or severity of a behavior or problem. When performing quantitative evaluation, first establish a baseline, which is a measurement of the target problem, prior to intervention. **Qualitative measures** are more subjective and reflective of the client's experience (information is gathered largely from observation and different forms of interviewing) and provide a view of whether progress is being made.

Engaging Clients in Review of Progress Toward Treatment Goals

The specific objectives and strategies that will support the selected interventions are outlined in an **intervention or treatment service plan** for the client. The intervention plan for the client should be reviewed at the beginning of treatment, as well as periodically during treatment. This will ensure the goals remain aligned with the client's strengths, needs, progress, and interests. Additionally, at the conclusion of services, the interventions should be reviewed to clarify what was/was not met and whether or not additional interventions are needed.

Clarifying the roles and responsibilities of the counselor, the client, and the client system in the intervention process can reduce the chance of miscommunication, misunderstanding, and interventions not working as intended. This clarification process can be developed during the intake process and initial sessions by actively listening to what the client hopes to achieve, and working together to develop a step-by-step intervention methodology. When possible, the stages, objectives, and milestones of the intervention should be documented in order to have an available reference point, drive accountability, and reduce any confusion around the expectations of all involved parties.

The **problem-solving approach** to interventions is a commonly used framework to cover these points. This is a seven-stage model that encourages active listening and engagement techniques (such as eye contact and other receptive body language); fostering trust and collaboration with the client (such as by showing genuine interest in the client as a person, rather than just in the context of the issues at hand); working together to identify the problem to be addressed and possible solutions; introducing allies in the resolution processes (such as clinical providers, a yoga or meditation teacher, or other experts that could help the client); developing a documented resolution plan and actively engaging all parties to follow it (such as through accountability cues, positive reinforcement, and celebrating small victories);

135

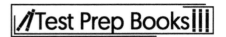

and support for sustaining the desired behaviors until the client is capable of terminating the intervention.

While one can be hopeful that the client and client systems will be cooperative and willing in this framework, that is not always the case. Clients may show distrust, anxiety, fear, or apathy, especially in the beginning. Often, the most important role of the counselor is building trust with the client and the client system. The counselor should continue to encourage a trusting, collaborative relationship until the time of service termination.

Client Self-Monitoring

Client self-monitoring can be a useful technique for turning subjective qualitative information into more quantifiable data. Clients may engage in self-assessment techniques and practices that include journaling, questionnaires, and evaluations. Clients collect data about goals, objectives, and the targeted behavior. This technique collects important information about client progress, but it also adds to clients' feelings of empowerment and self-determination as they become collaborators in treatment. Clients can either track information related to thoughts or behaviors or can use more formal charting techniques. Counselors should assist clients with defining and identifying which type of information to track and then demonstrate how to use the selected tracking technique. Self-monitoring methods serve several purposes. As clients become more invested in treatment, their awareness of strengths and areas in need of improvement may also increase. This will enable the client to monitor behaviors as they occur, allowing for the development of insight related to behavioral change.

Flaws in Goal Setting

Goal setting must be specific to each client and should be mutually agreed upon. Setting clear time frames that are supported by the counselor is essential to success. Goal setting may cause issues if goals are too ambitious or vague or have no identifiable benefit. It is also important to explore what motivation exists for a client to work toward a goal. If adequate motivation is present, the counselor also needs to consider what will happen if the goal is not met. In some cases, failure to meet goals can cause a client to become highly discouraged and unwilling to stick with the process of reformulating goals. During the process of working toward goals, a client may realize another goal is better suited. It's important to reevaluate goals during the process to help the client grow and embrace personal change.

Documentation and Report Writing for Collaboration with Other Providers and Client Support Systems

Counselors can provide a holistic level of care for their clients by collaborating with providers of other health-related services. For example, if a client suffers from depression, a counselor could contact the client's primary care provider (after receiving permission from the client by means of a signed HIPAA form) to discuss medical tests that might rule out organic causes of depression. Likewise, if the depressed client is obese, the counselor could work with the client's dietician to discuss dietary and exercise changes that might aid the client's recovery.

In all cases, it is important for counselors to keep comprehensive records of their interactions with other providers. Any test results and other communications obtained from these providers should be kept in the client's secure treatment file. If the counselor writes a report for another provider, it should provide only the minimally required information.

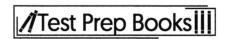

Discussing with Clients the Integration and Maintenance of Therapeutic Progress

The **problem-solving therapeutic model** serves to teach clients how to manage stressors that come in life. Often, clients do not possess skills that allow them to effectively navigate negative events or emotions without increasing personal harm. The goal of the problem-solving model is to teach clients the skills necessary to deal with negative life events, negative emotions, and stressful situations. In particular, goals of this model should be to assist clients in identifying which particular situations may trigger unpleasant emotions, understanding the range of emotions one might feel, planning how to effectively deal with situations when they arise, and even recognizing and accepting that some situations are not able to be solved.

The counselor, however, may be an instructional guide to facilitate problem solving for the client. Because problem-solving skills are one of the primary methods of resolving issues and often are skills that clients lack, the counselor may need to model them for the client so that the client can then develop their own skills. Counselors need to maintain empathy and congruence with the client during the problem-solving process, and even though they may have verbally instructed or modeled problem-solving methods, they need to maintain rapport in the relationship.

Educating Clients on the Value of Treatment Plan Compliance

There are times when clients may need extra encouragement from the counselor to adhere to treatment, so the counselor may need to contract with the client for additional motivation. Counselors should show empathy and offer clear communication of therapy parameters. Counselors may need to verbally explain the therapy process and explain the benefits of the therapeutic alliance, because often the clients have never before been involved in the therapeutic process. In the case of mandated clients, counselors often need to report to the client's legal agency concerning the therapeutic progress of the client, and the client needs to be made aware of the parameter of this report so that there is clarity of client responsibilities for the therapy and change process. Clients who are involuntary/mandated are often required to attend therapeutic sessions with the counselor, and their attendance is monitored. Mandated clients need to be made aware of this reporting, so that perhaps they are motivated to attend therapy on a regular basis.

Counseling Skills and Interventions

Aligning Intervention with Client's Developmental Level

A client's development level will vary from client to client, and it may even vary for the same client over the full course of an intervention. Therefore, the counselor should make no assumptions about the client's ability to cope, the way the intervention will be accepted and utilized, or any other aspect of the working relationship. These factors should be assessed upon intake and at regular intervals thereafter, the frequency of which may vary on a case-by-case basis.

Assessments should holistically take into account the client's development, including age, psychological factors, emotional factors, social factors, acute personal conditions (such as an impending divorce or recent refugee status) that may temporarily impact the client's functioning, and any other scope of development that may be appropriate for the client's need. For example, a client who has a history of violent behavior and a history of playing physical sports with extreme contact may find it beneficial to undergo neurological development assessments. By viewing the client through a holistic perspective, counselors can ensure interventions are appropriate across all domains of development; if so, the interventions are more likely to be effective and received positively by the client.

Aligning Intervention with Counseling Modality

Individual
Individual therapy can be an appropriate option for many reasons. A few considerations for choosing this modality would be if the client needs individualized treatment, requires scheduling flexibility, or prefers the privacy of individual counseling. Issues addressed in individual counseling are numerous and can include the same issues that would be focused on in family or group counseling, but in individual counseling the client is the priority. The counselor can decide with the client whether the client's goals and needs would best be met through individual therapy. Interventions such as exposure therapy and psychodynamic therapy work well in individual therapy as these interventions are unique to the client and allow them to progress and open up emotionally at their own pace in an intimate and safe setting.

Family Practice Approaches
One of the main goals of **family therapy** is to allow each family member to function at their best while maintaining the functionality of the family unit. When working with families, the counselor must:

- Examine and consider all systems affecting a family and each individual member to determine problems, solutions, and strengths, and also consider the functionality of the family subsystems.

- Respect cultural, socio-economic, and non-traditional family systems and not automatically define those systems as dysfunctional if they are not the norm. The overall and individual family functioning should be accounted for.

- Work to engage the family in the treatment, while considering the specific traits of the family (i.e., culture, history, family structure, race, dynamics, etc.).

- Assist in identifying and changing dysfunctional patterns, boundaries, and family problems.

138

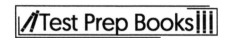

The following are important concepts in family therapy:

- **Boundaries**: Healthy boundaries around and within the family must exist for families to function effectively. The boundaries must be clear and appropriate.

- **Emotional Proximity and Distance**: These are the type of boundaries that exist within a family system.

- **Enmeshed**: Boundaries are unclear and pliable. Families that have very open boundaries within the family unit may have very fixed boundaries between outside forces and the family.

- **Disengaged**: Boundaries are rigid with little interaction and emotional engagement. Families that are disengaged within the family system tend to have very open boundaries around the family unit.

- **Family Hierarchy**: The power structure within the family. For families to function effectively, there must be a clear delineation of authority. There must be an individual or individuals who hold the power and authority in a family system. In a traditional family, this should ideally be located within the parental system.

- **Homeostasis**: Family systems should maintain homeostasis or remain regular and stable. When life events become too stressful and the family can no longer function as it normally would, the state of homeostasis is threatened. This is usually when many families seek help.

- **Alliances**: Partnerships or collaborations between certain members of a family. When alliances exist between some members of a family, it can lead to dysfunction (i.e., parent and child have an alliance that undermines the parental subsystem).

Couples Intervention/Treatment Approaches

Many couples enter treatment after experiencing long-standing problems and may seek help because all other options have failed. One of the goals of couples' therapy is to help clients develop effective communication and problem-solving skills so they can solve problems throughout and after treatment. Other goals include helping the couple form a more objective view of their relationship, modifying dysfunctional behavior/patterns, increasing emotional expression, and recognizing strengths. Counselors should create an environment to help the couple understand treatment goals, feel safe in expressing their feelings, and reconnect by developing trust in each other. Interventions for couples are often centered on goals geared toward preventing conflicting verbal communication and improving empathy, respect, and intimacy in a relationship. Therapeutic interventions, along with exercises, are designed to help couples learn to treat each other as partners and not rivals. **Cognitive Behavioral Therapy** is also used in working with couples. It uses cognitive restructuring techniques to help change distorted thinking and modify behavior.

Group Work

Individuals seeking counseling may benefit from group work in addition to, or in place of, individual counseling. **Group work** can be defined as a goal-directed intervention with small groups of people. Groups focus on nonpathological issues, such as personal, physical/medical, social, or vocational, and act to support and encourage growth. Groups are popular for addictions, eating disorders or weight loss, grief, anxiety, and parenting. They can be homogenous and share demographic information and goals or

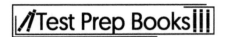

can be heterogeneous and diverse with multifaceted goals. Group members benefit from the process through sharing and the ability to learn new ways to react and cope with difficulties. It is essential that groups have a trained leader to help create structure, boundaries, and rules and keep the group on track.

The intention of group work is to improve the socioemotional and psychoeducation needs of the individual members of the group through the group process. There are two types of groups in social work: therapeutic and task groups. Task groups are created to perform a specific task or purpose. These groups differ in the amount and type of self-disclosure, confidentiality, and communication patterns. There are several types of treatment groups, including support, educational, and therapy groups. Groups can also be long-term or short-term, depending on the type and purpose.

Groups can be open or closed. **Open groups** are ongoing and allow for new members to enter at any time. Open groups are typically used for support and life transitions. There are challenges to this type of group, since the members are at different stages in the group process. The frequently changing membership can be disruptive to the group process because members may not feel as emotionally safe to share with others. **Closed groups** are time-limited, and new members can only join during the beginning stage. The advantages to this type of group are more engagement and better trust by the members, since the group process is more stable. A disadvantage is that if several members leave the group, the group process may not be as effective.

Aligning Intervention with Client Population

An intervention's success depends in part on whether the intervention plan is aligned with the individual's cultural experience and life experience. The intervention should be appropriate for the client's life. For example, counselors may specifically tailor the intervention for a veteran or a client with a physical or intellectual disability. All individuals are part of cultures with specific traditions, habits, and norms. These can vary by race, ethnicity, immigration status, income level, geographical location, or social status. It's important to take culture into context in order to show respect for the individual's way of life, tailor interventions to be easily understood, create trust and cooperation, and avoid wasting time or resources. Cultural contexts can be understood through researching the community, reading literature or periodicals from the area, and networking with people in the setting.

Counselors must be culturally competent to meet the needs of all clients. Counselors must also recognize the differences in individuals of the same culture and not use a cookie-cutter approach to deal with people of the same demographic group. When choosing interventions, treatment methods, and evaluation techniques, counselors must also consider the appropriateness of the selection for the client's cultural background. According to the NBCC Code of Ethics, counselors must show multicultural competence and should not engage in counseling techniques that may discriminate against groups based on gender, ethnicity, race, national origin, sexual orientation, disability, or religion.

Implementing Individual Counseling in Relation to a Plan of Treatment

Licensed professional counselors are obligated to provide their clients with time-limited and effective treatment methods. Time-limited treatments can actualize clients' treatment objectives in the fewest number of sessions possible. Effective methods have been established empirically through scientific research.

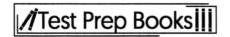

Once a counselor determines a diagnosis and understands the clients' treatment goals, they develop a treatment plan. The treatment plan is based on the diagnosis and a particular treatment method. For example, a counselor may choose to use Cognitive Behavior Therapy for a client diagnosed with depression because CBT has demonstrated efficacy in the treatment of depression. The treatment plan would follow CBT protocol, adjusted as necessary to fit the client's needs. The counselor would plan for a limited number of sessions to complete the treatment and would evaluate along the way whether the treatment is effective. If the treatment is not effective, it would be extended and/or altered.

Establishing a Therapeutic Alliance

An important element of the counseling relationship is the establishment of a **therapeutic alliance**, or collaborative effort between the counselor and the client, that will predict the success of the counseling experience. The relationship between the counselor and the client or client system is influenced by a number of components. These include the type of emotion that is shown by the parties during sessions, the general attitude toward the working relationship (e.g., positive, supportive), and the value each party places on the working relationship. The counselor should ensure that empathy, sympathy, and acceptance of the client and client system are shown during sessions to help foster a positive relationship. These aspects can be further supported by the counselor's initiative to build rapport with the client, such as through allowing the client to openly express feelings, work at a pace that feels comfortable, and encouraging them to shape and make decisions related to the intervention.

Generally, counselors who are inviting and interpersonally sensitive will be able to form a positive therapeutic alliance with the client. The working alliance can be assessed using a couple of tools. The Working Alliance Inventory is a self-reporting Likert questionnaire that explores how well the client's and counselor's thoughts about therapy are aligned. Both the counselor and the client answer more than thirty questions pertaining to counseling goals, first impressions, and the effectiveness of counseling sessions. The Barrett-Lennard Relationship Inventory is another tool used to measure congruence, regard, and empathy of a relationship. It is important for the therapeutic alliance to be established in the early counseling sessions to ensure the development of a positive working relationship.

When working with non-voluntary or involuntary clients who are mandated legally to seek treatment, the counselor must help the client overcome any negative feelings of anger or mistrust about treatment. With all clients, appropriate relationship building between the counselor and client is a necessary part of engagement and motivation. Clients must feel they are in a safe, empathetic environment. They also should experience a sufficient level of trust for the counselor in order for treatment to be effective. To create an effective treatment relationship, the counselor must project an attitude free of judgment, recognize the client's individual attributes, strengths, and abilities, and encourage the client's right to be an active participant in their own treatment.

Theory-Based Counseling Interventions

Modeling
Modeling is a technique used in therapy to allow clients to learn healthy and appropriate behaviors. Counselors "model" certain actions and attitudes, which can teach a client to behave in a similar fashion in their own life. Modeling is somewhat indirect. It is not suggested to the client to act in specific ways; rather, the counselor demonstrates desired behaviors, and the client begins imitating them.

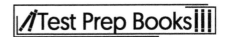

Reinforcement

Reinforcement is a tool of behavior modification, used to either encourage or discourage specific thoughts or behaviors. **Positive reinforcement** rewards desired behaviors, thus encouraging the client to continue them. Counselors can provide positive verbal reinforcements, for example, to a client sharing difficult feelings, which in turn will encourage the client to continue sharing. The term **positive** in this case does not refer to a "good" outcome but to the act of applying a reward, such as a positive reaction from the counselor. **Negative reinforcement** works to discourage unwanted thoughts or behaviors by removing a stimulus after a specific action. The negative does not make it "bad"—rather, it is the act of removing a negative stimulus to eliminate a specific thought or behavior.

Extinguishing

Extinguishing is the process of ending, or making extinct, a specific maladaptive thought pattern or behavior. Previously occurring behaviors were reinforced, and when reinforcement (either positive or negative) ceases, the behavior will eventually be extinguished. It may be a goal in counseling to extinguish unwanted thoughts or behaviors that are harmful or a hindrance to the client.

Cognitive Behavioral Techniques

Cognitive Behavioral Therapy (CBT) is typically a short-term treatment that focuses on transforming behavior by modifying thoughts, perceptions, and beliefs. Conscious thoughts affect behavior. Consequently, to promote consciousness of behavioral patterns in the client, the counselor (in the therapist role) will often assign homework in the form of exercises or journaling. The premise is that by identifying and reframing negative or distorted thoughts, the desired behavioral change can occur. CBT combines techniques and traits of both behavioral (positive and negative reinforcement) and cognitive therapies (cognitive distortion and schemas).

Cognitive restructuring is a concept used in CBT. The goal of cognitive restructuring is to help clients change irrational or unrealistic thoughts so that, ideally, change will lead to development of desired behaviors.

- The steps for cognitive restructuring are as follows:

- Accept that negative thoughts, inner dialogue, and beliefs affect one's feelings and emotional reactions.

- Identify which thoughts and belief patterns or self-statements lead to the target problems. Clients use self-monitoring techniques, including a log to track situations as they occur and the accompanying thoughts or feelings.

- Identify situations that evoke reoccurring themes in dysfunctional thoughts and beliefs.

- Replace distorted thoughts with functional, rational, and realistic statements.

- Reward oneself for using functional coping skills.

In-Life Desensitization

Desensitization is a behavior modification technique designed to replace an anxiety-producing stimulus with a relaxation response. Also known as systematic desensitization, it is a process to help the client manage fear or phobias. The client is taught relaxation techniques, whsich can include breathing,

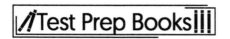
mindfulness, and muscle relaxation. Next, a "fear hierarchy" is created to rank stimulus from least to most fearful. The client is gradually exposed to the object or action that causes anxiety and then moves up the fear hierarchy and practices relaxation techniques. The goal is for the client to reach the most feared object or action and be able to react with calmness and control.

Addiction Issues

Addictions can be in the form of drugs, alcohol, or behaviors that cause financial instability and social impairment. It is important for counselors to distinguish when a behavior or addiction has become problematic for the client. Clients who continue to use substances or participate in behaviors despite legal or social consequences may require a counseling intervention. When assessing for substance abuse addiction, tolerance is an important aspect to consider. **Tolerance** is having to use more of the substance to obtain the same desired effects as before. Additionally, clients who continue taking substances to avoid withdrawal symptoms demonstrate dependence. After establishing a trusting relationship, counselors can encourage addiction recovery by helping their clients locate support groups, engage in twelve-step programs, secure social connections, and develop a relapse prevention plan. CBT helps clients focus on reducing problematic behavior that is associated with the addiction. The development of coping strategies, such as avoidance and self-control, helps to prevent a relapse. Counselors can assist clients with identifying and modifying cravings, triggers, and risky behaviors that can enable the addictions. Incorporating **motivational enhancement therapy** can encourage clients to address self-destructive behaviors and improve motivation to change.

Cultural Considerations

Culture refers to the way a group of people lives, behaves, thinks, and believes. This can include behaviors, traditions, beliefs, opinions, values, religion, spirituality, communication, language, holidays, food, valued possessions, and family dynamics, among other factors. Geography, social status, economic standing, race, ethnicity, and religion can determine culture. Culture can be found within any organized community, such as in a place of worship or workplace. The following are examples of specific types of culture:

- **Universal**: the broadest category, also known as the human culture, and includes all people

- **Ecological**: groups created by physical location, climate, and geography

- **National**: patterns of culture for a specific country

- **Regional**: patterns for specific areas of a country that can include dialect, manners, customs and food/eating habits

- **Racio-ethnic**: group that shares a common racial and ethnic background

- **Ethnic: group** that shares a common background, including religion and language

Cultural Skills

Counselors should be well versed in **cultural skills**. They must be able to apply interviewing and counseling techniques with clients and should be able to employ specialized skills and interventions that might be effective with specific minority populations. Counselors need to be able to communicate effectively and understand the verbal and nonverbal language of the client. They also should take a

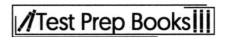

systematic perspective in their practice, work collaboratively with community leaders, and advocate for clients when it's in their best interests.

When working with clients from diverse backgrounds, counselors should be able to shift their professional strategies.

Family Composition and Cultural Considerations

In the United States, a long-standing definition of the family unit has been the nuclear family, which consists of a single man and a single woman (typically married to one another) and their immediate children. However, there are other concepts of family reflected in other cultures that can encompass alternate dynamics.

Families can consist of any small group of individuals that are related by blood or choose to share their lives together. These can consist of heterosexual or homosexual couples with or without children, single parent households, childfree households, homes with extended family all living under one roof, blended families involving step-children and step-parents, or lifelong partners that choose not to marry legally.

Culture and ethnicity play a large role in defining a family unit. For example, many Eastern cultures value living with extended family and consider everyone in the physical household to be a member of the immediate family unit.

American psychiatrist **Murray Bowen (1913–1990)** first established the family systems theory, which later served as the basis for family, or systems-focused, counseling. The **family systems theory** seeks to explain the high level of emotional interdependence that family members have with one another and how this interdependence individually affects each member of the family system. This theory states that the unique and complex cohesiveness that is found in family systems promotes positive behaviors like teamwork and taking care of one another; however, it can also cause negative behaviors, like anxiety or addictions, to diffuse from one person into the entire system.

The family systems theory is made up of eight distinct concepts:

- **Triangles**: refers to three-person systems, considered to be the smallest system that can still be stable. A third person adds extra support to manage intense emotions, tension, or conflict. The theory states that a two-person system cannot usually weather high levels of emotion, tension, or conflict over time.

- **Differentiation** of Self: how much an individual's personal beliefs differ from that of his or her group's beliefs. It is an important function of developing one's self. A strong self usually correlates with confidence and pragmatism, while a weak self usually correlates with an unhealthy need for approval from others.

- **Nuclear Family Emotional System**: referring to four different relationship patterns in this system. The patterns are marital conflict, dysfunction in one spouse, impairment in one or more children, and emotional distance, which refers to the fact that it occurs and how it affects the way problems are handled within the family.

- **Family Projection Process**: how parents project emotional conflict onto their children. The process can lead to pathologies in the child's psyche.

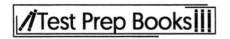

- **Multigenerational Transmission Process**: regarding the variance in differentiation of self between generations. The differentiation of self between parents and children over time leads to a widespread difference in beliefs between the oldest generation and the youngest generation of the family.

- **Emotional Cutoff**: regarding issue resolution. The act of failing to resolve issues between family members by reducing or eliminating contact with one another is emotional cut-off.

- **Sibling Position**: the importance of birth order and its influence on someone's functioning. It incorporates not only the birth order as it relates to how that person will function in workplaces and relationships, but also focuses on the birth order of each of the individual's parents and the influences those have on parenting styles.

- **Societal Emotional Process**: how the previous seven concepts hold true for any society. All families and societies will have progressive and regressive periods of development over time.

Important Terms

Affectional Orientation—a term used to describe one's romantic orientation toward a specific sex; an alternative term to *sexual orientation*

Alternative Family—any group of people that considers themselves a family unit but does not fall into the definition of a nuclear family

Emic—being aware of a client's culture and using counseling approaches accordingly

Empty Nest Syndrome—feelings of isolation, depression, or purposelessness that some parents may feel when their children move out of the family home

Ethnocentrism—a belief that one's culture is superior to another's

Ethnocide—purposely destroying another's ethnicity or culture

Ethnology—a branch of anthropology that systematically studies and compares the similarities and differences between cultures

Etic—an objective, universal viewpoint of clients

Gender Schema Theory—a theory by **Sandra Bem** in 1981 that describes how people in a society become gendered, especially through categories of information such as schemata

Heterogeneous Society—a society that is diverse in characteristics, cultural values, and language

High Context Culture—information is implicit and communicated through unspoken messages, with a focus on personal relationships and with fewer rules

Homogenous Society—a society that primarily consists of people with the same characteristics, cultural values, and language

Low Context Culture—information exchanged with little hidden meaning, with clear, explicit rules and standards, and relationships deemed less important than tasks

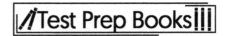

Modal Behavior—statistically, the most common and normative behaviors of a society

Nuclear Family—a family unit that consists of a married man and woman and their immediate children

Nuclear Family of Orientation—the family one is born into

Nuclear Family of Procreation—a family created by marriage and childbearing

Reciprocity—a social norm that says people should pay back what has been provided to them. This type of exchange relationship is used to build continuing relationships with others.

Sexual Orientation—an individual's sexual preference toward a specific gender

Stereotype—a preconceived notion about a group of people, not necessarily based in fact

Tripartite—awareness, knowledge, and skills of multicultural counseling

Systemic Patterns of Interaction

Systemic patterns of interaction are based on the belief that multiple factors impact the relationship between individuals. A client's social, familial, political, and cultural beliefs are all environmental factors that influence a current state of mind. This belief is part of the **systems theory**, which aims to conceptualize a client's issue based on their surroundings. The theory focuses on viewing individuals as their own system whose behaviors, thoughts, and emotions affect everyone in connection with them. In order to create a system that works for all members involved, counselors must help clients identify each person's expectations, behaviors, and desires. Using a systemic approach, insight into each member's role can help determine how that role affects the functionality of an entire group.

For example, a woman can be a nurturing mother at home, a disciplinary leader at work, and an encouraging friend within her social circle. All of these roles help to fulfill the overall system of interaction. Alternatively, there are negative interaction patterns that can strain communication and cause conflict among individuals. An example is individuals who rapidly escalate an argument with minimal provocation and have low frustration tolerance. This pattern is usually directed at another person who does not engage in shouting and will remain silent. Other individuals will attempt to control a situation by verbalizing threats of exposure, abandonment, or harm. Effective communication and constructive dialogue can help attain positive relationships and encourage clients to become an active participant within a system.

Family Member Interaction

Components of a Family History

Family history can provide insight into an individual's influences. The family unit is the most immediate system to which an individual belongs, so understanding it can provide invaluable perspective.

Counselors often use a genogram to understand the individual's family dynamic. A genogram is a visual chart that depicts an individual's familial relationships over a specified period of time by collecting relationship dynamics, attachments, interactions, and behavioral patterns. It can also aid clients with self-understanding and help the counselor choose appropriate assessments.

Inquiries about family history may explore:

- Ethnic and cultural background.

- Immigration status and experiences.

- Family composition (i.e., nuclear, blended, fostered or adopted children, divorced parents, co-parenting status).

- Socioeconomic status.

- Educational levels of family members.

- Employment status of family members.

- Personal and occupational goals and ambitions of family members.

- Achievements of family members.

- Traumas or loss experienced by any family members.

- Medical, financial, or domestic problems.

- Values held by each family member and the priority of each value.

- Any perceived favoritism experienced to certain children or adults.

- Roles held within the family.

Some of these topics may be sensitive to discuss and should be approached empathetically.

Family Theories and Dynamics

Family systems theory is an iteration of the basic systems theory. When seeking to explain the behavior of an individual, one must look also at the interrelationships of the individual's family. The assumptions of this theory are as follows:

- A family is a unique unit and is unlike any other family.

- A family is interactional, and its parts vary in their resistance to change.

- Healthy family development depends upon the family's ability to meet the needs of the family and the individuals comprising the family.

- The family undergoes changes that cause differing amounts of stress to each family member.

External Boundaries

External boundaries define the family and distinguish it from individuals and systems outside of the family. Boundaries in systems theory are not physical or tangible, but can be observed, in a sense, via a family's attitudes, rules, and use of space. Some families have **closed boundaries**. Families that use closed boundaries are characterized by having many rules about associating with non-family, physical barriers used to limit access to the family, rigid rules and values, few connections with others, and are

147

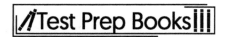

traditional and wary of change. Families that have **open boundaries** are characterized by having many connections to individuals outside the family, fluid rules, spontaneous decision-making skills, and minimal privacy. Uniqueness is valued more than tradition, and there is no fear of change. Open boundaries may lead to the family experiencing more chaos.

Internal Boundaries

Internal boundaries are rules that develop and define the relationships between the subsystems of the family. A **subsystem** might include the parents, the males of the household, or members of the family who share the same hobby. **Role organization** within a family is influenced by the size of the family, its culture and history, lifestyle, and values. In a healthy, well-functioning family, roles should be both clear and flexible.

As a family grows, rules develop that define how family members relate both to each other and to the world around them. Rules may be explicitly stated or implicitly understood. Families vary greatly in the type of rules that they have, as well as regarding whether rules can be easily discussed or modified.

Distribution of power in a reliable manner is important to the functioning of a family, though this distribution may change over time in response to changing needs of family members. Effective communication is also necessary for the family system. Roles, behaviors, and rules are all established through some type of communication. Communication can be open (clear and easy to understand) or closed (confusing and unclear).

Family Life Cycle

Family life cycle theories assume that, as members of a family unit, individuals pass through different stages of life. Although various theories will break down the stages somewhat differently, the following is a common conceptualization of the stages:

- **Unattached Young Adult**: The primary tasks for this stage are selecting a life style and a life partner. Focus is on establishing independence as an adult and independence from one's family of origin.

- **Newly-Married Couple**: The focus in this stage is on establishing the marital system. Two families are joined together, and relationships must be realigned.

- **Family with Young Children**: The focus in this stage is on accepting new family members and transitioning from a marital system to a family system. The couple takes on a parenting role. Relationships must again be realigned with the extended family (e.g., grandparents).

- **Family with Adolescents**: The focus here is on accommodating the emerging independence of the adolescents in the family. The parent-child relationship experiences change, and the parents may also begin to take on caregiving roles with regard to their own parents.

- **Launching Family**: The focus in this stage is on accepting the new independent role of an adult child and transitioning through the separation. Parents also must face their own transition into middle or older age.

- **Family in Later Years**: In this stage, spousal roles must be re-examined and re-defined. One focus may be the development of interests and activities outside of work and family. Another focus is on navigation of the aging process and losses that may occur.

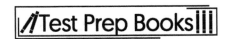

The basic family life cycle can vary significantly as a result of cultural influences, expectations, and particular family circumstances (e.g., single-parent family, blended family, multi-generational family).

Family Dynamics

Family dynamics are the interactions between family members in a family system. Each family is a unique system. However, there are some common patterns of family dynamics. The following are common influences on family dynamics:

- The type and quality of relationship that the parents have
- An absent parent
- A parent who is either extremely strict or extremely lenient
- The mix of personalities in the family
- A sick or disabled family member
- External events, particularly traumatic ones that have affected family members
- Family dynamics in previous generations or the current extended family

The following are common roles in the family that may result from particular family dynamics:

- The problem child: child with problematic behavior, which may serve as a distraction from other problems that the family, particularly the parents, do not want to face

- **Scapegoat**: the family member to whom others unjustly attribute problems, often viewed as "bad," while other family members are viewed as "good"

- Peacekeeper: a family member who serves to mediate relationships and reduce family stress

Effects of Family Dynamics on Individuals

There are many ways in which the family influences the individual socially, emotionally, and psychologically. All family systems have their own unique characteristics, with both good and bad functional tendencies. The family interactions are among the earliest and most formative relationships that a person has, so they define the relational patterns that the individual develops and utilizes with all subsequent relationships. Parenting styles, conflict resolution methods, beliefs and values, and coping mechanisms are just a few things that a person learns from their family of origin. It is also within the family that a person first develops an image of self and identity, often having to do with the role that they are given within the family system and the messages communicated by parents. If a child has a secure and healthy relationship with the family members, this will likely lead to overall wellbeing and emotional stability as an adult.

When it comes to physical or mental illness, the role that the family plays is critical in lowering risk factors and minimizing symptoms. A strongly supportive family will help a person function at the highest level possible. Oftentimes, family members can serve as caregivers or play less formal—but still critical—roles in supporting a person's health.

Religious and Spiritual Values

Religion is a potentially influential component of counseling that should be explored in the first sessions. A client's behaviors and values may be based on religious beliefs. Depending on the client's religion, their beliefs could either assist the client in creating change or they could hinder the process. Religion

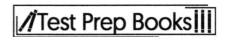

can be a valuable tool to help clients cope with stressful situations or to recover from lifechanging circumstances. Encouraging prayer or attendance to worship services as part of treatment can be beneficial for clients who find strength through their faith. It can be a reminder of the morals and values of their religion, which can motivate clients to commit to change. Although religion can be useful in counseling, it can also be part of the client's presenting problem. Exploring a client's religious beliefs and having knowledge of different religions can be crucial in developing a plan for treatment. For instance, if a client is struggling with an identity issue that is seen as a sin in their religion, an understanding of those beliefs will play a significant part in the counseling process. Respecting a client's religious beliefs and incorporating them into treatment will also help to build the therapeutic relationship.

Spirituality

Spirituality is sometimes mistaken for religion, but in fact, they are quite different terms. **Religion** is an organized system of beliefs that generally contain a code of conduct and often involve specific devotional or ritual observations. **Spirituality** is more abstract and includes participation in spiritual activities such as meditation, chanting, prayer, or unselfishly serving others. A spiritual person may or may not belong to a religious organization. Spirituality places emphasis on the growth and well-being of the mind, body, and spirit.

Studies have shown that persons who embrace spirituality tend to live both longer and happier lives. Several benefits of being a spiritual person include the following:

- The individual strives towards being a better person.
- There is an increased likelihood of connections with others.
- Spirituality offers hope to the hopeless through strong faith.
- It provides a path to heal from emotional pain.
- It helps reduce anxiety through meditation and other spiritual activities.
- The optimism that spiritual persons tend to have leads to greater life commitment.

Spirituality can be incorporated into the counseling process. A client's spiritual views may encompass their higher sense of purpose, meaning, the reason for existence, worldview, and sense of place in the universe. Counselors need to be aware of their own spirituality and be able to appropriately support a client without imposing or rejecting their spiritual views. Spiritual practices that can be helpful in counseling include meditation, prayer, mindfulness, and reflection.

Guiding Clients in the Development of Skills or Strategies for Dealing with Their Problems

Skills or Strategies for Dealing with Problems

An important aspect of counseling is helping people work through challenging events in their life. The counselor's role is to facilitate awareness and help clients resolve their internal conflicts. There are various strategies a counselor can use to guide clients to develop their own strategies for problem resolution. The first step is to ask the client what they are trying to accomplish with counseling and how committed they are to creating change. Understanding the presenting concern is a crucial aspect in developing a treatment plan and setting goals. A model of assessment known as the **DO A CLIENT MAP** takes a broad range of variables into consideration before establishing a treatment plan. The client map focuses on areas such as objectives, treatment models, resources, and timing. For example, a client dealing with anger issues will require certain steps in counseling to uncover the underlying cause of the

150

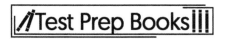
rage, such as unprocessed trauma, sadness, or fear. One key component of anger therapy is **emotional regulation**, which includes relaxation techniques to maintain control of uncertain situations. Other skills for anger management include skill development for crisis prevention and cognitive restructuring for balanced thinking patterns. Other examples include increasing self-awareness for clients with control issues, building trust in clients with paranoia, and cognitive restructuring for clients with social anxiety.

Counseling strategies will be dependent on the client's overall goals, motivation, and readiness for change. For example, a client wanting to overcome codependency issues may seek treatment when feelings of resentment and emptiness overpower their daily activities. Counselors may initiate interventions, such as placing the client in a support group that follows a twelve-step model. **Co-Dependents Anonymous (CoDA)** helps clients learn self-compassion and set personal boundaries. Once clients learn to develop self-care and communicate needs clearly, counselors can progress to evaluating therapy goals.

Cognitive and/or Behavioral Interventions
Cognitive Approaches
Cognitive approaches to the counseling process involve changing the way the client thinks in order to facilitate progress and problem-solving skills. Cognitive approaches tend to be evidence based and favored by insurance carriers, as they are efficacious for a variety of client issues, including substance use and personality disorders. Cognitive approaches focus on changing maladaptive thinking and cognitive distortions, and thus may help clients engage in behavior change. Cognitive distortions involve fallacious thinking patterns engaged in by the client, such as black-and-white thinking. Types of cognitive approaches may include cognitive behavior therapy, rational emotive behavior therapy, and solution focused brief therapy. There are many modalities of cognitive therapies and counselors should implement them when necessary.

Behavioral Approaches
Behavioral approaches, which originated with **Skinner and Pavlov**, include methods of changing and motivating client behaviors toward reaching constructive goals. The underlying concept is that if clients can change behavior, they may also alter the way they think. Skinner and Pavlov believed that all behavior is learned, and they believed in conditioning. Tokens may be awarded for positive behavioral changes in the client; this occurs in what is called a token economy. Cognitive behavioral therapies, which focus on both the cognition and the behavior of the client, are considered evidence based and are favored by managed care insurers.

Problem-Solving Approaches
The **problem-solving therapeutic model** serves to teach clients how to manage stressors that come in life. Often clients do not possess skills that allow them to effectively navigate negative events or emotions without increasing personal harm. The goal of the problem-solving model is to teach clients the skills necessary to deal with negative life events, negative emotions, and stressful situations. In particular, goals of this model should be to assist clients in identifying which particular situations may trigger unpleasant emotions, understanding the range of emotions one might feel, planning how to effectively deal with situations when they arise, and even recognizing and accepting that some situations are not able to be solved.

The counselor, however, may be an instructional guide to facilitate problem solving for the client. Because problem-solving skills are one of the primary methods of resolving issues, and often are skills

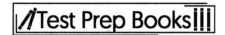
that clients lack, the counselor may need to model them for the client so that the client can then develop their own skills. Counselors need to maintain empathy and congruence with the client during the problem-solving process, and even though they may have verbally instructed or modeled problem-solving methods, they need to maintain rapport in the relationship.

Components of the Problem-Solving Process

When working with clients to develop problem-solving skills, counselors must first engage and prepare clients by discussing the benefits of improving such skills and encouraging clients to commit to the problem-solving process during the goal setting/contracting phase.

Steps in the problem-solving process:

- Step 1: Assess, define, and clarify the problem. As with goal setting, counselors should assist clients in clearly determining and defining the specific problem. Counselors should focus on the current problem and ensure clients do not become distracted by other past or current difficulties. Examine specific aspects of the problem, including behaviors and the needs of those involved.

- Step 2: Determine possible solutions. Counselors should lead discussion among participants to determine possible solutions and encourage client(s) to refrain from limiting options at this point. The purpose is for clients to gain practice in solution development. In the case of family work, all capable members should be allowed to offer solutions and should feel safe to do so without fear or criticism from other members.

- Step 3: Examine options and select/implement a solution. Counselors should assist clients in examining the benefits and drawbacks of each possible solution and choose an option that best meets the needs of those involved.

- Step 4: Evaluate and adjust. Counselors should help clients to determine the success of the solution. Client(s) can use a practical form of tracking solution effectiveness (charts, logs, etc.). If it is determined the solution is not working, the client can return to the solution-generating stage.

Rational Problem-Solving Process

Rational problem solving is based on facts and clear consequences. It is an analytical approach that relies on predictability and understood outcomes. The rational decision-making process has distinct steps to define a problem and then weigh and rank the decision-making criteria. Next, the client must develop, evaluate, and select the best alternative. It is also important to explore consequences as well as what might happen if no decision is made and no action is taken.

Intuitive Problem Solving

Intuitive problem solving is based on feelings and instinct. It is an approach based on emotions and a "gut feeling" about what might be the right decision. Although in some cases it may be the right way and result in the correct decision, it is important for the counselor and client to work together on understanding any problem and possible solutions. It is also important to know when to utilize rational decision making versus intuitive or when to employ both strategies.

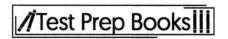
Strengths-Based and Empowerment Practice

Empowerment is a strengths-based modality, and the goal is that all clients should feel empowered based on their personal identities. Clients need to feel in control of most of their lives and circumstances, and this is what empowerment permits. Working from a strengths-based perspective empowers clients to facilitate change in their own lives. Counselors may seek to empower clients by focusing on strengths and bolstering clients' social constructs. Clients may need to be empowered from a racial, ethnic, religious, gender, or age perspective because they have suffered discrimination in these areas. Counselors may act as political advocates in these realms to combat social oppression affecting clients. The counselor should take into account the differences each client possesses due to their race, religion, or circumstance, and use these differences as strengths.

Teaching Coping Strategies to Clients

Teaching coping skills is an important role of the counselor in the therapeutic relationship. **Coping skills** enable individuals to manage stressful situations, solve problems, handle uncertainty, and develop resilience. Coping skills can include solution-focused problem solving, removing negative self-talk, learning mindfulness or other stress management techniques, and gaining support through friends, family, and community. Individuals may learn how to identify specific patterns to their feelings and behaviors, and thus, learn new and healthier responses. As there are many ways for individuals to develop and practice coping skills, counselors can provide options and unique plans for clients to best meet their needs.

Counselors may act in the role of teacher to instruct clients about coping and other skills. Coping skills may include relaxation techniques, deep breathing, time out, and improved communication skills. Common diagnoses that often require the instruction of coping skills include stress reduction, anxiety, and major depression. Clients may be able to utilize coping and acceptance skills for these diagnoses because they are frequently chronic, and clients will need to cope with them on an almost daily basis. Clients often need to learn a plethora of new skills to manage their issues and complex problems, and they and the counselor should collaborate on coping and other skills to manage these circumstances. Counselors can partialize and brainstorm with clients concerning coping and other treatment skills. Clients sometimes need detailed instructions in order to succeed with treatment goals. Clients need to be engaged in therapy outside of sessions and learn how to cope when the counselor is not present, so assigning clients' homework between sessions is a method of skills building. While the counselor may offer suggestions to the client for coping and other skills, the client is ultimately the most effective arbiter of their own treatment.

Finding Happiness

Happiness can be defined in many ways, and individuals may have challenges in arriving at a state where they feel entirely happy. Research on happiness shows that it is small things, like activities, and not hypothetical future events or material possessions that create the most happiness. Counseling can assist in helping individuals explore times when they felt happy and work on ways to increase and maintain their happiness. By asking clients about past happy times and what about those times made them feel happy, the counselor will be able to help clients explore how to feel happier in the present. It is important to recognize that future achievements may not produce desired happiness, such as "I will be happy when …". Rather, counselors should focus on helping clients appreciate what makes them happy in the present moment and how to use that happiness to feel more fulfilled each day.

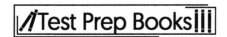

Steps in Skill Development

Clients frequently need to develop better coping strategies or improved social, communication, or life skills. Examples of skills that counselors may help clients develop include anger management, parenting, and substance abuse management. Skill training can take place in individual, family, group, or classroom formats. Steps in skill development include:

- Step 1: Skill identification. Identify and describe the skill(s) to be developed and how the client will benefit by acquiring the new skill(s). Engage clients and garner motivation to build skill development.

- Step 2: Demonstrate use of the skill. Give the client a visual example of what the skill looks like by modeling and performing role-play of the desired skill. This can be completed by a counselor and the client or in a family or group situation with another client.

- Step 3: Use of the skill outside of session and evaluation. The client should use the skill in everyday situations. The counselor can use sessions to discuss and evaluate a client's mastery of the skill and whether further skill development is needed.

Models of a Helper

Gerard Egan developed a model for helping outlined in his book, *The Skilled Helper*. Egan drew from several theorists, including **Rogers, Carkhuff,** and **Albert Bandura**, to create a **three-stage model for helping**. The phases of the model are identifying the present situation or scenario, defining the desired scenario, and developing a strategy to achieve it. The model provides a framework and map that clients can internalize for use when faced with a problem. It was designed to empower individuals to develop skills and confidence to solve problems outside of a helping relationship.

Imagery

Guided imagery can be a powerful tool in the counseling process. **Guided imagery**, which draws upon the mind-body connection, can be used to help the client alleviate anxiety, relax, and control or change negative thoughts or feelings. A counselor, who helps the client envision a place of relaxation and calm, guides the process. The counselor encourages the client to visualize and relax into the details of the image. Clients can also envision the successful outcome of a situation or imagine themselves handling a stressful situation. Once learned, clients can practice imagery on their own to help reduce stress and anxiety.

Role-Play

Role-play is a type of modeling and is also called behavior reversal. This technique enables clients to view the different ways a person may handle a challenging situation. It also allows a client to view a non-tangible behavior in a more tangible way. When clients practice skills and develop new and more productive methods of coping, they are able to take an active role in treatment, increasing their sense of empowerment and self-determination.

Assertiveness Training

Assertiveness training is an intervention that can be used in multiple settings with an assortment of interpersonal difficulties. This type of training helps individuals learn to express their emotions, thoughts, and desires, even when difficult, while not infringing on the rights of others. There are ways in which individuals can assert themselves, including saying no to a request, having a difference of opinion

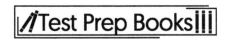

with another person, asking others to change their behavior, and starting conversations. Counselors must respect cultural differences when working with clients to develop assertiveness skills. For example, some cultures feel it is inappropriate for women or children to assert themselves. Role-play is an effective technique to help clients develop assertiveness skills.

Role Modeling

Role modeling, which offers the client a real-life view of desired target behaviors, can be an important tool to learn new skills. The counselor can request that clients demonstrate the behavior before modeling it, thereby allowing the counselor to assess a client's current skills and abilities. Counselors can demonstrate a coping model showing the skill or desired behaviors, including difficulties, anxieties, or challenges. The counselor can also demonstrate a mastery model, which shows confidence and competence with the desired behaviors. Each method has benefits and drawbacks. In coping mode, the client and counselor can process the interaction and identify improvements or changes that can be made to the desired behaviors or actions. There are several types of modeling:

- **Symbolic Modeling**: Client watches a visual representation of the modeled behavior (i.e., video, TV, images)

- **Live Modeling**: Client watches while a person performs the behavior

- **Participant Modeling or Guided Participation**: Client observes model performing behavior and then performs the behavior and/or interacts with the model

- **Covert Modeling**: Client visualizes the desired behavior

Promoting Relaxation

As part of the counseling process, clients may need to learn basic relaxation techniques, which can be simple to learn and practice. Stress can cause increased anxiety and tension; thus, relaxation techniques help reduce both mental and physical stress. Clients may present with racing thoughts, fatigue, or headaches; techniques such as awareness, breath work, and progressive relaxation can be of great benefit. Clients who have a reduction in their stress level may be more engaged in the counseling process and better able to manage difficulties outside of sessions. **Meditation** is a powerful relaxation tool to help build awareness and the ability to calm oneself. Relaxation can help diminish the activity of stress hormones in the body, reduce feelings of anger and frustration, lower heart rate, and improve confidence.

Guidelines for Giving Advice

There are two main types of advice: substantive and process. **Substantive advice** can be considered directive and may involve the counselor imposing their opinions onto clients. Process advice is more empowering and helps clients navigate options for solving their own issues. An example would be a client who is struggling with anxiety. Substantive advice would be the counselor telling the client he or she should practice deep breathing. **Process advice**, in the same example, would be teaching the client how relaxation techniques can lessen anxiety and providing examples. Counselors can offer process advice to help clients better understand their problems and possible solutions. Clients may ask for advice, and in some situations, it may be appropriate for the counselor to offer process advice; it is less likely that substantive advice should be given. Providing counseling is more complex than simply giving advice; thus, counselors should explore when, why, and how to give advice, if needed. As the goal of counseling is to help individuals gain a better self-awareness and competence, giving advice may

155

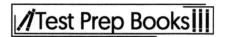

undermine the process by not allowing clients an opportunity to learn ways to solve their own issues both within and after counseling.

Helping Clients Develop Support Systems

As part of the intake process and initial sessions, counselors need to explore and understand clients' existing support systems. All individuals have varying degrees of social support, which can include friends, family, and community. Counselors can help clients evaluate their level of support and determine how the support system can help during counseling and after it has ended. It may be necessary to help clients find ways to develop additional support, such as through groups or organizations. A support system is necessary to provide help, encouragement, and care.

Structured and Unstructured Helping Relationships

Individuals can get help and support from many types of relationships, both structured and unstructured. **Structured relationships** include those with professional helpers, such as counselors, therapists, medical professionals, and counselors. These relationships have clear goals and are time-limited both in session and overall duration. Unstructured relationships also provide support but are more ambiguous and ongoing. These can include community support, groups, friends, family, and activities such as workshops or retreats.

Facilitating Clients' Motivation to Make the Changes They Desire

Characteristics of Willingness to Change

Entering into counseling can provoke anxiety, fear, and resistance to change. Clients may have both internal and external reasons to want or need to change but exhibit some unwillingness to do so. Clients with internal or intrinsic motivation understand that they need to change to move forward, grow, and achieve personal goals. External factors, such as mandated counseling, can be motivating, but may create additional resistance. Clients will be more motivated and willing to change when they have a vested interest in the process and believe they will achieve a successful outcome. Commitment to the process is essential, especially considering that counseling may not seem enjoyable or even interesting but may be necessary.

Motivation and resistance impact a client's readiness to change behavior. These are two crucial components to examine when developing an intervention plan. **High motivation** is indicated by self-confidence and self-efficacy, as the client believes they are capable of change. High motivation is also characterized by a client's desire to correct an identified problem, work toward a goal, and reliably show up for sessions. High motivation also shows in the client's belief that implementing a change will improve their overall quality of life.

Resistance can refer to any behavior that indicates the client does not want to work with the counselor or improve their personal situation. Resistance may be indicated by a client's refusal to show up on time, or at all, for sessions. A client involuntarily coming to sessions (such as by a court order) may state that there is no tangible problem to work on, or the client may state they feel no changes are occurring. Counselors should examine resistance holistically to ensure they are not contributing to it. For example, clients may exhibit resistance to counseling sessions if they do not feel comfortable with the counselor, if they do not understand the counselor, or if they are expected to work on issues they do not yet feel ready to address.

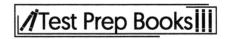
Readiness to change occurs in six stages: **pre-contemplation** (where an individual does not believe a need for change exists or is not self-aware), **contemplation** (where an individual recognizes a problem but is not ready to address it), **preparation** (where an individual recognizes a problem and sets the stage for change), **action** (where an individual takes active, involved steps to stop a problem), **maintenance** (where the individual commits to the desired behaviors), and **termination** (where the individual is able to regularly sustain the desired behaviors without relapse).

Motivation and resistance pertain to the individual's readiness to acknowledge and change behaviors. The more the individual feels ready to make a change, the higher the motivation and the lower the resistance. Some indicators of high motivation and low resistance include:

- Awareness and open acknowledgment of the presenting issue
- Willingness to list pros and cons of behavior change
- Willingness to make small steps toward and document outcomes of behavior change
- Acknowledgment that changing behavior is in the individual's best interest

Some indicators of low motivation and high resistance include:

- Lack of recognition of a present problem
- Hostility or apathy towards the counselor (which may be revealed by skipping sessions)
- Discussion of a presenting issue without openness to changing associated behaviors

Counselors can increase the client's motivation by discussing changes positively in terms that demonstrate benefit to the client's life, allowing the client to set his or her own goals and providing assistance only for those specific goals, highlighting the tools the client possesses to make changes, and acknowledging and respecting the client's fears about change.

Reassurance

Reassurance is an affirming therapeutic technique used to encourage and support clients. Reassurance can help alleviate doubts and increase confidence. Counselors use reassurance when a client experiences setbacks or an inability to recognize progress. Clients can be reminded of past successes to help bolster their ability to solve current problems. It is important that reassurance is genuine and not overused by counselors to pacify clients, but rather as a tool to validate and inspire continued growth.

Improving Interactional Patterns

Improving relationships for the client requires minimizing maladaptive interaction patterns. Interaction patterns that can harm a relationship include negative interpretations, shutting down, defending, complaining, and disapproving. A **validating style of interaction** is characterized by partners respecting each other's opinions and emotions, compromising, and resolving problems mutually. Volatile patterns lead to arguments and conflict, followed by reconciliation. The **avoiding style** is characterized by not dealing with problems at all. An example of a therapy method that attempts to improve interactional patterns is the Gottman Method. The **Gottman Method** includes assessment of the relationship and the development of a therapeutic framework with primary interventions. The areas addressed include conflict management, creation of a shared meaning, and development of friendship. The interventions assist with replacing negative conflict patterns with positive interactions to strengthen a relationship. The overall goal of this method is to achieve a sense of understanding, awareness, empathy, and interpersonal growth.

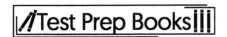

Providing Crisis Intervention

Phases of a Crisis Period
In 1964, psychiatry professor **Gerald Caplan** defined the recognizable phases of a crisis:

- Phase 1. This first phase consists of the initial threat or event, which triggers a response. The individual may be able to employ coping skills or defense mechanisms to avoid a crisis. The individual may experience denial.

- Phase 2. This second phase is the escalation, during which initial attempts to manage the crisis are ineffective and the individual begins to experience increased distress. The individual may employ higher-level coping skills to alleviate the increasing stress levels.

- Phase 3. The third phase is the acute crisis phase, during which anxiety continues and may intensify to panic or a fight-or-flight response. As stressful feelings continue to escalate, the individual experiences major emotional turmoil, possible feelings of hopelessness, depression, and anxiety. There are still attempts to problem-solve during this phase, and new tactics may be used.

- Phase 4. This final phase is marked by complete psychological and emotional collapse, or the individual finds a method to resolve the situation. the individual may experience personality disorganization and become severely depressed, violent, and possibly suicidal. There may be remaining emotional and psychological dysfunction or impairment if the coping mechanisms used were maladaptive.

Caplan theorized that individuals need to maintain homeostasis or remain in balance with their environment. A crisis is caused by an individual's reaction to a situation, not by an actual incident.

Crisis Intervention
Crisis intervention is typically a short-term treatment usually lasting four to six weeks and is implemented when a client enters treatment following some type of traumatic event that causes significant distress. This event causes a state of disequilibrium when a client is out of balance and can no longer function effectively. Counselors can either use generic crisis intervention models for varied types of crises or can create an individualized plan for assisting the client. The main goal of crisis intervention should be to help clients develop and use adaptive coping skills to return to the level of functioning prior to the crisis.

A crisis situation requires swift action and specially trained mental health personnel and can occur at any time in any setting. Albert Roberts proposed a seven-stage model to deal with a crisis and provide effective intervention and support. Roberts's stages are as follows:

- Stage 1. Conduct thorough biopsychosocial assessments of client functioning and identify any imminent danger to self or others.

- Stage 2. Make contact, and quickly establish rapport; it is important that the counselor is accepting, nonjudgmental, flexible, and supportive.

- Stage 3. Identify specific problems and the possible cause of crisis; begin to prioritize the specific aspect of the problem most in need of a solution.

158

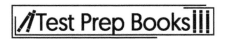
- Stage 4. Provide counseling in an attempt to understand the emotional content of the situation.

- Stage 5. Work on coping strategies and alternative solutions, which can be very challenging for an individual in crisis.

- Stage 6. Implement an action plan for treatment, which could include therapy, the 12-step program, hospitalization, or social services support.

- Stage 7. Follow up and continue to evaluate status; ensure that the treatment plan is effective and make adjustments as needed.

Critical Incident Stress Debriefing

Designed to support individuals after a traumatic event, **Critical Incident Stress Debriefing (CISD)** is a structured form of crisis management. Specifically, it is short-term work done in small groups but is not considered psychotherapy. Techniques used include processing, defusing, ventilating, and validating thoughts, experiences, feeling, and emotions. CISD is best for secondary trauma victims, not primary trauma victims. For example, in cases of workplace violence, any employees who witnessed an event or who were indirectly impacted could benefit from CISD. Employees who were first-degree victims would need more individualized, specialized care and therapeutic intervention. It is important that CISD is offered as quickly as possible after an event; research has indicated it is most effective within a 24- to 72-hour time frame and becomes less effective the more time lapses after the event. CISD can be managed by specially trained personnel and could include mental health workers, medical staff, human resources, or other professionals. Trained Crisis Response Teams can be ready or quickly available to provide support directly following a traumatic situation.

Crisis Intervention Process
ENGAGE AND ASSESS

Counselors participate in client engagement by helping to de-escalate volatile emotional states through establishing rapport, using empathy, employing emotional management techniques, and accessing outside systems (family, friends, and support groups). Additionally, the counselor assesses the crisis situation to determine the level of care required (general triage may include intensities ranging from one to three) and how the client has been impacted.

SET GOALS AND IMPLEMENT TREATMENT

Goal setting should occur in collaboration with a client's treatment plan. Intervention strategies, tasks, and timeframes should correspond with the desired goal and objectives. The primary goal should be to assist clients in returning to pre-crisis functioning. However, there will likely be additional and related goals and tasks as the plan of action is implemented.

EVALUATE AND TERMINATE

Counselor concludes treatment and evaluates completion of goals. It is important to discuss with the client what coping skills have been developed and how they might be able to use those skills for future crises and challenges.

Transference and Defense Mechanisms

Transference

Transference is a concept from psychoanalysis that refers to the process of the clients transferring any feelings toward others onto the counselor. These feelings are likely unconscious, as they arrive from

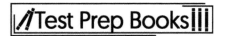

childhood experiences and relationships. For example, the counselor may remind clients of their distant parent, and the clients will project feelings about that parent onto the counselor. Transference can be very powerful, although both positive and negative forms exist. Positive or good transference allows clients to work through issues with the counselor, who is safe and nonreactive. Clients can project negative feelings or emotions onto the counselor, thus being able to resolve them in the absence of the parent or individual. Negative or bad transference exists when clients project negative emotions and become angry or hostile toward the counselor. This type of transference can create a blockage and diminish the effectiveness of therapy. It is the role of the counselor to understand and manage transference as it arises in the relationship. Transference can also occur for the counselor with clients. Supervision and consultation are both helpful and necessary should this occur.

Defense Mechanisms

Sigmund Freud's *psychoanalytic theory* focused on the conflicts, drives, and unacceptable desires in the unconscious mind and how they affect a person. One method of dealing with unconscious conflicts is through *defense mechanisms*, which are the mind's way of protecting a person from unacceptable thoughts. Here are some of the most common defense mechanisms:

- *Repression* is when a person suppresses thoughts or memories that are too difficult to handle. They are pushed out of the conscious mind, and a person may experience memory loss or have psychogenic amnesia related to those memories.

- *Displacement* takes place when someone displaces the feelings they have toward one person, such as anger, and puts it on another person who may be less threatening. For example, someone may express anger toward a spouse, even if they are really angry with a boss.

- *Sublimation* is when the socially unacceptable thought is transformed into healthy, acceptable creativity in another direction. Pain may become poetry, for example.

- *Rationalization* is when unacceptable feelings or thoughts are rationally and logically explained and defended.

- *Reaction formation* occurs when the negative feeling is covered up by a false or exaggerated version of its opposite. In such a case, a person may display strong feelings of affection toward someone, though internally and unconsciously hate that person.

- *Denial* is refusing to accept painful facts or situations and instead acting as if they are not true or have not happened.

- *Projection* is putting one's own feelings onto someone else and acting as if they are the one who feels that way instead of oneself.

Facilitating Trust and Safety

The nature of the counseling relationship necessitates that clients trust and feel safe with their counselors. Clients reveal personal information to their counselors, and they must be able to trust that the counselor will not spread that information. They should also feel confident that their counselor is reliable, responsible, knowledgeable, and competent to handle their innermost thoughts, feelings, and experiences.

160

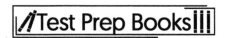

Counselors can facilitate trust with their clients by explaining that they are bound by confidentiality (with some exceptions having to do with harming others or themselves). This allows clients to feel secure when disclosing information that they would not share elsewhere.

Additionally, counselors gain their clients' trust when they respond appropriately to the disclosure of difficult material. When counselors show compassion, care, and concern instead of judgment and condemnation, clients are more likely to develop trust and feel safe.

Building Communication Skills

An individual can communicate verbally and non-verbally through body language or silence. Interviews, two-way casual conversations, and written or verbal standardized assessments can help the counselor determine the individual's communication skills. **Role-playing** a specific situation can help the counselor determine how an individual communicates in certain contexts. Assessing the individual's personal, family, social, or cultural context can also provide valuable insight to communication skills and help validate an assessment.

Counselors use verbal and nonverbal communication techniques to engage clients in completing treatment goals. Verbal communication is vital to the counselor/client relationship, and counselors should be skilled at greetings, summarization, reflection, and the conveyance of new information to the client. The client may misconstrue a counselor's body language if it does not represent openness and trust. Likewise, the counselor needs to be adept at analyzing the client's body language in order to move forward. Clients use both verbal and nonverbal communication to convey their story to the counselor, and communication techniques used by the counselor can be modeled to teach the client improved communication. Clients should be instructed to recognize their own communication techniques in the context of the relationship with the counselor. Clients who are withdrawn or isolated may need especially sensitive communication with the counselor in order to better communicate verbally and nonverbally.

In order to build a strong helping relationship with the client, the counselor must learn to use effective verbal and nonverbal techniques. These skills are necessary throughout the treatment process and especially during assessment and engagement.

Developing and Facilitating Conflict Resolution Strategies

Counselors may engage in conflict resolution with clients by acting as a mediator or advocate. **Mediators** work with clients to intervene in the conflict and develop helpful solutions that reflect all parties involved. For example, the counselor may act as a mediator in family or couples therapy conflicts. Counselors may also work with clients on developing their own conflict resolution skills through methods such as reflection, role-playing, and empty chair techniques. Counselors may also encourage clients to practice the use of *metacommunication*, which is communication about the behaviors and reactions of their regular and possibly dysfunctional method of interactions or communication. Sometimes the client is in conflict with the counselor and transference issues must be resolved before progress can be made. Counselors and clients need to be in collaboration concerning treatment goals and modalities so that conflict is reduced.

In some cases, agencies contract with mediation services outside the agency to assist clients in resolving conflicts. Professional mediators are trained in mediation techniques and are paid by the agency for

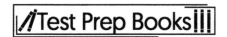

their services. They can be the final step of resolution when the agency cannot resolve client conflict. Child protective services agencies sometimes use professional mediators to reduce or eliminate conflict in cases involving juveniles.

Developing Safety Plans

Safety plans are problem-solving tools clients can follow when they are unable to think clearly or care for themselves. Counselors can help clients identify tasks to perform when crisis intervention is needed. Safety plans will be dependent on the reason clients require them. Clients with suicidal ideation, victims of domestic violence, and individuals with mood disorders can benefit from establishing a safety plan. There are a couple of components to a safety plan that should be created in collaboration with the client. Counselors and clients must first be able to recognize the signs of danger.

Clients who verbalize intent to self-harm or harm others are exhibiting signs of a crisis and require intervention. It is also important to be able to identify what the client is able to do on their own to mitigate the negative thoughts and manage stress. Initiation of coping strategies, such as meditation, music, and exercise, that can de-escalate harmful thoughts should be included. Another component to incorporate is the identification of resources. Clients and counselors can work together to create a list of friends, family, or professional resources to be contacted in crisis situations. The goal of a safety plan is to be client-centered, realistic, and achievable.

Facilitating Systemic Change

Counselors can apply the principles of systems theory to create change when working with families. An important concept of this theory is the idea that one part of a family system affects and changes other parts of the system.

Homeostasis is a concept that refers to families' resistance to change and their pressure to maintain balance and the status quo. Counselors must use techniques to disrupt the homeostasis of a family in which problematic behaviors exist. For example, in a family with a parentified male child, a counselor might physically move the boy away from his mother and father and place him across the room, while placing the mother and father next to each other. This maneuver has the potential to disrupt the system. It is designed to help the married couple create stronger boundaries around their marriage, thereby excluding the child from the husband-wife dyad.

Counselors can also facilitate systemic change by having clients draw genograms to show generational patterns. These diagrams visually depict family patterns of marriage, substance abuse, violence, divorce, etc. across multiple generations. They are designed to show families' negative and positive patterns and may give them motivation to begin intentionally creating new patterns.

Providing Distance Counseling or Telemental Health

Telemental health is an evolving form of counseling. Since the COVID-19 pandemic, telemental health services have become more prevalent, but the rules and regulations are not firmly established and may differ from state to state. While some insurance companies have started to pay for these services due to no-contact regulations during the pandemic, it is not certain if this will continue to be a covered practice post-pandemic.

Telemental health includes video conferencing, phone calls, chat, text messages, and emails. Individuals,

162

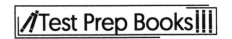

couples, families, and even groups can benefit from these services. Counselors who utilize telemental health must ensure that their devices and software are secure and do not allow recording.

Providing Education Resources

Counselors often don multiple roles in their profession, one of which includes providing information and assisting with access to educational services. When providing educational services, the counselor must determine what skills, information, or knowledge needs to be acquired, as well as the capabilities of the client and the amount of time available for the development of new skills. The provision of education may be done in individual, family, or small group classes, or large group forums. Counselors may also recommend resources such as books, articles, or websites that may help clients acquire new information.

Clients with substance addiction issues can benefit from resources that provide education on common addictions, locate rehabilitation centers near their area, or provide intervention hotlines in case of a crisis. Websites such as addictionresource.com and drugabuse.gov provide an array of information for clients seeking education and additional resources. Clients who experience depression can benefit from outside engagement when counseling sessions do not occur. These clients are at a high risk of suicide and may require multiple resources. Organizations such as the **National Alliance on Mental Illness (NAMI)** provide support groups, advocacy, and educational articles to bring awareness and help clients experiencing emotional distress. Clients whose safety is at risk due to domestic violence also require a vast amount of resources. The **National Domestic Violence Hotline** offers pathways to creating a safety plan, education on recognizing the signs of domestic violence, and a list of regional organizations to help those in need.

Providing Psychoeducation for Clients and Groups

Psychoeducation refers to any form of training or instruction that is provided to clients and the client system as a part of understanding mental health or psychological issues and treatments. Its goal is to support clients experiencing mental illnesses, their families, and their networks while eliminating the stigma that has been associated with mental health issues for decades. Psychoeducation methods include explaining potential causes for specific mental health issues, understanding the challenges of specific mental health issues, explaining how support systems can acknowledge and cope with not only a client's mental health condition but also their own caregiving stress, and teaching coping skills, building resiliency, and overcoming obstacles in ways that are accessible. This form of education can occur in group settings, seminars or webinars, and in individual or family sessions. It can also be presented through newsletters, other media, and formal courses.

It may be offered in-home, online, in hospitals or other healthcare facilities, in community centers, or at conference venues. It is not considered treatment, but it is a beneficial complement to clinical care. It promotes positive and inclusive language, eliminates shame and fear around mental illnesses, creates educational value, fosters network support and understanding, and acknowledges a variety of feelings and responses to mental health conditions. Psychoeducation techniques are associated with reduced inpatient and hospitalization rates for clients with mental health conditions. Psychoeducation is correlated with clients' self-reported feelings of acceptance and increased family support. Family and friends self-report a better understanding of their loved one who may have a mental health condition, a better understanding of their role in providing positive support and care, the ability to draw healthy

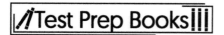

boundaries for themselves, and relief from learning and utilizing self-care techniques that reduce caregiver stress. g

Summarizing

Summarizing is an active listening and rapport-building technique. The counselor listens to the content provided by the clients and summarizes the essential points of the conversation. This process can help isolate and clarify the essential aspects of issues and ensure that both the client and the counselor can focus on the most critical tasks. Additionally, summarization can be helpful in goal setting or at the end of a session.

Reframing or Redirecting

A technique used by counselors to help clients create a different way of looking at a person, situation, or relationship is known as **redirecting** or **cognitive reframing**. This technique helps clients look at situations with a different perspective. For example, reframing thought processes can be effective in counseling teenagers who do not always agree with parental decisions. Anger that results from imposed curfews or punishments for underperforming academically can be redirected by having the client empathize with their parents and analyze the reasons for the restrictions. Effective reframing should acknowledge the client's feelings and help interpret the situation in a different manner. For example, clients who experience fear of failure can use that emotion to reframe their thought process into a positive one. Encouraging them to use fear as a form of awareness as opposed to a paralyzing emotion can help clients look at their situation with a different mindset.

Facilitating Empathic Responses

Empathy is considered an essential counseling skill. It is used not only to initially build trust but also throughout the counseling process. The process of empathy is used to help the counselor understand the client's viewpoint. It is more complex than sympathy, which is somewhat passive and a sense of feeling bad for another person. Empathy focuses on gaining insight into the client's experience to offer effective means to deal with any issues or concerns. Although psychologist Edward Titchener was the first to use the term, it is strongly associated with the client-centered approach of **Carl Rogers**. Rogers believed empathy extended beyond understanding a person's situation; it involved the counselor imagining him or herself in that situation. This level of empathy requires genuineness, acceptance, and a small measure of vulnerability on the part of the counselor.

Self-Disclosure

In rare cases, it may be appropriate for counselors to self-disclose to clients. It is important to remember that the therapeutic process is to help clients, not indirectly benefit counselors. First and foremost, counselors should consider the intent and who will benefit from their self-disclosure. It is not appropriate for clients to be burdened with counselors' emotions, as it could shift the atmosphere and power dynamic of therapy. Counselors can disclose an emotional reaction to content from clients, provided it is for the benefit of the clients. Counselors should be cognizant of their clients' level of functioning and issues prior to any purposeful self-disclosure to ensure professional boundaries are maintained.

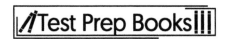

Constructive Confrontation

For many clients, there comes a point when goals aren't being reached in counseling. The counselor needs to recognize when progress isn't being made and observe (through active listening) any inconsistencies that are holding the client back. This includes listening for any contradictions the client makes regarding their behaviors or feelings. These inconsistencies may be the cause of conflict in the client's life. The client may say one thing but do another, or they may say two opposing things. The counselor will need to confront the client about these inconsistencies, but it needs to be done carefully. It is important that a therapeutic and trusting relationship is established before the counselor attempts any confrontation. The client could interpret the counselor's questioning or comments as criticism. The client needs to be approached with empathy to show that the counselor has sincere interest in revealing and understanding their conflicting actions and/or words. When pointing out contradictions, it is best to reflect back what the client has said and delicately inquire about discrepancies. If the client is open to analyzing how this affects their ability to make changes, they may reach a new level of self-awareness and begin to move forward in therapy.

Counselors should be sensitive to the needs of clients they work with. Some clients will respond better than others to confrontation, and the counselor needs to have the skills to identify how and when confrontation should occur. Culture and gender may be a factor in how confrontation will be received. The counselor should also be mindful of the language that is used. Accusatory or harsh language will be met with resistance, while encouraging and positive words are more likely to aid in the therapeutic process. If the confrontation is met with denial, the counselor will need to approach the problem in a different manner at a different time.

Facilitating Awareness of Here-and-Now Interactions

Here-and-now in counseling refers to using the present interactions between the counselor and client or between group members to resolve issues and change behaviors in clients. The idea behind this technique is that interactions or feelings that clients experience during counseling sessions reflect interactions and feelings that occur outside of counseling and that, by addressing them at the present moment, new behaviors and methods of interaction can be learned. In order for here-and-now interactions to be therapeutic and effect change, the counselor has to be aware of these opportunities for working through issues as they arise. After addressing the problem and working through it together, the counselor must summarize what has happened and make the client aware of how this interaction was handled and how this more productive and healthy method can be used to change behaviors and interactions in their daily life.

Counselors who follow the **theory of Gestalt therapy** place an emphasis on the present as opposed to the past or the future. Past experiences are not ignored but are used as milestones for change and growth. For example, clients who are unable to fulfill their interests due to unfinished business can benefit from incorporating the Gestalt method. The counselor can assist the client with redirecting their energy in a positive manner and creating adaptive ways to function despite negative past experiences. Examples of positive energy include optimistic statements, compassionate actions, and self-care. The **Empty Chair Technique** is an exercise that encourages dialogue between the client and an empty chair beside them. The chair should symbolize another person in the client's life, themselves, or a part of themselves in order to engage thoughts, behaviors, and emotions. Role reversal is essential so that the client is able to focus on immediate experiences and work through different aspects of conflicting situations.

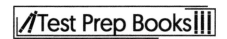

Linking and Blocking

Blocking is the act of the group leader stopping unwanted behaviors from members that may be harmful or hurtful or violate confidentiality. This helps to set appropriate standards for how the group should behave. With linking, the group leader relates members' stories or situations to enhance interaction and cohesion of the group.

Management of Leader–Member Dynamics

Broadly speaking, anything that impacts the group can be considered dynamic. The word **dynamic** means change, activity, or progress. Thus, a group is constantly adapting and evolving. **Dynamics** are the interrelationships between the members, which include the leadership style, decision-making, and cohesiveness. **Cohesiveness** is the degree to which the group sticks together. There are two types of cohesion: task and social. Task is the level at which the group works to achieve a common objective. **Social cohesiveness** refers to the interpersonal relationships within the group.

There are three main styles of leading groups:

- **Autocratic**: This leader is authoritarian and sets clear rules, boundaries, and goals for the group. This type can be beneficial in situations where there are time or resource limitations, constant changes to membership, or the need to coordinate with other groups. This type of leadership can create resentment and dissatisfaction, as it is unilateral and strict.

- **Democratic**: This leader is considered the fairest by taking into consideration ideas and choices of the group. Not to be confused with the political usage, these leaders do not wield specific power or prestige; rather, they work to maintain a participatory style and harmonious atmosphere.

- **Laissez-Faire**: This is the most relaxed style of leadership; group members are responsible for all aspects of decision-making. Laissez-faire is an absence of leadership, which works best with motivated, self-directed members.

Modeling Giving and Receiving Feedback

Clients can benefit from counselors not only by the specific techniques they use, but also by observing how their counselors interact with them. The interactions between counselors and clients within sessions can demonstrate appropriate ways for clients to give and receive feedback in their lives outside of counseling sessions. For example, a client who is shy and unassertive could benefit from receiving genuine feedback about her interactional style in a way that is non-critical yet straightforward. Her observations about how the therapist gently and honestly speaks truth to her could give her courage to accept feedback from others without taking offense. The counselor could also demonstrate how to receive feedback by asking the client if she is satisfied with the progression of therapy. The openness of the counselor to receive feedback could exemplify how to accept feedback from others.

Impact of Extended Families

Clients with extended families often have concerns with invasions of privacy, unsolicited advice, and frequent criticisms. It is important for counselors to guide clients toward responding positively to uncontrollable behaviors. Setting boundaries is an important part of maintaining privacy. For example,

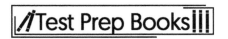

extended family members who often interfere with activities of daily living may cause a disruption in routine. Clients should be encouraged to voice their concerns and explain their emotions to the family member in order to reach an understanding. When conflicts between individuals arise, including a third person creates **triangulation**. Counselors should encourage clients to address their concerns directly with the person involved in the disagreement and avoid sharing frustrated feelings with a third person. Individuals who find themselves following routines they are unhappy with can become resentful and repress their anger. These clients should be encouraged to break the pattern and communicate alternative solutions that work for the entire family.

Containing and Managing Intense Feelings

When there is a difficult situation or crisis, extreme emotions are usually involved. If possible, a client should be guided through relaxation techniques to help calm them down. Oftentimes, a calm and neutral party who can facilitate a conversation or listen to the client empathetically, but without feeding the emotion, will automatically de-escalate the situation. Confrontation or matching the client's emotions will escalate the situation. Allowing the client to communicate the situation fully may help them to become less emotional and more focused on the facts. At this point the client may be able to focus on the next steps and specific tasks that need to be done. If possible, help the client to regain emotional control so that extreme options such as restraints are unnecessary.

Influence of Family of Origin Patterns and Themes

The family that a person grew up with is considered to be that person's family of origin. This can be their biological parents and siblings, grandparents, aunts and uncles, adopted parents, or any other people who raised them and were part of the household that the person grew up in. Whether biological or not, every family has patterns of interactions that are passed on to the next generation and affect aspects of the family members' lives such as relationships, self-worth, and regulation of emotions. Everything from religious beliefs to how anger is dealt with are established early in life by the influence of the family of origin.

When working with a client to understand and change present behaviors and patterns, the counselor can explore the patterns and interactions of the family of origin to identify the source of any dysfunction. There are numerous issues, such as anxiety, intimacy problems, and abuse, that can be attributed to these patterns and interactions that occur early in life. By exploring behaviors learned from the client's family of origin, the counselor can help the client unlearn old family behaviors and learn new and acceptable habits and responses, form better concepts of self, and change the types of relationships that they tend to gravitate toward.

Social Support Network

An individual's **social support network** consists of the family, friends, and community groups that the client can turn to when in need of any kind of support. **Support** can be provided in many ways, such as listening to problems, giving advice, sharing resources, assisting with financial responsibilities, or running errands. Having a social support network makes difficult circumstances easier to bear. Individuals who do not have a support system tend to suffer from more mental and physical health problems than those who have a support system. A positive network of support can alleviate feelings of loneliness and can provide motivation for healthy changes and continued progress towards goals. An important consideration when looking at a client's support system is whether the individuals in that

167

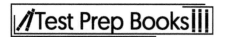
system provide a positive or negative influence. Counselors should be aware of the possibility that the system of support that a client has may include friends or family who perpetuate the issue that the client is trying to overcome. Therefore, counselors should be aware of the impact that each client's social support network has on their progression through counseling.

Structured Activities

Counselors have many theoretical approaches from which to choose, and within those approaches is a vast assortment of structured activities they can utilize to help clients meet their treatment goals. Recent research reflects the positive benefits of journaling and gratitude exercises for clients struggling with different types of diagnoses. For instance, gratitude has demonstrated efficacy in treating depression; therefore, counselors can encourage their clients to write a list of things they are grateful for every day.

Counselors can also have their clients complete genograms. **Genograms** are diagrams of family structures that include several generations. Clients are instructed to draw "maps" of their family history that include information such as marriages, births, deaths, occupations, divorces, suicides, drug and alcohol abuse, child abuse, etc. These can show clients generational issues existing within their families. Therapists can then work with clients to uncover destructive patterns in their immediate families and find ways to stop them.

The **empty chair technique** is a common therapeutic activity. This technique requires the client to sit across from an empty chair and have a dialogue with a person in their life or with some part of themselves. The therapist then has the client switch chairs and speak from the other perspective.

Therapists can also have clients write letters that are not intended to be given to the recipients. These letters can be written to people who are living or dead. This technique allows clients the opportunity to express their thoughts and feelings without facing the intended recipients when it may be unsafe or impossible to do so.

Interactions in Groups

Promoting and Encouraging Interactions Among Group Members

It is the role of the counselor to encourage all members to participate in the group process. Members serve different roles in the group and can change their roles as the group progresses. Roles can be defined as functions the individual members of the group are fulfilling or performing that facilitate the group process. Clients typically take on various roles during group treatment. There are both functional and nonfunctional roles. **Functional roles** assist the group and include the energizer, harmonizer, tension reliever, and gatekeeper. **Nonfunctional roles** can disrupt and hinder the group and include the interrogator, dominator, monopolizer, aggressor, and recognition seeker. Other roles include victim, scapegoat, and follower, who are not overtly negative but do not assist in positive group functioning.

The counselor must be aware of the roles of each individual and how those roles are affecting the group, so interventions can be made when necessary. The counselor can solicit feedback from each member of the group throughout the group process. The counselor can use blocking to stop unwanted behaviors from members that may be harmful or hurtful or violate confidentiality. Counselors should encourage positive interactions between group members and guide and encourage members to assume positive roles that benefit themselves as individuals and the group as a whole. To enhance interaction and

168

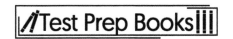
cohesion of the group, the counselor can use the technique of linking by relating members' stories or situations. Members who have similar issues can assist one another in therapy.

Promoting and Encouraging Interactions with the Group Leader

Counselors should encourage their clients who are in group therapy to interact with the group leader. The leader is there to not only facilitate the group, but also to help the group members get as much out of the group as possible. Groups may have multiple leaders. Co-leadership is widely used in group therapy sessions and is found to have many beneficial aspects. **Co-leadership** may be used as a way to train therapists to lead groups and is found to have positive impacts, especially in larger groups. Having two leaders can help ensure that all members get attention, can actively participate, and assist the group in accomplishing more. Co-leadership can be detrimental if leaders do not get along or cannot form a cooperative and united management team for the group.

Phases in the Group Process

Phases in the Group Process

Several theories outline the developmental stages of a group. One of the most well-known is **Bruce Tuckman's four-stage model**: forming, storming, norming, and performing. **Forming** is the stage where the group members are just beginning to get acquainted and may be anxious and less vocal. **Storming** involves conflict, discord, and struggles to agree upon a leader. **Norming** is the agreement stage, during which a leader is chosen and conflicts begin to resolve. **Performing** is the point at which the group becomes effective at achieving defined tasks. A fifth stage, **Adjourning**, was added, which defines the point at which the group terminates.

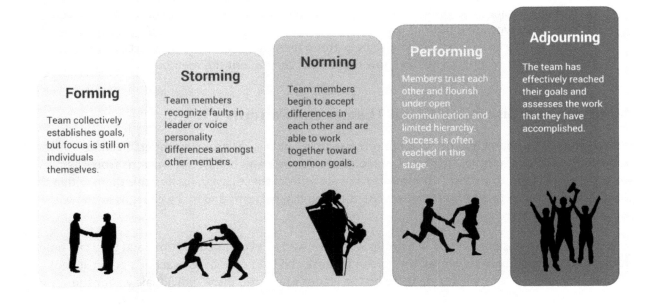

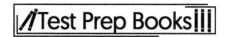

Other group development theories include that of **Irvin D. Yalom**, whose three-stage model included orientation, conflict/dominance, and development of cohesiveness. **Gerald Corey**'s stages included initial, transition, working, and termination. All three theories share similar progressions of the group process. A general method of categorizing the group process is the beginning, middle, and end stages. Each stage is classified by different activities, processes, and tasks:

- **Beginning Stage**: Counselors determine the group's purpose, members, objectives, and other logistical tasks (time, location, etc.). Group formation occurs at this stage as new members come together. The counselor fosters a safe and trusting environment by establishing acceptable group norms. As group members become more comfortable, conflicts arise as power and control behaviors emerge. Group roles and alliances begin to form. The counselor's role is to help guide the group through these challenges and process any conflicts that arise within the group.

- **Middle Stage**: This stage is where most group work is done. Members share information, openly address issues, and work through conflicts. Some groups do not make it to this stage for several reasons, including member dynamics and a lack of investment of the group members. Group cohesion or the connectedness of the members is extremely important at this stage. The role of the counselor is to help members focus on methods and the meaning of communication, working through group differences and confronting members when necessary. Counselors should also help develop more intensive levels of cohesiveness while building on member individuality.

- **End Stage**: Group members come to resolutions on the issues addressed during the group process. Members may have strong reactions to termination, especially if there was a high level of cohesion developed during the group process. The counselor should lead the group in discussing feelings about termination and be aware of negative reactions that may surface. When these types of emotions occur, counselors should address any challenges that arise with members. The counselor should also help group members identify and reflect on the skills learned in the group process and how those skills can benefit the members with future challenges.

Identifying and Discussing Group Themes and Patterns

Groups can take on characteristics that are often seen in families. As group members become comfortable with one another, their true personalities emerge and behavioral patterns from their families of origin tend to surface. Counselors can take note of these dynamics and use them within the group setting in a way that helps members see their familial patterns and make changes in line with their treatment goals.

For example, if there is one person in a group who is viewed as everyone's favorite and who can do no wrong, then this person likely played the role of favorite child at home or as teacher's pet in school. Another example is a person who wants to be the leader's favorite; these individuals vie for the counselor's attention and attempt to curry favor by the way they respond to the leader.

The counselor must be sensitive to all types of themes appearing in the group and be sure not to succumb to the subtle pressure to keep members in the roles they have played all their lives. Instead, the counselor's job is to identify these patterns and use them as therapeutic tools for transformation.

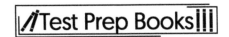

Creating Intervention Based on the Stage of Group Development

Groups have different stages of development, but not all groups go through every stage. The stages are:

- 1. Forming/pre-affiliation
- 2. Storming/power and control
- 3. Norming/intimacy
- 4. Performing/differentiation
- 5. Adjourning/termination

In each stage, the leader is responsible for creating certain elements that will help the group function productively and transition successfully to the next stage.

For example, in the forming/pre-affiliation stage, a group leader could help a group function properly by actively easing members' concerns about being part of the group. The leader would also intervene if any conflict arose because conflict would be counterproductive in the early stage of group formation.

Another example of group leader intervention can be found during the performing/differentiation stage. In this stage, the group is more productive, has established a sense of security and trust in the leader and in each other, and members are more willing to engage in honest feedback. A group leader in this stage might encourage member-to-member empathy by directing one person to talk with another member who is angry to try and understand why the person is feeling that way.

Challenging Harmful Group Member Behaviors

For a therapy group to be successful, leaders must fill crucial roles that change depending on the stage of the group's development. One important duty of the leader is ensuring that group members are safe from harmful group interactions.

Sometimes a group member will behave in a destructive manner or say hateful things to other members. The therapeutic group is one in which the potential for conflicts exists, and leaders know that some conflict is productive and necessary when diverse people share intimate details about their lives. However, when a group member becomes aggressive or hostile to another member in a damaging way, the leader must confront the member. This must be done in a way that is straightforward, caring, and professional. The leader must stop the aggressive behavior and also attend to the offended member.

Interaction of Members Outside of the Group

Groups are designed to fulfill different tasks. **Supportive groups** (those used for severe mental illness or medical conditions) sometimes encourage interaction outside of the group. Forming genuine friendships outside of the group could be beneficial for members. **Psychodynamic groups** (those designed to affect personality changes while focusing on relationship issues and interpersonal dynamics) often prohibit outside group involvement. This is done to prevent interference with therapy goals. **Cognitive behavioral groups** (designed for treating symptoms of psychiatric conditions or for acquiring new coping skills) also discourage members from interacting outside the group. **Self-help groups** (designed around themed life issues such as AA or grief support groups) often encourage members to interact outside of the group. The therapeutic purpose of the group determines whether members are allowed to have contact outside of the group.

Core Counseling Attributes

Awareness of Self and Impact on Clients

The process of acquiring values is important for counselors to keep in mind when working to understand where their own values and their clients' values originated. Counselors should be aware of their own moral codes, values, biases, and prejudices to avoid conflict with the treatment they are providing to clients. The process of acknowledging and controlling personal values in counseling practice is called *value suspension*. **Self-awareness** is a vital part of ensuring that one's personal values and beliefs do not intrude on the counselor/client relationship. It may be necessary to seek consultation from a supervisor or colleague in situations where one's personal values or beliefs conflict with those of the client and when those feelings cannot be resolved. In extreme cases where consultation and self-reflection cannot remedy the conflict, termination of the counselor/client relationship and referral to another therapist may be necessary.

Professional Boundary Issues

Conflicting values occur when the counselor's values and knowledge about best practices are at odds with the client's values, history, relationships, or lifestyle. **Vicarious trauma** may happen when a counselor experiences symptoms of trauma after listening to a client's experience. These symptoms may arise due to the counselor sharing a similar history of trauma. Boundaries may be difficult to maintain if the counselor feels that they need to rescue the client due to an unhealthy attachment to positive results in practice. This is termed the **rescuer role**. Professional boundaries may also be difficult to set and maintain if there is poor teamwork between colleagues in the counseling organization. This is evident when counselors assume the roles of other team members because they believe they are not fulfilling their responsibilities to the client.

Motives for Helping Others Through Counseling

Just as clients are motivated to seek counseling to resolve issues and/or improve their lives, counselors exhibit motivation to help others. Counseling, as a profession, allows an opportunity to positively impact the lives of individuals and help improve society. It is important as part of professional development for counselors to explore their motivation to join the profession. Some graduate programs may require individuals to receive counseling as part of their education to ensure they have adequately addressed their own issues and prevent using the clients to get their own needs met. In some specific areas of counseling, such as addictions, it is more common for counselors to have experienced addiction and recovered, thus motivating them to assist others.

Genuineness and Congruence

The term **congruence** is associated with the person-centered work of Carl Rogers. Congruence can be defined as genuineness on the part of counselors, in that there is agreement on their words and actions. Counselors display congruence when their body language, affect, and words correspond to demonstrate genuine concern for the client. Lack of congruence is revealed when counselors express concern but at the same time seem bored, disinterested, or use language that does not indicate a true understanding of the client. Counselors who are nonreactive or act as a blank screen for clients are not expressing congruence. Rogers considered congruence to be essential for effective counseling.

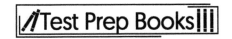

Counselors need to be congruent—in agreement and harmony—with client feedback and encourage clients' self-direction. Counselors and clients begin treatment by enhancing congruence in communication so that mutually agreed upon goals may be developed for the client. The counselor should be invested in the therapeutic relationship and able to participate in a way that assists the client in becoming more self-aware. If a counselor is not congruent with the client, then treatment progress may be hindered and the client should be referred to another counselor who is a more appropriate fit.

Knowledge of and Sensitivity to Gender Orientation and Gender Issues

The term *gender* refers to a range of physical, behavioral, psychological, or cultural characteristics that create the difference between masculinity and femininity. *Gender identity* is a person's understanding of his or her own gender, especially as it relates to being male or female. *Sexual orientation* is a more complex concept as it refers to the type of sexual attraction one feels for others. This is not to be confused with *sexual preference*, which refers to the specific types of sexual stimulation one most enjoys.

Types of Sexual Orientation

- **Heterosexual**: An individual who is sexually and emotionally attracted to members of the opposite gender, also known as "straight"

- **Homosexual**: An individual who is sexually and emotionally attracted to members of the same gender, sometimes referred to as "gay" or "lesbian"

- **Bisexual**: A male or female who is sexually attracted to both same and opposite gender sex partners

- **Asexual**: An individual who has a low level of interest in sexual interactions with others

Types of Gender Identity

- **Bi-gender**: An individual who fluctuates between the self-image of traditionally male and female stereotypes and identifies with both genders

- **Transgender**: A generalized term referring to a variety of sexual identities that do not fit under more traditional categories, a person who feels to be of a different gender than the one he or she is born with

- **Transsexual**: A person who identifies emotionally and psychologically with the gender other than that assigned at birth, lives as a person of the opposite gender

Those who are transgender or transsexual may be homosexual, heterosexual, or asexual. Being transgender can be defined as identifying as a gender other than the gender one was assigned at birth. Publicly sharing that one is transgender can be difficult for some individuals. Transgender individuals may live in a community where their identity is not positively accepted or is misunderstood, and they may feel shamed or ridiculed. It may be a difficult experience for close family members to understand the perspective of a transgender individual, which can affect the cohesiveness of family relationships and the family unit. Transgender individuals may also feel a lack of acknowledgement when others fail to use the correct pronouns or respect other identity wishes.

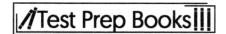

Some transgender individuals choose to medically transition to the gender they identify as. This is a procedure that requires physical, emotional, and psychological support. Individuals not receiving support during their transition can experience extreme feelings of sadness, isolation, and lack of belonging. Medically transitioning individuals also undergo hormonal changes in addition to surgical procedures, and these can cause unexpected feelings and reactions in the individual. There are also medical risks that go along with both the surgical and hormonal procedures of transitioning that the individual has to be aware of and manage. Finally, after the transition is complete, individuals may struggle with living as someone who is relatively unfamiliar to their friends, family members, and colleagues. The transgender person may or may not experience support and acceptance in these groups and relationships, and some group members may even act aggressively toward the transgender person. If this is the case, it may be helpful to find support groups where transgender individuals can find not only friendship and community, but also guidance on how to navigate their new life, society, friends and relationships, and medical recovery.

Knowledge of and Sensitivity to Multicultural Issues

Cultural Awareness

Counselors must be adept at working with diverse populations. **Diversity** includes race, culture, gender, ethnicity, sexual orientation, socioeconomic status, religion, and age. As part of the profession, counselors will provide services to individuals and families with whom they have no cultural similarity. Thus, it is essential for counselors to develop and maintain a level of cultural competence. The first step is for them to engage in self-awareness and gain an understanding of their own identity, including their belief systems and biases. As part of the counseling process, counselors should be able to acknowledge differences and communicate to clients with trust and credibility while demonstrating mutual respect. They should engage in ongoing professional development to gain skills and awareness of differing cultural needs and, from an ethical standpoint, to ensure they are providing competent services. To maintain credibility and trust, counselors must clearly define issues and goals for counseling, taking into consideration cultural variations.

Counselors need to be culturally aware in their attitudes and beliefs. This requires a keen awareness of their own cultural background and gaining awareness of any personal biases, stereotypes, and values that they hold. Counselors should also accept different worldviews, be sensitive to differences, and refer minority clients to a counselor from the client's culture when it would benefit the client.

Counselors need to have the appropriate knowledge of different cultures. Specifically, counselors must understand the client's culture and should not jump to conclusions about the client's way of being. Throughout their careers, counselors should be willing to gain a greater depth of knowledge of various cultural groups and update this knowledge as necessary. This includes understanding how issues like racism, sexism, and homophobia can negatively affect minority clients. Counselors should understand how different therapeutic theories carry values that may be detrimental for some clients. Counselors should also understand how institutional barriers can affect the willingness of minority clients to use mental health services.

Techniques for Working with Clients from Diverse Backgrounds

When working with clients from diverse backgrounds, counselors should be able to shift their professional strategies. Below are techniques and strategies counselors should keep in mind when working with clients of different cultures:

174

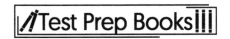
- Have appropriate attitudes and beliefs, gain knowledge about the client's background, and learn new skills as needed.

- Encourage the client to speak in his or her native language and arrange for an interpreter when necessary.

- Assess the client's cultural identity and how important it is to the client.

- Check accuracy of any interpretations of the client's nonverbal cues.

- Make use of alternate modes of communication, such as writing, typing, translation services, and the use of art.

- Assess the impact of sociopolitical issues on the client.

- Encourage the client to bring culturally significant and personally relevant items.

- Vary the helping environment to make it conducive to effective work with the client.

The following strategies can be used when working with clients with various religious backgrounds:

- Determine the client's religious background in the beginning sessions.
- Check personal biases and gain information about the client's religion.
- Ask the client how important religion is in his or her life.
- Assess the client's level of faith development.
- Avoid making assumptions about the religion.
- Become familiar with the client's religious beliefs, important holidays, and faith traditions.
- Understand that religion can deeply affect the client unconsciously.

Communication

Being educated on diverse populations is crucial to increase understanding and avoid discrimination. While education can be helpful in learning to communicate effectively, it is also important to ask questions and clarify anything that may be confusing when communicating with someone from another culture. Counselors also should be aware and observant when communicating with a client to make sure that communication on both sides is fully understood.

Counselors should have basic understanding of the ways in which communication norms can vary across cultures. Counselors should exhibit cultural competence with regard to communication as demonstrated by the following:

- Their awareness of both nonverbal and verbal communication differences

- Their ability to use language that is appropriate and respectful to different cultures

- Their recognition of personal strengths and limitations in communication

- Their willingness to actively remove barriers that may inhibit effective communication with individuals from different cultures

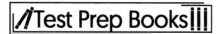

Nonverbal communication can be a common source of misunderstanding in cross-cultural communication. Different cultures place different emphasis on these aspects of nonverbal communication:

- Levels of appropriate assertiveness
- Use of facial expressions and physical gestures
- Appropriateness of physical touch in communication
- Personal space and seating arrangements

There are cultural differences with regard to conflict as well:

- In the U.S., participants in a conflict are typically encouraged to resolve the conflict directly.

- In other cultures, conflict is viewed as an embarrassment that should be dealt with as privately and quietly as possible.

Disclosure of personal information and openness with regard to feelings are uncomfortable in some cultures, and it may be considered inappropriate to ask direct questions with regard to these topics.

Decision-making styles also vary across cultures:

- Delegating vs. making decisions
- Majority rule vs. consensus

Sometimes there will be communication difficulties between the counselor and client, most notably with language or cultural differences that hinder straightforward communication. It is ethically imperative that all clients have access to adequate language assistance, including the option of a translator, so that those with limited English proficiency are still receiving the same level of care. The optimal situation is for clients to have a counselor who can speak to them directly in their first language, and this should be arranged whenever possible. However, this is not always feasible and a translator must be used. In cases where interpreters are necessary or are requested by the client, they should be professional and trained interpreters, rather than family members or non-professionals. They must also understand and agree to the rules of privacy and confidentiality. Counselors should make sure their communication is simple and easy to understand and also make sure to clarify what the client is saying if there is any confusion. Counselors should also familiarize themselves with the cultural backgrounds of the clients they work with to better understand their unique perspective and to minimize misunderstandings.

Cautions and Broad Statements Regarding Cultures

It is important not to use information about culture, race, and ethnicity in a stereotypical or overgeneralized manner. There are vast differences within groups. For example, group members holding a traditional viewpoint are likely to identify very strongly with their group and to reject the practices of other groups. In contrast, other individuals may be acculturated into a dominant group culture and may not identify with their culture of origin. With that caution in mind, some broad statements may be made

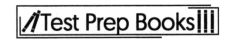

to help counselors gain a better understanding of the ways in which race, culture, and/or ethnicity can influence behavior and attitude:

- Native Americans: Core values include sharing, honor, respect, interdependence, obligation to family, group cohesion, and co-existence with nature.

- Latinos: There is enormous variability among the various Latino groups due to the differences in their histories and cultural experiences. Values include family, avoidance of conflict, respect for others, religiosity, and patriarchy.

- Asian Americans: Great diversity among groups should be noted, as this is a very broad category. Typically shared values across Asian cultures include family honor, deference to authority and to elders, humility, and avoidance of confrontation.

- White Americans: Personal preferences or desires frequently supersede those of the family unit. Values may include capitalism, individuality, and freedom.

- African-Americans: Extended family is held as very important; women are viewed as the center and strength of the family unit. Church and the extended church community may play a large role in an individual or family's life. There is a distrust of government and authority figures.

- Pacific Islanders and Native Hawaiians: Values include the interconnectedness between all people, not just family, that is related by blood, community, and sharing. They are often polytheistic, with a belief that spirits exist in animals and in objects.

Conflict Tolerance and Resolution

Helping clients deal with conflict requires resolution of negative emotions that result when individuals do not agree on a topic. **Emotional detours**, such as dominating or avoiding a situation, the inability to make decisions, and overaccommodating, can lead to emotional disturbances, including anger, anxiety, compulsions, and depression. Clients should be encouraged to express their initial positions, explore their underlying core concerns, and create a mutually agreed-upon plan that meets the expectations of all people involved. Conflict resolution is dependent on good communication. Obstacles such as threats, forceful opinions, and unsolicited advice can block effective communication. Counselors should also assess patterns of interaction, mediate effective dialogue, and block negative communication. The conflict resolution process begins with identifying concerns and establishing the importance of the confrontation. Taking turns defining the problem and acknowledging others' opinions can help build alternative solutions that satisfy conflicting ideals.

Empathic Attunement

Empathy is being able to relate to client circumstances and direction without the counselor actually experiencing it themselves. Sympathy differs from empathy in that sympathy is compassion for the client without having experienced the client's state of being. Empathy involves "being with" the client in their time and frame of mind. It involves connecting to the client on a visceral level while still maintaining some objectivity. Attunement occurs through listening to and watching the client. By tuning in to the client's words and body language, the counselor begins to experience empathy. The client's body language may reveal emotions that aren't being verbally communicated.

177

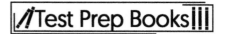

These emotions are usually subconscious, but sometimes they are emotions that the client doesn't feel safe sharing. Attunement to these unarticulated emotions, when expressed back to the client, can be a powerful way of showing the client they are in a place of safety and understanding. While working with a client, it is important to stay attuned to the changes in emotion and to pick up on the degree of comfort that the client has with moving forward and examining the emotions. In addition to feeling what the client is feeling, attunement can help the counselor guide the client through therapy at the rate that is most comfortable and effective for the client. Because empathy is the framework on which the counseling practice is built, it is imperative that counselors be empathetic with their clients. Those who cannot be empathetic should seek additional supervision or counsel in order to do their work effectively or refer the client to another counselor.

Empathic Responding

One of the most effective skills for encouraging clients to share and explore their emotions in counseling is **empathic responding**. The goals of empathic responding are for the client to know that the counselor understands exactly how they feel and to ultimately uncover the real significance and roots of their emotions. The counselor must have a deep sense of self-awareness in order to recall their own emotions from past experiences that enable the empathic response. Empathic responding is more than the counselor merely hearing the client and feeling pity for them, letting them know that they feel bad or happy for them, or telling them how awful, confusing, or stressful a situation must be. Empathic responding involves reflecting the emotions that the client expressed back to them and explaining the reasons for those feelings in a way that shows that the counselor can imagine being in the client's place.

It is crucial for the counselor to use words that describe precisely what the client is experiencing. This is not a time for problem-solving or judging the client's emotions. This is a time for the counselor to step away from their own perception of the client's problems and to step into the client's frame of reference and feel the same thing the client is feeling. When a counselor can show that they are simultaneously feeling the same emotions as the client without any judgment, the client should have no fear of being correct or incorrect in their expression of emotions. In this environment of true understanding and acceptance, the client will be more open to sharing their feelings. As the client's emotions are labeled accurately, the counselor and the client can deeply analyze and pinpoint the origins of the emotions and begin therapeutic change.

Fostering the Emergence of Group Therapeutic Factors

Counselors can foster the emergence of therapeutic factors to help the group successfully accomplish its goals. One of the most important initial therapeutic factors in group therapy is the promotion of cohesion, and counselors can accomplish this in several ways. For example, group leaders can promote cohesion by responding well when someone challenges their authority. The leader might ask the group if they agree with the challenge and what they think could be done differently to help the group. This, in turn, can help members bond with each other. Group leaders can also encourage empathy among members by calling upon individuals to check in with those who become emotionally dysregulated during sessions.

Counselors can promote therapeutic factors by helping members deal with conflicts appropriately. Instead of fearing conflict, the group can learn how to disagree without violating relationships within the group. The leader is often an important figure during conflicts because they monitor and provide space for safe discussions.

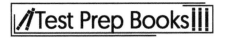

Counselors can also facilitate the emergence of therapeutic factors by showing care for all group members. When the leader demonstrates equal care for everyone in the group, members will likely feel safe to disclose more personal information. Not only does this encourage deeper disclosure, but it also provides the group members with an example of how they should act towards one another.

Additionally, counselors can provide insight to members about their behaviors and interchanges with each other. Counselors can use the group setting as a microcosm of the members' real-life situations by bringing about changes within the group that will result in outside transformations.

Non-Judgmental Stance

When interviewing a client, a counselor must be careful to eliminate all personal bias from their language. This relates to all subtle negative phrasing related to race, ethnicity, socioeconomic status, gender, gender identity, life choices, disability, or psychological disorders. The job of the counselor is to support the client without bias, always promoting the client's self-identity. Phrases or expressions that demean or stereotype a particular group of people should never be used. Similarly, labeling someone can be hurtful, especially in cases where that label has a negative connotation or stigma attached to it. Sometimes it may even be appropriate for the counselor to ask the client how they wish to be identified or addressed. Inclusive and affirming language should be used when talking about all groups of people and especially when talking to or about the client. Terms that are known to be offensive or degrading should always be avoided.

Counselors should treat all clients of all backgrounds with open-mindedness, without judgment, and with the client's desired intervention outcomes at the center of all interactions. Counselors may work with clients of different cultures, and counselors should respect the opinions and boundaries that these differences bring to treatment.

Counselors can communicate support and a nonjudgmental attitude through an open posture and eye gaze that shows interest but not intimidation.

Importance of Nonjudgmental Support

Support is a broad term for the way in which a counselor provides assistance and care to clients. Nonjudgmental support helps clients to open up, identify issues and the need for counseling, and set personal goals. A counselor can support a client by providing reassurance, acting as a sounding board, and simply listening without reaction. For the client, support from the counselor can allow a sense of being temporarily unburdened, which can facilitate healing. Support groups allow for peers or individuals experiencing similar issues (such as single parents and those struggling with addiction or eating disorders) to provide companionship and comfort through shared experiences.

Positive Regard

Carl Rogers believed that clients can begin to make changes independently once they experience positive regard from the counselor. **Positive regard** means that the counselor puts aside any judgment and embraces the client as a person of worth, not defining the client by their actions or expressions of emotions or beliefs. Counselors can show positive regard by allowing clients to speak freely about their behaviors, feelings, or thoughts without responding critically to what the client has said. The counselor should be able to communicate an understanding that the client is behaving or experiencing emotions

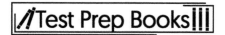
to the best of their ability. This freedom from judgment then allows the client to be more accepting of themselves and more confident in their decisions to create change.

Respect and Acceptance for Diversity

Clients may come from all backgrounds. It is important that counselors do not make any prior negative judgments regarding the personality or life of any client. Each individual has worth. It is essential for counselors to be mindful of any personal prejudices or biases and employ empathy and sensitivity when working with the client.

The client must be allowed to disclose details of a situation to determine influences from his or her culture. This can be done by conducting an interview with the client about his or her background, customs, personal beliefs, values, and relationships. Appropriate group interviews with key members in the client's life can also provide additional verbal and nonverbal information.

It is recommended that in order to be effective, counselors engage in ongoing professional development to gain skills and awareness of differing cultural needs and ethical standpoints and to ensure they are providing competent services. To maintain credibility and trust, counselors must honor the client's motives and goals for the session, taking into consideration cultural variations.

Listening, Attending, and Reflecting Skills

Active Listening and Observation
Active listening is crucial to the relationship- and rapport-building stage with clients. Counselors must be fully engaged in the listening process and not distracted by thoughts of what will come next or intervention planning. The counselor must not only hear the audible language the client is offering but must also look at the nonverbal behaviors and the underlying meaning in the words and expressions of the client. Nonverbal behaviors include body language, facial expressions, voice quality, and physical reactions of the client. Using certain facial expressions, body language, and postures shows that the counselor is engaged and listening to the client.

Counselors should display eye contact and natural but engaged body movements and gestures. An example would be sitting slightly forward with a non-rigid posture. As with all communication techniques, counselors should be aware of cultural differences in what is appropriate, especially related to direct eye contact and posturing. Other aspects of active listening include head nodding, eye contact, and using phrases of understanding and clarity (e.g., "What I hear you saying is . . ." and "You (may) wish to . . .") Counselors may verify they understand the client's message by paraphrasing and asking for validation that it is correct (e.g., "What I hear you saying is …").

Identifying the Underlying Meaning of Communication
Clients use both verbal and nonverbal communication during treatment. Counselors must develop the ability to interpret communication congruency or develop the ability to assess both types of expressions simultaneously to understand client messaging accurately. Clients may use facial expressions, gesturing, eye contact, tone of voice, or other ways to express feelings nonverbally. Counselors must notice whether the nonverbal communication reinforces or conflicts with verbal messaging.

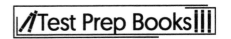
Silence

Silence can be an effective skill in therapy but must be used carefully, especially in the early stages of the process. Initially, clients may be silent due to many factors, such as fear, resistance, discomfort with opening up, or uncertainty about the process. Counselors who use silence in initial sessions must ensure clients do not perceive the counselor as bored, hostile, or indifferent. As counseling progresses, clients may gain additional comfort with silence and use it as a way to reflect on content, process information, consider options, and gain self-awareness. Newer counselors may have more difficulty with silence, as they may believe they are not being helpful if they are not talking. Silence is also viewed differently by culture, so cultural awareness is important in understanding and using it as a therapeutic tool.

Summarizing

Counselors may paraphrase and echo clients' verbal statements to acknowledge their feelings. **Summarizing** may involve reflecting back the statements made by the client to clarify what the client has said. Counselors also must summarize communication in order to provide sufficient records of the session. Further, during the end of the session, the counselor may wish to clarify goals and homework assigned for the next week so that the client is clear on the changes that need to take place.

Attending

Attending is the act of the counselor giving clients their full attention. Attending to the client shows respect for their needs, can encourage openness, and can create a sense of comfort and support in the counseling process. There are several ways for counselors to attend actively to clients, including maintaining appropriate eye contact, using reassuring body language and gestures, and monitoring their tone and expressions. Counselors can communicate support and a nonjudgmental attitude through an open posture and eye gaze that shows interest but not intimidation. They should use a caring verbal tone and facial expressions, which indicate attention to what their clients are saying and can be used in addition to silence to create a positive environment for counseling.

Reflecting

Reflecting is a basic counseling skill designed to build rapport and help clients become aware of underlying emotions. Counselors "reflect back" what a client says, both to indicate they are attending and also to analyze and interpret meanings. Reflecting is more than simply paraphrasing a client's words, as it involves more in-depth understanding and an attempt to elicit further information. An example would be a client stating, "I'm not sure what to do about my current relationship. I can't decide if I should stay or leave." The counselor would reflect by stating, "It sounds like you are conflicted about what to do; this is a difficult decision to make," and follow up with a probing question or allow time for the client to process and react.

The following are additional counseling skills:

- **Restatement**: Clarification through repeating back the client's words, as understood by the counselor

- **Reflection**: Restatement of what the counselor heard from the client, emphasizing any underlying emotional content (can be termed **reflection of feeling**)

- **Paraphrasing**: Repeating back a client's story while providing an empathic response

- **Summarizing**: Reiteration of the major points of the counseling discussion

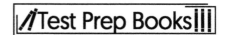

- **Silence:** Moments during which neither the client nor the counselor speaks; can be used for reflection but may indicate resistance from the client

- **Confrontation:** Technique in which the counselor identifies discrepancies from the client in a supportive manner (counselor may also ask for clarification to determine if content was misheard prior to exposing possible inconsistencies)

- **Structuring:** Used to set goals and agree upon plan for counseling; also used within sessions to make effective use of time and respect boundaries

Errors

Reflecting is one of several active listening and rapport-building skills but should not be overused. It is essential that the counselor be able to offer back meaningful restatements and not simply repeat back what is heard. It is also important that the counselor accurately reflects any feeling and does not project or misinterpret. In some cases, misinterpretation can help the client further clarify and is not detrimental to the relationship. By using reflection and clarification, any errors can be corrected. Even when errors occur, when the counselor clarifies what the client means, it communicates that the counselor is invested in understanding the client. From a cultural awareness standpoint, the counselor should be sensitive to any differences and ensure there is a level of trust prior to engaging in more in-depth reflection.

Methods of Facilitating Communication

Counselors may facilitate communication with the client by verbally encouraging communication or by addressing the client with constructive information concerning the case. Counselors need to recall information concerning the client from session to session in order to facilitate communication and move forward with the client. Clarifying the client's feelings and statements helps to ensure the counselor understands what is being communicated as well as lets the client know that the counselor is engaged and actively listening. Development of trust with the client may facilitate additional communication, and counselors should be sensitive to the trust-building process because it is the cornerstone of the helping relationship. Counselors may provide clients with homework outside of a session that facilitates communication during the next session.

Mandated clients, including court-ordered clients or clients ordered to counseling from child protective services, may face challenges in communicating with the counselor because they do not choose to be in treatment. Developing trust with these clients to facilitate communication is especially important for progress to be made. It's helpful to acknowledge the client's feelings and possible frustration about the mandated treatment. Clients who require out-of-home placement need clear communication with the counselor to clarify what is happening and make appropriate psychological adjustments to their circumstances.

Furthering and close/open-ended questions are additional communication techniques that are beneficial in counseling:

- **Furthering:** A technique that reinforces the idea that the counselor is listening to the client and encourages further information to be gathered. This technique includes nodding of the head, facial expressions, or encouragement responses such as "yes" or "I understand." It also includes accent responses, whereby counselors repeat or parrot back a few words of a client's last response.

182

- **Close/Open-Ended Questions**: Depending on the timing or information the counselor is seeking to elicit from the client, one of these types of questions may be used. Close-ended questions, such as "How old are you?" will typically elicit a short answer. Conversely, open-ended questions, such as "What are your feelings about school?", allow for longer, more-involved responses. Open questions are more likely to provide helpful information, as they require the client to express feelings, beliefs, and ideas. Open questions often begin with "why," "how," "when," or "tell me …". Counselors do need to be aware of the limitations of asking questions. Any questions asked should have purpose and provide information that will be meaningful to the counselor and the relationship. Curiosity questions should be avoided, as well as asking too many questions, which may feel interrogating to the client. A counselor can ask follow-up questions for clarification as needed. The counselor should provide the client adequate time to answer questions and elaborate but also allow time for the client to talk freely.

Case Studies and Practice Questions

Case Study #1

Part One

Intake

<u>Client</u>

Age: 21

Sex: Female

Gender: Female

Sexuality: Heterosexual

Ethnicity: White

Relationship Status: Single

Counseling Setting: Outpatient—on campus counseling office

Types of Counseling: Individual

Presenting Problem: Issues with body image, episodes of binge eating, and excessive exercise interfering with the quality of life

Diagnosis: F50.2 Bulimia nervosa, Moderate

Presenting Problem:

The client is a 21-year-old, single, white female who signed up for counseling due to issues with body image, episodes of binge eating, and excessive exercise interfering with her quality of life. She is a college student at Johns Hopkins University. She lives with her two roommates in a small, on-campus apartment and has been working as a waitress at a local restaurant for six months. She has experienced difficulty with body image issues since she was a teenager. Ever since she started working as a waitress, she has been exercising rigorously three times a day. She will often show up late to class and work because of her strenuous and lengthy exercise routine. During the day, she will not eat. On weekends, instead of spending time with her friends or studying for exams, she maintains her exercise routine and busy work schedule. Concerned with her habits, her roommates encouraged her to seek assistance from an on-campus counselor. Once there, she explained to the counselor that her schedule just does not allow for her to "eat at normal times."

Mental Status:

Your client appeared well-groomed and put together. Her hair, nails, and clothing appeared clean and polished. She expressed she was nervous to come to counseling and appeared fidgety and uncomfortable. She did admit she does not eat enough, and she is "tired of equating her self-worth" to her body's appearance. She admitted to having an unhealthy relationship with food. During the day she

184

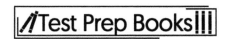

will not eat at all, but in the evenings, she will consume exorbitant amounts of food to make up for it. She admitted this binge eating cycle occurs daily. After she has finished eating, she feels an intense wave of guilt because she always consumes more than she originally planned to. When seeing other women that appear to be skinnier than her, she feels extremely insecure and depressed. She admitted to wishing she was skinnier and more beautiful when she looks in the mirror.

Family History:

Your client identified her family as "very close" and stated that they spend a lot of time together. She is an only child of two parents, her mother and father. Though her parents live out of state, she keeps in contact with both parents and spends holidays with them. Her father is often busy with work, but he calls weekly to see how school is going. She stated that she is closer to her mother, and they have a strong relationship. She did reveal that her mother has always put pressure on her to be perfect when it comes to grades as well as physical appearance. She stated her mother "always wants what's best for me." Upon further reflection, the client has realized her mother holds her to an impossible standard when it comes to looks and size. When asked if her mother has a healthy relationship with food, your client noted that her mother hasn't eaten in front of her often. When they do eat together, her mother won't eat much, and she mentions how much the client is eating. She has asked the client questions like "Are you sure you are hungry?" or "Don't you want to fit into your prom dress?"

1. Which of the following, disclosed during intake, confirms your client's diagnosis of bulimia nervosa instead of anorexia nervosa?
    a. Going long periods of time without eating
    b. Body image and self-esteem issues
    c. Excessive exercise
    d. Episodes of binge eating excessive amounts of food

2. What information revealed by the client would confirm the client's Bulimia Nervosa is moderate in severity?
    a. The feelings of guilt associated with binge eating episodes
    b. Several binge eating episodes each week
    c. The amount of exercise the client does
    d. Being late for work and school

3. When a client has an eating disorder, other mental health conditions may also be present. What is the simultaneous, but independent, presence of two or more medical conditions in a patient called?
    a. Codependence
    b. Diagnosis
    c. Comorbidity
    d. Morbidity

4. Based on the Mental Status Exam, what other mental health diagnosis may be co-occurring with the client's Bulimia Nervosa?
    a. Depression
    b. Schizophrenia
    c. Bipolar disorder
    d. Dissociative identity disorder

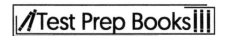

5. What information from the presenting problem suggests the client's disorder is affecting other areas of their life?
   a. The client exercises multiple times a day
   b. The client feels guilty after eating
   c. The client is working and attending college
   d. The client has been consistently late to school and work

Part Two

Second session, three days after the initial intake:

Your client arrived late for her second session. She was wearing yoga pants and a T-shirt, stating she was late because "she lost track of time at the gym." Her mannerisms and demeanor indicated she was rushed and anxious. When you asked how being late to appointments or obligations such as work or school makes her feel, she reported that it makes her feel "anxious and embarrassed." While continuing to build trust, you utilized your time with the client to determine what has added to her feelings of anxiety and depression. She described her compulsion to exercise for extended periods of time, even when she knows it will make her late. She also stated that she often feels depressed after cancelling plans with her friends. Sometimes she cancels plans with friends to stay home and eat large amounts of food in private. She doesn't want to eat in front of her friends. She described being embarrassed of her eating habits and her body. You expressed empathy and introduced the concept of treatment plans and her counseling homework moving forward. Based on previous experience with clients with Bulimia Nervosa and other eating disorders, you determine the best form of psychological treatment. This form of treatment involves recognizing and changing unhelpful ways of thinking and learned patterns of unhelpful behaviors. Recognizing and challenging the client's thought processes and behavior patterns will be the first steps.

6. One of the most important predictors of success in therapy is the:
   a. Mental health diagnosis of the client
   b. Experience level of the counselor
   c. Therapeutic alliance
   d. Ability to follow directions

7. What form of psychological treatment did the counselor determine would be best for the client?
   a. Cognitive behavioral therapy
   b. Art therapy
   c. Psychoanalytic therapy
   d. Humanistic therapy

8. If a client comes to you with an eating disorder, and you have no experience or training in this area, ethically you should:
   a. Tell the client you can help her with her issues of self-esteem or depression
   b. Continue to research the topic further and keep the client
   c. Refer the client to another counselor who is trained and experienced in this area
   d. Ask the client if there are other issues she would like to focus on instead

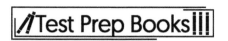

9. Which of the following statements best expresses empathy for the client?
    a. "Next time you are going to cancel plans with your friends, think about how bad it makes you feel."
    b. "Thank you for sharing that with me. I understand how upsetting it is to miss out on quality time with your friends."
    c. "I'm hearing that you are depressed when you stay home and miss time with your friends."
    d. "Why do you say you want to spend time with your friends, but continue to cancel plans with them?"

Part Three

Fourth session, three weeks after the initial session:

The client was punctual and her body language and facial expression was much more relaxed this session. She reported that she has been sticking to her counseling homework. Using Cognitive Behavioral Therapy, you have been working together to recognize and correct unhealthy thoughts and behaviors. Last session she wrote down several thoughts and behaviors she would like to work on. She noted she would like to eat smaller portions when she is hungry throughout the day instead of binge eating, would like to work out once a day instead of excessively, and would like to participate in more social activities with friends. This session you check in to see how her progress is in each of these areas. She reported that she has been getting to work and school on time, and only works out once a day now. She has been able to stop herself from working out excessively. She also reported that she is eating smaller meals during the day and has only had one binge eating episode this week. While this is a great deal of progress, she admits she still feels depressed and anxious most days. She has not increased her social activities and still feels isolated from friends. Some thoughts she has experienced are that she is "a burden to her friends" and that they "don't really want to hang out with me," even though they invite her out frequently and tell her they want to be there for her and support her. You continue to be authentic and genuine with your client, to build trust and enhance the therapeutic relationship. You discussed her progress and encouraged the great strides she has made so far.

10. Identifying distorted perceptions about food, learning how to eat healthy portions when hungry, and managing compulsive behaviors such as excessive exercising are:
    a. Different levels of treatment
    b. Concurrent treatment
    c. Barriers to client goal attainment
    d. Realistic treatment goals

11. When a therapist is real, authentic, and genuine with their clients, it is called:
    a. Congruence
    b. Empathy
    c. Reflection
    d. Positive Regard

12. Which of the following is an example of amplified reflection?
    a. "I understand you feel like a burden to your friends sometimes. That must be really difficult."
    b. "Your friends aren't supportive and never want to spend time with you."
    c. "You feel like your friends don't want to spend time with you."
    d. "Why do you feel like your friends don't want to hang out with you?"

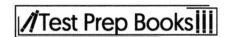

13. What term refers to Adler's belief that all people wish to belong?
    a. Introversion
    b. Extraversion
    c. Compensation
    d. Social connectedness

188

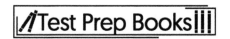

Case Study # 2

Part One

Intake

<u>Client</u>

Age: 25

Sex: Male

Gender: Male

Sexuality: Heterosexual

Ethnicity: White

Relationship Status: Single

Counseling Setting: Outpatient—community counseling office

Types of Counseling: Individual

Presenting Problem: Drinking excessively is interfering with quality of life and personal relationships

Diagnosis: F10.20 Alcohol use disorder, Moderate

Presenting Problem:

You have been assigned to a 25-year-old, single, male client who started counseling due to recent issues with alcohol. He is also experiencing a lack of motivation and frequent disagreements with family members. He recently graduated from law school but has yet to find employment. His school debts are in the hundreds of thousands of dollars. He laughs when he talks about this, saying, "This will never get paid off." He has openly admitted that he regularly drinks alcohol, which he claims got him through all his years at law school and helps him cope with the stresses of life. When asked about his drinking, he brags about how much he can drink without feeling the side effects. He reports that he tries his best to control the number of drinks he consumes a day, but he finds it difficult. He often loses track of how many drinks he has had once he starts drinking.

Mental Status:

The client was dressed in pajama pants and a wrinkled T-shirt. His clothes looked like he slept in them. His hair and beard were long and unkempt. His untidy appearance was consistent with his current low mood and recent lack of motivation. He reported that he has not been able to focus on applying for jobs. He often feels overwhelmed and exhausted at the prospect of filling out applications or going to interviews. He admitted that he wants to find work, but that he just needs to take a break after so many years of hard work and long hours in school. He said drinking helps him to unwind and relax. It also distracts him from his worries, so he often drinks every afternoon and into the late evening. Your client revealed that in the past few months he has been feeling down and has been sleeping almost 12 hours a night, which is much more than usual.

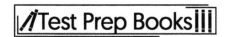

Family History:

Your client recently moved home to live with his mom and dad. He had not lived with them since he was in high school, and this change has been very difficult. He reported that he used to get along with both parents. When he would visit them, he would hang out with his dad and watch sports and have a few drinks. Your client expressed mild irritation with regards to his mother's insistence that he wake up earlier and work harder on getting a job. His father has lost his temper with him recently, telling him to "lay off the booze" and "get his life together."

1. What information determines the level of severity in alcohol use disorder?
    a. Number of drinks consumed weekly
    b. Number of months the client has been drinking excessively
    c. Number of symptoms the client exhibits
    d. The client's feelings about drinking

2. Which part of intake showed that the client has continued alcohol use even though it is causing social or interpersonal problems in their life?
    a. Family history revealed that he is having issues with family members due to his drinking
    b. Mental status revealed that he has been sleeping much longer than usual
    c. Mental status revealed that he has been feeling more down than usual
    d. Family history revealed that he used to watch sports and have a few beers with his father

3. When the client brags about how much he can drink without feeling the side effects, this is evidence of which symptom of alcohol use disorder?
    a. Withdrawal
    b. Tolerance
    c. Binge drinking
    d. Social and Interpersonal problems

4. The client was laughing when he stated that his school debt was in the hundreds of thousands of dollars and would never get paid off. When the counselor points out the client's inconsistent behavior, what is that verbal response called?
    a. Paradoxical intervention
    b. Active listening
    c. Accurate empathy
    d. Confrontation

Part Two

Second session, one week after the initial intake:

The second session was originally scheduled three days after intake. The client decided to cancel that session because "the appointment was too early in the morning." He scheduled this session for the afternoon so he would have time to sleep in. He indicated he felt "exhausted and emotionally drained" even though he reported he had slept for twelve hours the previous night. He disclosed that he has still been binge drinking every day, but he excused the behavior, saying, "my college friends drink all the time too." He mentioned that he does not see his friends often anymore and his relationship with his parents is suffering. This session, you concentrated on building trust. You continued to delve into the issues that have contributed to the client's increase in alcohol consumption. Your client expressed that he has been overwhelmed with school and internships for the past few years. He now feels like he

190

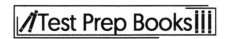

deserves a break and cannot even think about applying for jobs or interviewing. You express empathy and discuss the consequences of substance abuse and how it can affect all areas of the client's life negatively. During this session, you have the client complete a true/false questionnaire to determine the level of severity of his alcohol use disorder based on how many symptoms the client is experiencing. After determining the severity of his condition, you will be able to better create a treatment plan.

5. The client is sleeping much more than usual, has a low mood, and lacks motivation. These are indicators that the client may also be suffering from what mental disorder?
    a. Major depressive disorder
    b. Generalized anxiety disorder
    c. Post-traumatic stress disorder
    d. Borderline personality disorder

6. The client does not want to accept that his daily binge drinking is a problem, stating "my college friends drink all the time too." There are times when individuals refuse to acknowledge the reality of certain situations in their lives. What is this coping mechanism called?
    a. Repression
    b. Denial
    c. Compensation
    d. Sublimation

7. During this session, the client expressed concern for his relationships with his friends and parents. Which of the following is a time-limited, focused, and evidence-based approach to treat mood disorders like depression, that focuses on improving the quality of a client's relationships and social functioning?
    a. Talk therapy
    b. Humanistic therapy
    c. Cognitive behavioral therapy
    d. Interpersonal psychotherapy

8. How would you reflect the client's feelings of burnout that are preventing them from moving forward?
    a. "After years of hard work and long hours, you feel like you deserve a break."
    b. "Tell me more about how you feel when you think about applying for jobs."
    c. "Your drinking is preventing you from moving forward with your job search."
    d. "How do you expect to move forward if you won't even apply for jobs?"

9. The counselor determined the client has alcohol use disorder. To determine the level of severity and create an appropriate treatment plan, the counselor administers a true/false test with what type of recognition items?
    a. Multipoint
    b. Free choice
    c. Fill in the blank
    d. Dichotomous

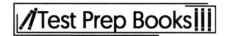

Part Three

Fourth session, three weeks after the initial session:

The client appeared to be more well-groomed this session. He was wearing clean clothes and had shaved his beard. When he arrived, his body language was closed, and he would not make eye contact. After a series of short answers and evasive responses, the client admitted that he had not completed his homework since the last session. When asked why he did not prioritize his homework or treatment plan, he stated that he "didn't think it would help me stop drinking." Later, he reported that he was ready to stop drinking now. This came as a surprise after he had not completed his assignment and had not seemed to accept his drinking as a serious issue in the previous session. The client asked if everything in counseling would be kept confidential. Once confidentiality was explained, the client told a story about his drinking the previous weekend. He admitted to going out to the bar because his parents would no longer tolerate his drinking at home. He ended up driving under the influence and woke up in his car in a cornfield on the side of the road. When he woke up the next morning, he didn't remember how he got there. This incident scared him, and he realized that his drinking might be a bigger problem than he originally thought. He stated that he is ready to focus on getting better. You continue to concentrate on empathy and active listening to build trust and enhance the therapeutic relationship. You discussed next steps in the treatment plan, collaborating to create realistic goals together.

10. In terms of confidentiality, what does it mean when a counselor states that privileged communication is qualified?
    a. All communication with the counselor is confidential.
    b. Details can be shared with the client's family members.
    c. Exceptions may exist.
    d. The counselor doesn't have to share anything the client says.

11. What term describes the client's tendency to fight or challenge the therapeutic process?
    a. Projection
    b. Resistance
    c. Rationalization
    d. Collaboration

12. Before the client blacked out and drove under the influence of alcohol, he refused to see his drinking as a serious issue. What is it called when a client suddenly becomes aware of a factor in their life that was previously unknown?
    a. Repression
    b. Introjection
    c. Denial
    d. Insight

13. Which is an example of active listening by the counselor?
    a. "If I'm understanding correctly, you've realized that your drinking is a serious issue that you would like to work on. Is that an accurate characterization?"
    b. The counselor nodding to illustrate that she is listening.
    c. "If you realized your drinking is a serious issue, then why didn't you complete your homework?"
    d. The counselor actively writing in their notebook to remember important details.

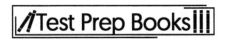
Case Study #3

Part One

Intake

<u>Client</u>

Age: 50

Sex: Female

Gender: Female

Sexuality: Heterosexual

Ethnicity: White

Relationship Status: Single

Counseling Setting: Outpatient—community counseling office

Types of Counseling: Individual

Presenting Problem: Experiencing extreme sadness, low energy, and feelings of isolation

Diagnosis: F32.1 Major depressive disorder, Moderate

Presenting Problem:

Your new client is a 50-year-old, recently divorced woman. She decided to start counseling because she has been experiencing extreme sadness over the past three years. These feelings of sadness have only increased over time. She finds it very difficult to get out of bed every morning and cannot wait to return home from work so she can lie right back down. On the weekends, she stays in bed most of the day. She has not been spending time with friends or coworkers anymore. She mentioned that her coworkers have noticed her change in mood over the past couple of years, often asking her if she is feeling okay or even telling her that she looks like she is going to cry. She avoids going to lunch with coworkers so she doesn't have to answer their questions. She will occasionally go on social media sites like Facebook, but she has admitted that doing so often leads to feelings of isolation. She has come to her initial session hoping to receive help in improving her energy levels and general interest in life and socializing, which have nearly disappeared.

Mental Status:

Upon arrival, your client was clean and put together. She was moving slowly and appeared to be exhausted and experiencing some pain. She complained about the stiffness in her joints and general aches and pains. She said that she lacks the motivation to exercise and does so rarely, instead spending a lot of time in bed. She reported that she rarely has any energy to do anything other than general daily routines, including going to work, making dinner, and showering. Due to the client's mental status and symptoms, you administered an assessment to determine the severity of the client's depression.

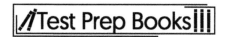

Family History:

Your client went through a divorce recently. She was married for 25 years and feels lost without sharing a home with her husband and engaging in their daily routines. She has admitted that they weren't happy for many years, but she still feels like the divorce means she is a failure. She grew up with both parents in the home until they got divorced when she was 12 years old. She always promised herself she wouldn't get a divorce and that she would always do her best to make her relationship work. Her father moved out of state after the divorce and started a new family. Her mother went through years of depression after the divorce. She remembers coming home from school to find her mother in bed during the day. She recognizes she is dealing with her divorce in a similar way but stated "at least I get up to take a shower and go to work every day."

1. Negative or stressful circumstances can trigger depression. What major life event mentioned during intake may have triggered the client's depression?
    a. Her parents' divorce
    b. Loss of job
    c. Her father moving out of state
    d. Her recent divorce

2. The client's coworkers have noticed her change in mood, often asking her if she is feeling okay or telling her that she looks like she is going to cry. Which symptom of depression is present based on these statements?
    a. Depressed mood that is observed by others
    b. Weight loss or gain
    c. Decreased concentration
    d. Fatigue

3. What disorder must be excluded when determining the diagnosis of major depressive disorder?
    a. Generalized anxiety disorder
    b. Schizophrenia
    c. Obsessive-compulsive disorder
    d. Post-traumatic stress disorder

4. The client shared her family history, including that her mother had depression after her own divorce. Based on this information, what is the likely cause of the client's depression?
    a. Genetic factors
    b. Environmental factors
    c. Both genetic and environmental factors
    d. Substance abuse

5. The counselor administered The Patient Health Questionnaire-9 (PHQ-9), where the DSM criteria are scored based on whether the client is experiencing symptoms, ranging from 0 points for "not at all" to 3 points for "nearly every day." What type of assessment is the PHQ-9?
    a. Diagnostic test
    b. Summative evaluation
    c. Norm-referenced rest
    d. Performance appraisal

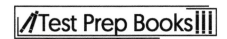

Part Two

Second session, one week after the initial intake:

Your client appeared to be in a similar mood to the first session. She was still well-groomed, her hair was clean and styled, and her nails were painted. She mentioned that she had gone to work each day that week, but she continued to go straight home to go to bed. She expressed that she would like to do more with her days than just go to work and lay in bed, but "that's all I have the energy to do." She reported that when she forces herself to stay up, she just wanders around the house thinking about her divorce and her ex-husband. They do not speak anymore, which is a big change in her life. She mentioned that during the week, when she would come home from work, her husband was the only other person she interacted with. The client said she went to counseling right after the divorce at the suggestion of her friends and family. After a couple of sessions, she decided to stop going because she was not seeing any progress. Now that it has been another year and nothing has improved, she decided to try counseling again. You explained to the client that counseling, especially talk therapy, is very helpful with clients in similar situations, but it is important to stick with it for more than a few weeks for it to be effective. There are also other options you can discuss, such as medication-assisted therapy. This session, you started the process of working together with the client to establish treatment goals and objectives.

6. Who famously invented talk therapy, which is also known as psychotherapy and focuses on exploring and ultimately changing negative thoughts, emotions, and behaviors?
    a. Erik Erikson
    b. Alfred Adler
    c. Carl Jung
    d. Sigmund Freud

7. Medication-assisted therapy consists of both medication and counseling or behavioral therapies for treatment. How effective is medication-assisted therapy?
    a. It has been shown to be ineffective
    b. It has been shown to be effective with people with emotional and behavioral problems
    c. It has been shown to work significantly better than talk therapy alone
    d. It has been shown to interfere with the effectiveness of talk therapy

8. What is the network of people who provide an individual with practical or emotional assistance?
    a. Support system
    b. Family
    c. Friends
    d. Counselor

9. What is the process of working together with the client to establish treatment goals and objectives?
    a. Codependence
    b. Therapeutic relationship
    c. Collaboration
    d. Helping relationship

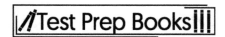

Part Three

<u>Third session, two weeks after the initial session:</u>
Your client seemed to be in a better mood than both previous sessions. Her body language was more open. At the end of the second session, you and the client had determined some realistic goals for counseling. Short-term goals included taking steps toward building up her social circle and exercising more to help manage her pain and boost her mood. As homework, she was supposed to reach out to two friends over the phone and make plans to see one of these friends in person for coffee. To start her exercise routine, she was assigned to take a short walk each day after work, even if it is only for 15 minutes. The client reported that she was able to take a short walk three days this week. You offered support and encouraged the client to continue the good work. The client revealed she did not complete all her homework from last week, as she did not call any friends or make plans with them. She stated that "I didn't feel ready to meet up with friends," and "I can see my friends once I'm feeling better."

The client continues to think about her divorce most days after work. She keeps thinking about negative experiences in her marriage and ways she could have acted differently to save her marriage. She knows her marriage was bad at times, but she cannot help focusing on the good parts and minimizing the flaws of her husband. Both of these ways of thinking are making it difficult for her to move on.

10. What is the process that focuses on the achievement of a time-limited goal and measures the degree to which that goal has been achieved?
   a. Goal setting
   b. Goal attainment scaling
   c. Resistance
   d. Rationalization

11. Which statement is an example of the counselor using self-disclosure?
   a. "It sounds like you are having a difficult time reaching out to friends or family right now. You feel like you aren't ready."
   b. "You don't want to see your friends or family."
   c. "When I went through my divorce, I had trouble getting motivated to work out or see friends too. One thing that really helped was spending time with my friends and family."
   d. "I know someone who went through a divorce, and it really helped them to spend quality time with friends and family."

12. The client is minimizing her ex-husband's faults and focusing only on his positive traits. What is the defense mechanism used when individuals create an ideal image of someone by focusing on their positive traits and ignoring their faults?
   a. Idealization
   b. Denial
   c. Regression
   d. Displacement

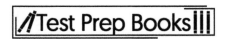

13. What form of cognition results in emotional discomfort due to fixation on troublesome events from the past or the present?
    a. Repression
    b. Rumination
    c. Introspection
    d. Sublimation

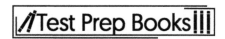
Case Study #4

Part One

Intake

<u>Client</u>

Age: 8

Sex: Female

Gender: Female

Sexuality: N/A

Ethnicity: White

Relationship Status: N/A

Counseling Setting: Outpatient—pediatric therapy office

Types of Counseling: Individual

Presenting Problem: Acting out at home and school, often distracted, fidgeting, interrupting, and arguing with both parents and teacher

Diagnosis: 314.01 Attention-deficit/Hyperactivity disorder

Presenting Problem:

You have been assigned to an 8-year-old female client. Over the past year, she has been acting out both at home and in school. She interrupts her teacher and classmates throughout the day and can't seem to sit still. Her teacher has indicated that the client is argumentative and challenges everything she says. During group activities or lessons, she often looks out the window and does not answer when called on. She has also had great difficulty calming down at night and is only averaging 8 to 9 hours of sleep each night. Her parents and teacher are concerned about the changes they've seen in the client. When they ask her what is going on, she seemed irritated and refuses to answer any questions.

Mental Status:

Your client arrived with her parents and baby brother. She was well-dressed, clean, and looked like an overall healthy child. She was holding her mother's hand and stood behind her mother. Once she became more comfortable, she started walking around the office looking at different toys and books. When her mother asked her to sit down, she continued to roam around the room. At the mother's insistence she sat in a chair briefly, started fidgeting and got back up to walk around. She appeared to be distracted and restless.

Family History:

Your client lives at home with her mother, father, and newborn baby brother. Before her brother was born, she was an only child. Her parents reported the change in her behavior began one year ago, which

198

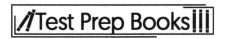

was around the time her mother and father let her know she would soon be a big sister. At home, she argues with her parents and does not want to sit down long enough to get her homework done. When she does try to complete work, she fidgets while she sits. When her mother sits with her and tries to get her to focus, she often must ask her the same questions repeatedly to get her to pay attention or answer. She loves playing with her baby brother and giggles when she makes him laugh.

1. Based on the symptoms mentioned during intake, what type of ADHD does the client have?
   a. Inattentive type
   b. Hyperactive-impulsive type
   c. Combined type
   d. Mild type

2. When is it common for children to act out or have struggles at school?
   a. When they have a life change, such as a new sibling
   b. When they have a disorder such as autism, ADHD, anxiety, or a learning disorder
   c. It is only common in oppositional defiant disorder
   d. Both A and B

3. Related to the growth and development of the brain, ADHD is one of the most common disorders of this type in children. What category of disorders is characterized by differences in the development of the nervous system and the brain impacting several areas of functioning including emotions, learning, and memory?
   Neurodevelopmental disorders
   Psychotic disorders
   Anxiety disorders
   Personality disorders

4. Which disorder that is commonly comorbid with ADHD should the counselor consider further based on the client acting argumentative and challenging her parents and teacher?
   a. Anxiety disorder
   b. Major depressive disorder
   c. Obsessive-compulsive disorder
   d. Oppositional defiant disorder

5. What symptom of ADHD is illustrated by the client frequently interrupting her classmates and teacher?
   a. Hyperactivity
   b. Impulsiveness
   c. Lack of attention
   d. Distractibility

Part Two

Second session, one week after the initial intake:
Your client arrived with her mother to her second counseling session. This session you divided the time between talking to the child and talking to her mother. The client was still clingy to her mother when they first arrived. When you spoke to your client alone, she continued to roam around the room or fidget in her chair. She answered many of your questions and seemed interested in talking to someone

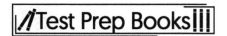
who wanted to know more about her. You focused on building the relationship, trust, expressing empathy, and helping her feel comfortable. The client reported that she likes being a big sister but stated "I wish my mommy would pay attention to me" and "the baby gets all the attention." Her mother mentioned that the client has been clingier lately, sometimes crying or throwing toddler-like tantrums when she is dropped off at school and has reverted to the old habit of sucking her thumb. Since she is 8 years old, this is a major concern for her mother. Her behavior at school has not improved and her mother doesn't know what to do next. You discuss next steps in treatment. Parent training is a very effective method that helps parents learn how to praise successfully, encourage desirable behaviors, and implement agreed-upon consequences for undesirable behaviors. This helps the child to modify their behavior and enjoy more positive interactions with parents. You assign the parents homework of spending one-on-one time with the client each day, as well as practicing positive forms of communication and acknowledging the client's feelings (positive or negative).

6. The client has reverted to old behaviors like tantrums and sucking her thumb. Common in children, what is the defense mechanism that occurs when you "escape" to an earlier stage of development?
   a. Repression
   b. Displacement
   c. Regression
   d. Compartmentalization

7. What is the ability to recognize and manage your emotions, behaviors, and reactions? For example, calming down after something exciting or upsetting happens.
   a. Self-regulation
   b. Separation anxiety
   c. Cognitive behavioral therapy
   d. Social skills

8. The counselor suggested that the parents spend uninterrupted one-on-one time with the client each day. This will help facilitate which healthy attachment style that is characterized by trust, comfort, and a positive connection with the caregiver?
   a. Disorganized attachment
   b. Avoidant attachment
   c. Anxious-resistant attachment
   d. Secure attachment

9. Select the psychologist who described attachment as "a lasting psychological connectedness between human beings."
   a. John Bowlby
   b. Lev Vygotsky
   c. Erik Erikson
   d. B.F. Skinner

Part Three

Fourth session, three weeks after the initial session:
Your client seemed to be more comfortable with talking to you and the routine of coming to counseling. She did not hide behind her mother when she arrived, and she ran over to her favorite chair. Her behavior at school has started to improve as well. She still wants to move around at her desk, so she has

200

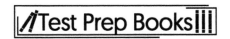

learned to stand at her desk or sit with a fidget toy. These adaptations have helped her to release energy without roaming around the room interrupting other students. She still has trouble focusing on tests at school or homework at home. Her mother reported that she has started to have more positive interactions at home. Her mother and father have utilized the skills learned in parent training. They have practiced positive reinforcement for behaviors, positive communication like empathy and reflection, and planned one-on-one time each day. The client said, "I feel special when I get time with mommy." The client has learned to identify and express feelings more instead of throwing tantrums or acting out. You recognize the progress and encourage them to keep up the good work. You explain that consistency and routine are key for progress to continue.

10. What do you call adjustments made in a system for an individual based on a proven need? Allowing the client to stand at her desk or have a fidget toy would be an example.
    a. Operant conditioning
    b. Reasonable accommodations
    c. Reinforcement
    d. Physical outlet

11. The client has excess amounts of energy and wants to stand and move around during class. This is an example of which of the following common symptoms of ADHD?
    a.   Lack of attention
    b. Distractibility
    c. Impulsiveness
    d. Hyperactivity

12. Which statement below is an example of the parents practicing empathy?
    a. "Don't be jealous of your baby brother, you know we love you."
    b. "You don't need to feel sad, it's a happy day."
    c. "From what I'm hearing, you feel sad and left out when I pay attention to your baby brother."
    d. "Why don't we play a game? That will put you in a better mood."

13. What is another treatment option for ADHD, when behavioral therapy and parent training do not have the desired effect of lessening the child's symptoms?
    a. Stimulants
    b. Antidepressants
    c. Depressants
    d. Steroids

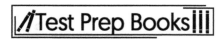

Case Study #5

Part One

Intake

<u>Client</u>

Age: 18

Sex: Female

Gender: Female

Sexuality: Heterosexual

Ethnicity: Asian

Relationship Status: Single

Counseling Setting: Outpatient—community counseling office

Types of Counseling: Individual

Presenting Problem: Rarely leaves home or interacts with anyone outside of immediate family, fear of new situations and interactions caused by language differences

Diagnosis: F40.10 Social anxiety disorder

Presenting Problem:
Your client is an 18 -year-old female who has just emigrated from Japan to United States with her parents and her older brother. She speaks very little English and presents herself as a very quiet and reserved person. Her brother has recently enrolled in college classes. Your client has not registered for any classes yet, despite her high academic achievements in high school. In Japan she was a great student, participated in extracurricular activities, and socialized with friends often. Since she arrived in the United States, she rarely leaves the home.

Mental Status:
Your client looked well put together, in crisp jeans and a blue blouse. She appeared to be shy, looking down and speaking quietly. She reported that she decided to come to counseling because she has been feeling anxious at the prospect of attending school or making new friends in the United States. She has not signed up for college courses, attempted to get a job, or talked to new people. When prompted to explain why, the client expressed her great fear at attempting to meet people or take classes using a language that she hardly understands. She admits it is isolating at times. When asked about her social life, she reported that she spends a lot of her time talking with friends and family back home.

Family History:
Your client lives at home with her mother, father, and older brother. Her mother and father do not speak English, and when she goes out with them, she feels pressured to translate and communicate with

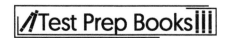

others on their behalf. For example, she takes her mother to the grocery store each week. She does not know much of the English language herself, so even this weekly outing is stressful. She noted that only interacting with friends online and spending most of her time at home is contributing to her feelings of isolation. However, she said that she would prefer to stay in the comfort of her home, where she feels safe, and take care of her parents and brother.

1. Which of the following terms refers to the ability of a counselor to understand how their own culture affects their relationship with a client who is from another culture or has a different belief system?
    a. Cultural competence
    b. Cultural considerations
    c. Culture shock
    d. Adjustment stage

2. Which of these disorders is NOT commonly comorbid with social anxiety disorder?
    a. Generalized anxiety disorder
    b. Avoidant personality disorder
    c. Narcissistic personality disorder
    d. Panic disorder

3. What is the mental state where an individual feels at ease and in control of their environment?
    a. Personal growth
    b. Comfort zone
    c. Danger space
    d. Learning zone

4. People with social anxiety disorder often worry about being embarrassed or judged by others. What is a common reaction to this feeling?
    a. Avoiding anxiety-producing social situations
    b. Feeling intense fear and anxiety in certain social situations
    c. Often feeling relieved once they arrive at a social gathering
    d. Both A and B

5. Which term is defined as a client psychologically allowing themselves to open up to a counselor from a different culture by sharing their thoughts and feelings?
    a. Therapeutic alliance
    b. Self-disclosure
    c. Therapeutic surrender
    d. Helping relationship

Part Two

Second session, one week after the initial intake:

Your client arrived at her second session on time, and she appeared well groomed. She presented as very quiet and shy. You began the session with small talk about her family and friends back home. Building rapport, trust, and learning more about the client is crucial to building a strong helping relationship. You discussed the difficulties of moving to a new culture where one does not know the language well. She reported that she feels isolated when she stays home and often helpless when she goes out to complete even small tasks. It has been difficult for her to adjust to life in a new city, finding

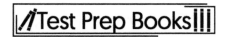

her way around, and to the new culture and way of life. She worries about the expectations of others, not knowing how to act in new situations in a new country. She feels more comfortable staying in the house, so she doesn't have to struggle or feel anxious. When asked to describe what happens in an uncomfortable situation, she stated that she becomes hot, flushes, feels like her heart is beating fast, and sometimes even starts to shake. She is most concerned with what the other people are feeling and if she is making them uncomfortable. You supported her, expressing empathy and understanding. At the end of the session, you discussed treatment options, including cognitive behavioral therapy and medications.

6. What standards is the client describing when she said she has difficulty navigating and understanding the rules in a new country, including the social expectations of others?
    a. Laws
    b. Cultural adjustments
    c. Culture shock
    d. Cultural norms

7. Symptoms of mental health disorders may present differently for different cultures. Which of the client's reported symptoms is different than those typically found in Western Culture?
    a. Blushing and overheating
    b. Rapid heartbeat
    c. Worry about making others uncomfortable
    d. Shaking

8. Homesickness, helplessness, disorientation, and isolation are all symptoms of what phenomenon that often occurs when someone moves to a new, unfamiliar environment?
    a. Culture shock
    b. Social anxiety disorder
    c. Social phobia
    d. Adjustment period

9. In Japan, individuals often focus on the wants and needs of the group instead of the wants and needs of each individual. What is this type of culture defined as?
    a. Western culture
    b. Eastern culture
    c. Individualistic culture
    d. Collectivist culture

Part Three

Fifth session, four weeks after the initial session:
Your client has become more talkative and open with you over the past couple of sessions. One method that has been helpful in addressing her social anxiety is developing positive methods for her to use in stressful situations, including controlling her breathing, progressive muscle relaxation, and paying attention to her senses. She has been utilizing these behaviors and sticking to the treatment plan. The client is cooperative and is making great efforts to move forward. You have focused on cognitive behavioral therapy to address and correct unhelpful thoughts, paired with a method of therapy where the client confronts a feared social situation repeatedly until their anxiety decreases. This has included taking small steps, such as going alone to a coffee shop to order a drink and a snack once a week. Last

204

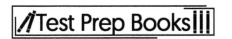

week she was also assigned homework to go to the grocery and ask for help when she could not find something on her list. She succeeded in completing these tasks and was proud of her success, admitting that she felt quite happy ordering for herself and getting out in the world. These positive feelings are natural reinforcers, making it more likely for her to continue this activity in the future. You discuss her success and work together to plan future treatment goals. You determined a good future goal would be to meet a new friend and spend 30 minutes talking at a coffee shop.

10. What are the positive methods a person uses to deal with stressful situations, allowing them to confront an issue head on, take action, and resolve problems in a healthy way?

    a. Coping mechanisms
    b. Reframing
    c. Challenging negative self-talk
    d. Coping skills

11. What is the method of therapy in which an individual confronts a situation that causes feelings of fear or anxiety repeatedly until their level of anxiety decreases?
    a. Positive reinforcement
    b. Exposure therapy
    c. Negative reinforcement
    d. Systematic desensitization

12. The client felt happy and proud of herself after completing each task, such as her weekly outing to the coffee shop down the street. She was also rewarded with a favorite drink and pastry. These "rewards" are a form of which type of positive reinforcement?
    a. Tangible reinforcers
    b. Social reinforcers
    c. Natural reinforcers
    d. Token reinforcers

13. What are the methods that change negative thought processes by interrupting and redirecting thought patterns that have become destructive or self-defeating?
    a. Goal setting
    b. Self-empathy
    c. Cognitive restructuring
    d. Reflection

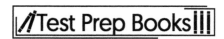

Case Study #6

Part One

Intake

<u>Client</u>

Age: 27

Sex: Female

Gender: Female

Sexuality: Heterosexual

Ethnicity: Black

Relationship Status: Married

Counseling Setting: Outpatient—community counseling office

Types of Counseling: Individual

Presenting Problem: Worry, anxiety, and lack of sleep interfering with quality of life

Diagnosis: F41.1 Generalized anxiety disorder, Severe

Presenting Problem:

The client is a 27-year-old woman from Manhattan, New York. She is newly married and has a newborn baby girl. The client is currently unemployed, and her husband is working two jobs to make ends meet. She worries every day about the family's finances, retirement, and the baby's well-being, and she can't seem to calm herself down. When asked about going back to work, she immediately begins to cry at the thought of leaving her newborn baby in the care of a complete stranger. Sometimes her worrying has even gotten in the way of her concentration. The client reported that she has also been experiencing prolonged muscle tension and bouts of indigestion. At her initial visit, the client asked for help getting to sleep at night and staying asleep, and she has expressed the desire to generally "feel better."

Mental Status:

Your client appeared to be tired and in a state of anxiety and nervousness. She was fidgeting with her sweater and admitted to being extremely exhausted. She said she has trouble falling asleep and staying asleep at night. This is contributing to her anxious and worried thoughts—the more tired she is, the more difficult it is to deal with these worries. When asked what her main concerns are, she said she is mostly worried about money, the family's future, and her baby. She used to be the breadwinner of the family. She worked in publishing for several years. In recent years, her lack of sleep and anxiety began to affect her career. When she became pregnant, she decided to take time off from work. She does have plans to return to work once she "feels better." She began searching for work but found there are not many openings in her field. When she finds jobs to apply to, they often do not utilize her skills and experience. The salaries of these positions reflect this, and do not provide enough money to pay for

206

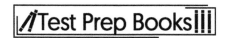

childcare. She worries so much about her baby that she cannot comprehend leaving her child to go back to work.

Family History:
Your client is recently married to her husband. She met her husband in college, and they have been together for five years. A few months after the wedding, she found out she was pregnant. She has a newborn baby daughter. With her husband working two jobs, she is responsible for almost all her daughter's care. This is contributing to her exhaustion. Her husband has expressed concern about his wife doing all the childcare and not sleeping at night. He has suggested that his mother, who lives only twenty minutes away, could help with childcare a couple of times a week. The client is so worried about leaving her daughter in someone else's care, she does not even want his mother to help. The client reported that her parents live back home in Ohio. They visited when the baby was born, but do not live close enough to visit often. She talks to her mother on the phone but does not want her mother to worry. She tells her everything is going great, even though deep down she knows she needs more help. She doesn't want her parents to know she has been feeling this anxious and has started to attend counseling.

1. Maslow's hierarchy of needs is one of the best-known theories of motivation, stating that actions are motivated by certain physiological needs. Which level of Maslow's pyramid would include the need for a stable career?
    a. Self-actualization
    b. Esteem
    c. Safety needs
    d. Love and belonging

2. What type of family is characterized by both parents being employed?
    a. Traditional family
    b. Nuclear family
    c. Child-free household
    d. Dual-career family

3. The client is concerned with taking steps back in her career and accepting a low-paying position that does not utilize her education and experience. What is it called when a worker is engaged in a position that is below their skill level?
    a. Unemployment
    b. Underemployment
    c. Overemployment
    d. Leisure

4. Common in people with generalized anxiety disorder, what is the sleep disorder in which an individual struggles to fall asleep or wakes up often?
    a. Insomnia
    b. Panic disorder
    c. Night terrors
    d. Sleep apnea

207

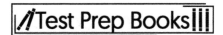

5. The client does not want her parents to know she is attending counseling, as her family has a negative view of counseling and seeking help for one's mental health. What are the culturally based attitudes and beliefs that can have a negative effect on how an individual views themselves, other people, and society as a whole?
   a. Cultural norms
   b. Culture shock
   c. Social norms
   d. Cultural stigma

Part Two

Second session, one week after the initial intake:

Your client arrived at this session with her baby. She explained that her husband was working his second job, so she didn't have anyone to watch her daughter. This session, the client completed the Generalized Anxiety Disorder Severity Scale. This test measures the presence and severity of generalized anxiety disorder by assigning numerical values to symptoms or behaviors associated with anxiety. The client expressed that her symptoms of anxiety have increased over the years, and it has been affecting her life. She noted that she is unable to work or seek employment and no longer has a social life. In past years, she was able to do both of those things. She doesn't spend much time with her husband or see her friends. Most of her time is spent at home with the baby. What used to feel like normal worries have become much more severe. You discuss treatment options and long-term and short-term goals. Long term, the client expressed she would like to eventually start socializing again and get back to work. Short term, she would like to focus on sleeping better and controlling her emotions better. She said, "When I feel anxious or worried, I want to be able to control those emotions and calm myself down before they spiral out of control."

6. What kind of data does the Generalized Anxiety Disorder Severity Scale collect?
   a. Qualitative data
   b. Nominal data
   c. Psychometric data
   d. Quantitative data

7. How did the birth of the client's daughter, her recent marriage, and loss of employment affect the client?
   a. These major life events led to an increase in the severity of her anxiety.
   b. These major life events distracted her from her previous anxiety.
   c. These major life events had no effect on her anxiety.
   d. These major life events significantly lessened her anxiety.

8. Worry is said to reside in the mind, often be temporary, and lead to the use of problem-solving skills to address issues. How is anxiety different than normal worry?
   a. Anxiety can have physical symptoms such as heart palpitations, indigestion, or muscle tension.
   b. Anxiety compromises the ability to function in daily life.
   c. Anxiety is more persistent.
   d. All of the above

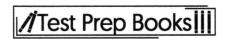

9. The client stated, "When I feel anxious or worried, I want to be able to control those emotions and calm myself down before they spiral out of control." What is the ability to control or manage your emotional state called?
   a. Mindfulness
   b. Emotion regulation
   c. Interpersonal effectiveness
   d. Distress tolerance

Part Three

Fourth session, three weeks after the initial session:

The client arrived at this session alone and reported her daughter was with her mother-in-law. The client appeared to be more rested. Over the last three sessions, you have addressed some of the immediate concerns of the client, one being the sleep issues she has been experiencing for some time. It is important to address this issue, as the lack of sleep and ensuing exhaustion only increase the symptoms of anxiety. The client expressed that the sleep medication has been helping her fall asleep and stay asleep for longer. In combination with the sleep medication, you have addressed her behavior surrounding bedtime, including nighttime routine, drinking caffeine at night, duration of sleep, and when to take sleep medication.

Another short-term goal was to work on controlling the client's thoughts and emotions better. Through the use of a specific form of cognitive behavioral therapy, you have been able to work on the client's ability to manage her emotions. You've been teaching her methods for connecting with the present moment and noticing passing thoughts without being controlled by them. This treatment encourages individuals to acknowledge that they have anxiety, but work on making positive changes to manage their anxiety at the same time. The client has been working hard toward treatment goals and has made steps forward. She reported that she has been able to leave the baby with her mother-in-law twice a week, and she has used the new methods she has learned in counseling to control her anxiety. You continued to build the therapeutic relationship, practiced active listening and empathy, and collaborated with the client for next steps in treatment planning.

10. In addition to sleep medication, what other medications are typically prescribed for a client with generalized anxiety disorder?
   a. Antipsychotics
   b. Depressants
   c. Antidepressants
   d. Stimulants

11. What term refers to behaviors surrounding bedtime, including one's nighttime routines, such as drinking caffeine at night, duration of sleep, and schedule for sleep medications?
   a. Sleep habits
   b. Sleep hygiene
   c. Insomnia
   d. Sleep disturbances

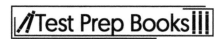

12. Based on the description, what specific type of cognitive behavioral therapy is the counselor using with the client?
   a. Rational emotive behavior therapy
   b. Acceptance and commitment therapy
   c. Cognitive behavioral play therapy
   d. Dialectical behavior therapy

13. What is the ability to connect with the present moment and notice passing thoughts without being controlled by them?
   a. Meditation
   b. Self-soothing
   c. Mindfulness
   d. Active listening

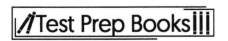

Case Study #7

Part One

Intake

<u>Client</u>

Age: 62

Sex: Male

Gender: Male

Sexuality: Heterosexual

Ethnicity: White

Relationship Status: Divorced, single

Counseling Setting: Outpatient—community counseling office

Types of Counseling: Individual

Presenting Problem: Low energy, anger issues, and poor communication skills causing difficulties at work and in personal relationships

Diagnosis: F60.81 Narcissistic personality disorder

Presenting Problem:
The client is a 62-year-old single and very successful man from Houston, Texas. He has been experiencing bouts of low energy over the past several months which are interfering with his work and personal affairs. He is known at the office and at home for exploding into a rage at any perceived slight or disagreement. If family members or coworkers are not complimentary of him and in agreement with him, he cuts them off or has an outburst. More recently, he has become more withdrawn at work. His personal physician has suggested that the client take some time off from work or gradually reduce his number of hours, but he is reluctant to make any changes. He is the sole owner of his business and explained that he alone has made his fortune, and that without him, the entire business would collapse. When asked about personal relationships, the client reported that he has had two failed marriages and even more failed relationships. On his initial visit, he repeated over a dozen times that he was very successful and that all he needs to keep going is to regain his energy and figure out a way to get his children and his employees to give him more credit and respect for his accomplishments and generosity.

Mental Status:
Your client was well-dressed and presented as very self-involved and lacking empathy for others. When discussing what brought him to counseling, he was very focused on the perceived problems of his coworkers and family members. He did not take responsibility for any of the issues going on in his life and reported feeling like most people did not understand or appreciate him. He shared that he has heard people at work describing him as difficult and self-centered. He didn't agree with this perspective

211

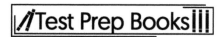
and said that the coworkers were just jealous of him. He was often exasperated talking about the slights of others and how he isn't appreciated at work and home.

Family History:

Your client has had issues keeping any close friendships or family relationships. He reported this is through no fault of his own and listed off several occasions where the other person was responsible for making him angry. When asked about his divorces, he placed the blame on the women he was in relationships and marriages with, saying the women were not in his intellectual bracket, did not understand him, and didn't see how amazing and special he truly is. He has three grown children, and he stated that they are ungrateful for all his financial support. He has not been very involved in their lives, saying he has been too busy and focused on his success and his business.

1. The client repeated over a dozen times that he is very successful and rich. This is an example of which symptom of narcissistic personality disorder?
   a. Being interpersonally exploitative
   b. Grandiose sense of self-importance
   c. Feelings of jealousy and belief others are jealous of them
   d. Narcissistic rage

2. The client expected coworkers to always speak about him in a positive light, automatically agree with him, and comply to any demands without question. This is an example of which symptom of narcissistic personality disorder?
   a. Preoccupation with fantasies of extreme power, success, and brilliance
   b. Lack of empathy
   c. Sense of entitlement
   d. Belief that they are "special" and unique

3. Taking out frustrations on others and withdrawing at work are both symptoms of what type of work-related stress that is common in those with narcissistic personality disorder?
   a. Unemployment
   b. Stressful work environment
   c. Job performance
   d. Burnout

4. Which is NOT true in regards to dating and relationships for those with narcissistic personality disorder?
   a. Narcissists struggle to truly love others
   b. Narcissists are only interested in how their partner will meet their needs
   c. Narcissists often make understanding their partner's thoughts and emotions a priority
   d. Narcissists often make partners feel ignored, uncared about, and unimportant

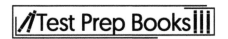

5. Is narcissistic personality disorder more common in women or men?
   a. Males are diagnosed with this disorder more often than females.
   b. Females are diagnosed with this disorder more often than males.
   c. There are no gender differences in the prevalence of this disorder.
   d. There haven't been enough studies on narcissistic personality disorder and gender to determine this.

Part Two

Third session, two weeks after the initial intake:

During the previous session, you focused on building the relationship with your client and actively listening to the client's thoughts and emotions. When a client often places the blame on others and does not take responsibility for their actions, it is important to focus on foundational listening, attending, and reflecting, rather than determining whether something they are doing is good or bad. The best treatment plan for those with narcissistic personality disorder is psychoanalysis or talk therapy. During this session you explored the client's childhood, friendships, and relationships. The client reported that his father was often absent, spending most of his time at work. His parents held him to a high standard, but even when he reached those standards, they did not show that they were proud of him. He remembered desperately trying to get his father's approval, but he rarely noticed him. He stated that both of his parents lacked warmth and were not affectionate with him as a child. His mother was often hot and cold, often showing him affection only in front of others. He remembered that as a child, he would wonder what was wrong with him or why he wasn't good enough for his parents to give him love and attention. The client mentioned that he has had difficulty forming friendships or relationships, but repeatedly placed the blame on other people. He failed to understand how his often-selfish behaviors or angry outbursts have led to losing his relationships.

6. The client expressed that his emotional needs for affection, support, attention, and competence were ignored by his parents. What is it called when the parents or guardians fail to meet these emotional needs during childhood?
   a. Childhood trauma
   b. Childhood emotional neglect
   c. Physical abuse
   d. Self-preservation

7. Common in those with narcissistic personality disorder, what is it called when someone lacks confidence about who they are and what they do, often feeling incompetent, unloved, or inadequate?
   a. Envy
   b. Absence of admiration
   c. Sense of entitlement
   d. Low self-esteem

8. During this session, the counselor focused on foundational listening, attending, and reflecting instead of whether what the client was saying was good or bad. Select the term that refers to the counseling method that focuses on just the facts and "everything as it is."
   a. Nonjudgmental stance
   b. Active listening
   c. Constructive confrontation
   d. Accurate empathy

213

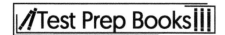

9. What symptom of narcissistic personality disorder is illustrated by the client's inability to identify or understand the feelings and needs of others?
    a. Sense of entitlement
    b. Arrogant attitude
    c. Envy of others
    d. Lack of emotional empathy

Part Three

Fifth session, four weeks after the initial session:

The client has started to gain an understanding of how his behavior affects others. He admitted his quick temper and self-centeredness have led to him not having close relationships with family members, friends, and coworkers. Over the last two sessions you focused on teaching the client how to communicate with others more effectively, recognize how others are feeling, and what they are thinking. He shared a situation at work, where a coworker disagreed with him. He would have typically felt slighted and had an angry outburst. Through methods he has practiced in counseling, he was able to take a step back and consider another perspective before acting. Practicing empathy and learning affective communication strategies are two of the main goals for the client.

This session you focused on recognizing his own maladaptive behaviors and defense mechanisms. He volunteered that he is often quick to anger or quick to blame or place responsibility on others. He reported that he is motivated to change the way he communicates and that he hopes to rebuild his relationships with his children. He has realized that he is getting older, and he is going to be alone for the rest of his life if he doesn't make changes now.

10. What is the learned behavior where individuals constantly blame others for the shortcomings and failures in their life?
    a. Denial
    b. Projection
    c. Victim mentality
    d. Displacement

11. What defense mechanism is characterized by learning to overachieve in one area to make up for failures in other areas, thus protecting from feelings of inadequacy, insecurity, and unlovability?
    a. Repression
    b. Overcompensation
    c. Compartmentalization
    d. Rationalization

12. The client has started to practice the understanding that other people have their own thoughts, feelings, and motivations that do not revolve around him. These are the first steps in developing what important life skill that most narcissists lack?
    a. Mindfulness
    b. Compassion
    c. Sympathy
    d. Empathy

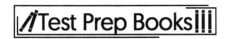
13. What is the therapeutic method used to help achieve a positive outcome when confrontation is necessary, through teaching improved communication, self-awareness, and reduced conflict?

  a. Constructive confrontation
  b. Authenticity
  c. Congruence
  d. De-escalation

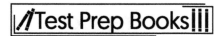
Case Study #8

Part One

Intake

Client

Age: 85

Sex: Male

Gender: Male

Sexuality: Heterosexual

Ethnicity: White

Relationship Status: Married, Widowed

Counseling Setting: Outpatient—community counseling office

Types of Counseling: Individual

Presenting Problem: After wife's death, client is experiencing lack of sleep, feelings of extreme sadness, and persistent focus on wanting his wife back, which are disrupting his life and daily activities

Diagnosis: Prolonged grief disorder

Presenting Problem:

Your new client is an elderly man in his mid-80's. Sixteen months ago, he lost his wife of almost sixty years. The client expressed he was hesitant to come to his initial counseling appointment. He finally consented due to his daughter's persistence. She is concerned with the amount of time and level of grief that her father is experiencing. The client recently lost his driving license after an at-fault accident, and he does not sleep or eat well. When asked why he decided to come to this appointment, he responded that he wants his wife back and his old life back.

Mental Status:

The client appeared to be exhausted and had a low mood. His posture was slumped, and he had a flat affect and tone of voice. When speaking about his deceased wife, he often appeared tearful. He spoke repeatedly of his wife and the way life "used to be." He repeatedly mentioned that he wished for nothing more than to be with his wife again. He also feels some guilt and responsibility, often wondering "what I could have done differently so that she would still be here today." He reported that he has not been sleeping and this exhaustion contributed to his car accident.

Family History:

Your client is recently widowed after being married to his wife for almost sixty years. He stated that she was the love of his life and best friend. Without her, he feels lost and isolated. Many other family members have passed away, including both of his parents and his two siblings, who have been gone for

216

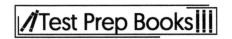

several years. He stated that his daughter is the only one he has left. He admitted that he wouldn't have started counseling if it weren't for the persistence of his daughter. She is married with two grown children, but he said he doesn't want to be a burden to his daughter. As he recently lost his license, he feels like he is losing his independence. His daughter must pick him up to take him to the grocery store, doctor's appointments, and any other outing. The client expressed everything was easier when his wife was here.

1. What is the strong physical and emotional reaction to the loss of someone or something that may include feelings of extreme sadness and intense longing to be with that person?
   a. Mourning
   b. Bereavement
   c. Denial
   d. Grief

2. Also common following the loss of a loved one, prolonged grief disorder shares key similarities to what other mental health disorder?
   a. Generalized anxiety disorder
   b. Major depressive disorder
   c. Social anxiety disorder
   d. Bipolar disorder

3. The client mentioned missing his wife and wanting to be with her again several times during intake. Which primary symptom of prolonged grief disorder is illustrated here?
   a. Marked sense of disbelief about the death
   b. Strong yearning for or persistent preoccupation with the person who passed away
   c. Avoidance of reminders the person is dead
   d. Intense emotional pain related to the death, including anger or sorrow

4. The client has been feeling guilty and feels that if he had done something differently, his wife would still be alive today. This is an example of what kind of thinking?
   a. Wishful thinking
   b. Magical thinking
   c. Counterfactual thinking
   d. Critical thinking

5. What is it called when you have constant, repetitive, or obsessive thoughts about a person or idea that interferes with normal mental functioning?
   a. Rumination
   b. Emotional numbness
   c. Avoidance
   d. Acceptance

Part Two

Second session, one week after the initial intake:
The client appeared to be experiencing exhaustion and a low mood, similar to the initial session. You discussed the idea of working together as a team to determine goals for treatment. When asked what his long-term goals are for counseling, he reported that he is still hesitant as he knows it will not "bring

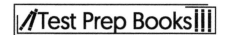

my wife back to me." He reported that his main goal would be to find a way to be with his wife again. Until then, he said he wishes he could have his normal life back. This session, you prioritized developing a level of comfort through building the trust and a positive relationship with the client. The client talked about how he has been feeling exhausted and is having trouble falling asleep and staying asleep. You discussed the benefits of sleeping medication on a temporary basis to get the client back on a better sleep schedule. He was visibly relieved at the possibility that he will be able to get more sleep and that it could contribute to him feeling better soon. This is a good option for the client, as controlling obsessive thoughts is more difficult when you are exhausted. He expressed that he misses his wife every day and doesn't feel like himself, stating "I feel as though a part of me died with her. I don't know who I am without her."

6. What term refers to the counselor and client working as a team to decide on the goals for counseling and the steps to reach them?
    a. Therapeutic alliance
    b. Client goal attainment
    c. Collaboration
    d. Treatment plan compliance

7. What is it called when a client is hesitant to participate in or take steps toward meeting demands of the therapeutic process?
    a. Reluctance
    b. Barrier to goal attainment
    c. Termination
    d. Resistance

8. During this session, the client said "I feel as though a part of me died with her. I don't know who I am without her." This is an example of which symptom of prolonged grief disorder?
    a. Suicidal thoughts or actions
    b. Sleep disruption
    c. Persistent preoccupation with the deceased
    d. Identity disruption

9. What is an example of an at-risk behavior that is prevalent in both prolonged grief disorder and major depressive disorder?
    a. Homicide
    b. Suicidal thoughts or actions
    c. Alcohol or drug abuse
    d. Relationship violence

Part Three

Fourth session, three weeks after the initial session:

The client arrived at the session with an improved mood and appeared to be more well rested. He reported that he had been taking his sleep medication for the past two weeks and had started sleeping an average of eight hours a night. He stated that this has made it easier for him to function and to control his thoughts and behaviors better. During the last session, you discussed the client's treatment plan, determining the best form of treatment to address many of the symptoms of prolonged grief disorder. This method of treatment includes cognitive restructuring and reframing, as well as

218

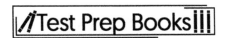

challenging unhealthy thought and behavior patterns such as obsessively focusing on the past. It is also important for the client to take steps toward resuming some normal activities. This session, you work together with the client to set a new goal. The client is going to schedule a time each week to spend quality time with family, and another time to see friends. The client stated that this week he is going to schedule a lunch with an old friend on Wednesday and he is going to visit his daughter and grandchildren on Friday. He said he is looking forward to these plans.

10. What therapeutic technique being utilized with the client involves challenging unhealthy thought and behavior patterns such as obsessively focusing on the past?
    a. Talk therapy
    b. Cognitive behavioral therapy
    c. Dialectical behavioral therapy
    d. Exposure therapy

11. When someone is overwhelmed by loss, it is common to experience irrational self-scripts or feelings of false guilt. What method do counselors use to identify these thoughts, challenge them for accuracy, and help clients replace those thoughts with more functional and realistic ones?
    a. Role playing
    b. Evocative language
    c. Reframing
    d. Cognitive restructuring

12. Which stage of grief involves acknowledging the impact that the loss has had on one's life and the ability to stop wishing for everything to be exactly as it used to be?
    a. Acceptance
    b. Denial
    c. Bargaining
    d. Depression

13. The counselor complimented the client on making plans with friends and family members and taking positive steps toward reaching their counseling goals. What term describes the degree to which a client conforms to treatment advice and methods to reach their counseling goals?
    a. Treatment plan compliance
    b. Goal setting
    c. Reassurance
    d. Collaboration

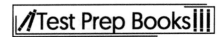

Case Study #9

Part One

Intake

<u>Client</u>

Age: 43

Sex: Female

Gender: Female

Sexuality: Heterosexual

Ethnicity: White

Relationship Status: Single

Counseling Setting: Outpatient—community counseling office

Types of Counseling: Individual

Presenting Problem: Anger issues impacting interpersonal relationships, risky behaviors and violent outbursts affecting quality of life

Diagnosis: F60.3 Borderline personality disorder

Presenting Problem:

Your new client is a 43-year-old single White female. She is reluctant to attend counseling and stated that it has never helped her before. She stated that she is willing to give it one more try. Your focus this session is to begin building a positive therapeutic relationship with the client and discuss the client's background and mental health history. Ever since she was in her twenties, she has struggled with anger issues which have made it difficult for her to form interpersonal relationships both romantically and platonically. Every time there is a minor inconvenience or conflict, she feels an intense anger and takes it very personally. Sometimes this anger is so strong, she initiates intense verbal arguments and does not want to speak to the person ever again. The client reported that she is capable of stopping herself from being physically violent with others during her outbursts. She has an extensive history of seeking mental health treatment but has not experienced any improvement.

Mental Status:

The client seemed defiant and out of focus. She had a chip on her shoulder, admitting that she did not think counseling would work for her. In the past she has tried individual counseling many times, and following a violent altercation in the past, she tried inpatient therapy for several weeks. She admitted that her angry outbursts have led to the loss of many relationships and jobs alike.

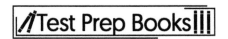

Family History:

Your client reported that she does not have close relationships with family members. During her teens and twenties, she had a lot of arguments with her parents and sister. She doesn't speak with her parents often. She said when she does talk to her mother on the phone, she can tell she is disappointed in her. She knows her mother is concerned for her well-being, as she is always asking if she has gotten help or is doing better. The client stated she would rather not talk to her mom and "feel her judging me." She described her relationship with her sister as volatile. They have been through some phases where they are close and others when they argue and don't speak for long periods of time. She said she is not currently speaking with her sister.

1. What is another name commonly used to describe borderline personality disorder?
   a. Bipolar disorder
   b. Emotional dysregulation disorder
   c. Oppositional defiant disorder
   d. Manic depression

2. Borderline personality disorder is often misdiagnosed as what mental health disorder, which has many similar symptoms, including mood instability?
   a. Narcissistic personality disorder
   b. Schizophrenia
   c. Generalized anxiety disorder
   d. Bipolar disorder

3. What is the name of one of the most troubling symptoms of borderline personality disorder, which is described as intense, inappropriate anger?
   a. Borderline rage
   b. Reaction formation
   c. Passive aggression
   d. Assertiveness

4. What are common triggers for anger and violent outbursts in those with borderline personality disorder?
   a. Disagreements
   b. Separations
   c. Rejections
   d. All of the above

5. What is a common fear in those with borderline personality disorder, leading to symptoms such as being overly sensitive to criticism, difficulty trusting others, difficulty making friends, and taking extreme measures to avoid rejection or separation?
   a. Social situations
   b. Negative evaluation
   c. Abandonment
   d. Failure

221

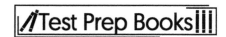

Part Two

<u>Second session, one week after the initial intake:</u>
The client appeared to be in a more energized or manic state this session. Her speech was rapid, and she did not stop at appropriate intervals. Her thought patterns seemed erratic, but she was more openly sharing her thoughts and feelings. In the previous session, she mentioned her anger issues have led to issues in her family relationships and romantic relationships. When asked how her mental health has affected her quality of life in other ways, she mentioned several impulsive behaviors that are negatively impacting her life. The client reported that occasionally she will disappear for days. During this time, she has been known to engage in sex with strangers. Previous relationships have been ruined over this impulsive sexual behavior. Sometimes she will spend excessive amounts of money or go on last minute trips, and she has racked up a significant amount of credit card debt. The client stated that she often feels differently days later and wonders why she participated in these behaviors. She remembers looking back and wondering what she was thinking at the time.

6. Often part of a manic episode, what is it called when someone is speaking more rapidly, often switching from one train of thought to another, with the extreme need to share their thoughts, ideas, and comments?
    a. Interrupting
    b. Pressured speech
    c. Narcissistic monologue
    d. Hyperverbal speech

7. What term refers to the dysfunctional preoccupation with sexual fantasies, urges, or behaviors that are difficult to control?
    a. Impulsivity
    b. Sexual dysfunction
    c. Hypersexuality
    d. Lack of sexual desire

8. The client's disappearing for days, excessive spending, and risky sexual behaviors are all evidence of what symptom of bipolar disorder?
    a. Manic episode
    b. Depressive episode
    c. Hyperactivity
    d. Risky behavior

9. Borderline personality disorder involves a longstanding pattern of which behavior?
    a. Distinct episodes of mania lasting days or weeks
    b. Changes in mood that are not triggered by conflicts in interactions with other people
    c. Distinct episodes of depression lasting days or weeks
    d. Abrupt, moment-to-moment swings in moods, relationships, self-image, and behavior

Part Three

<u>Fourth session, three weeks after the initial session:</u>
During the previous session, you discussed the client's personal goals for counseling. You also determined the best treatment method for the client, which will include the practice of core

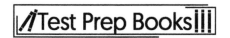

mindfulness and developing skills for interpersonal effectiveness, emotion regulation, and distress tolerance. This session you spoke about how these methods will help the client deal with everyday interactions with friends and family and help them to develop the skills to maintain interpersonal relationships. During the session, you noticed that she has scars and lesions all over both of her arms. When you inquire about them, she mentioned how she recently got into a fight with her sister. She reacted by cutting herself so she can "feel something other than anger and emptiness." You express empathy for what the client is experiencing. You then utilize this opportunity to discuss impulsive and emotion-driven behaviors and positive ways to cope with negative emotions. You teach the client "what" skills, where the client can observe, describe, and participate fully in the present moment, and "how" skills, where the client can focus on the present moment with a non-judgmental mindset, focusing on one thing at a time, and in an effective manner.

10. What therapeutic technique involves core mindfulness, interpersonal effectiveness, emotion regulation, and distress tolerance?
    a. Psychotherapy
    b. Cognitive behavioral therapy
    c. Dialectical behavior therapy
    d. Transference-focused therapy

11. For individuals with borderline personality disorder, emotions can be intense and volatile leading to dysfunctional behaviors. What are the skills and strategies for enhancing control over personal emotions?
    a. Distress tolerance
    b. Emotion regulation
    c. Interpersonal effectiveness
    d. Coping skills

12. The counselor taught the client which strategy for coping with impulsive and emotion-driven behaviors, using "what" skills and "how" skills?
    a. Emotional detachment
    b. Emotional dysregulation
    c. Psychosocial skills
    d. Mindfulness

13. What is the deliberate, self-inflected destruction of body tissue without suicidal intent, including cutting, burning, biting, or scratching skin?
    a. Nonsuicidal self-injury
    b. High-risk behaviors
    c. Suicidal behavior
    d. Suicidal ideation

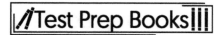
Case Study #10

Part One

Intake

<u>Client</u>

Age: 9

Sex: Male

Gender: Male

Sexuality: Heterosexual

Ethnicity: White

Relationship Status: Single

Counseling Setting: Outpatient—pediatric counseling office

Types of Counseling: Individual and family

Presenting Problem: Defiant, angry, and uncooperative behavior that affects his school and home life, inability to control emotions and conduct behavior in a socially appropriate manner

Diagnosis: F91.3 Oppositional defiant disorder

Presenting Problem:

Your new client is a 9-year-old boy who is in fourth grade. Over the past year, his parents and teachers have noticed a drastic change in his behavior. The client's teacher has reported that whenever the client is asked to stop doing what he wants to do, or to start doing something he doesn't wish to do, he begins to throw things in the classroom. It started with smaller items like pencils but has escalated. He has now thrown books off the shelves and has even attempted to rip posters off of the walls. His teacher is concerned for his safety and the safety of other students. She noticed that this behavior has also affected his relationships with friends at school. After witnessing his frequent outbursts, other students do not want to sit with him in class or play with him at recess. The school and his parents are quite concerned and wish for the client to receive the help he needs to function in a more socially and emotionally appropriate manner.

Mental Status:

The client has been exhibiting increasingly defiant and uncooperative behavior at home and in school. What started as verbal refusal to normal requests, such as picking up his room or finishing his homework, has escalated to more violent outbursts and throwing things. His parents and teachers did not notice the shift in behavior until this school year. The client is not able to control his emotions in socially acceptable ways, leading to difficulties with friends, family life, and school.

224

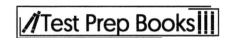

Family History:

The client's home life has been suffering this year. He lives with his mother, father, and little sister. At home, his parents have only noticed this behavior when his mother asks him to do chores, start his homework, or brush his teeth. He is especially bothered if he is in the middle of another activity, like viewing a tablet or playing a game. He will attempt to hit his mother or throw clothes, schoolbooks, and bathroom items on the ground or directly at his mother. When his father interacts with him, there never seems to be any conflict. When asked if the client has any family history of oppositional defiant disorder, his mother noted that his uncle has had mental health problems, including antisocial personality disorder.

1. The client's refusal to cooperate or comply with small requests from his teacher and mother illustrate which symptom of oppositional defiant disorder?
   a. Often angry and resentful
   b. Often deliberately annoys others
   c. Often actively defies or refuses to comply with requests from authority figures
   d. Often blames others for their mistakes or misbehavior

2. Based on the client's history, what is one factor that may be linked to his oppositional defiant disorder?
   a. Genetics
   b. Environment
   c. Biological defect
   d. Brain injury

3. When parents are not able to get their child's oppositional defiant disorder under control, it may escalate to what disorder in their teenage and adult years, with symptoms including aggression toward people and animals, destruction of property, deceitfulness, and theft?
   a. Borderline personality disorder
   b. Antisocial personality disorder
   c. Bipolar disorder
   d. Conduct disorder

4. What disorder, defined by symptoms of impulsivity, hyperactivity, inability to focus, and irritability is almost always comorbid with oppositional defiant disorder?
   a. Sensory processing disorder
   b. Attention-deficit/hyperactivity disorder
   c. Conduct disorder
   d. Autism spectrum disorder

5. Which of the following is NOT true when diagnosing an individual with oppositional defiant disorder?
   a. Level of severity is determined by how many areas of life are negatively affected
   b. Individual must exhibit four of the eight criteria for at least six months
   c. Must negatively impact their functioning at work, school, or home
   d. Client must be a male between the ages of eight and twelve years old

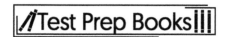

Part Two

<u>Second session, one week after the initial intake:</u>
You decided to spend the majority of this session speaking to the client alone, talking about their emotions and behaviors at school and at home. When his parents were not in the room, he was cooperative and would answer specific questions when asked. He was allowed to explore the room and play with toys as long as he participated in the conversation. He seemed to understand this rule and participated very well. The client admitted that he has not been a good listener at school and at home. When asked for an explanation for his recent behavior, the client often blamed the teacher, other students, or his mother. You focused on building trust, expressing empathy, and explaining what you would be doing in counseling in terms he could understand. You collaborated to determine the client's goals for counseling.

His parents joined the session for the final fifteen minutes. You explained that you will continue individual sessions to build a comfort level with the client before moving on to family sessions as well. You explained that you will be working with the parents and teaching them techniques to help their child improve his behavior and learn new social and emotional skills. You emphasized the importance of making clear cut rules, being consistent, and rewarding desired behaviors.

6. Found to be extremely successful with children with oppositional defiant disorder, what is the treatment method that involves teaching parents techniques to help their children improve behaviors and learn new skills?
   a. Cognitive behavioral therapy
   b. Dialectical behavior therapy
   c. Parent management training
   d. Psychotherapy

7. What is the treatment method that works with oppositional defiant disorder by replacing symptoms like defiance and irritability with calming thoughts and positive strategies?
   a. Social skills training
   b. Cognitive behavioral therapy
   c. Mindfulness
   d. Play therapy

8. What is an unrealistic therapeutic goal for a child with oppositional defiant disorder?
   a. Correct and replace all negative, defiant, or uncooperative behaviors
   b. Teach emotional management strategies and social skills
   c. Reduce intensity and frequency of defiant and hostile behaviors toward adults
   d. Terminate temper tantrums and replace them with calm, respectful compliance to adult directions

9. What term, described in B.F. Skinner's theory of operant conditioning, refers to when a response or behavior is followed by a reward, leading to repetition of the desired behavior?
   a. Negative reinforcement
   b. Punishment
   c. Extinction
   d. Positive reinforcement

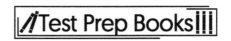

Part Three

Fourth session, three weeks after the initial session:

During the previous session, you started to work on social skills training for the client. You continue to teach the client creative problem solving during this session. You encourage the client to talk about conflicts with his teacher, friends, or family members and weigh options for responding. The client tells you about a conflict with his teacher in class this week. When free play time was over, the teacher asked him to put away his toys and sit at his desk. The client threw his toys and refused to sit down. You discussed more socially acceptable methods to deal with this conflict. You acted out the part of the teacher and the client was able to practice problem solving and choosing a healthier reaction to the teacher's request.

You have also been working with the client's parents on rewarding positive behaviors, correcting negative behaviors, and using clear and consistent rules at home. With these clear rules and consequences, his parents have reported his behavior at home is already improving. He has been more cooperative when asked to complete his homework or items from his chore list. When he completes these tasks, he is given a reward, such as a special treat or playing with his favorite game. You have trained his parents to show social skills and problem-solving skills at home as well. Through observing these behaviors, the child will learn new social skills without direct instruction.

10. What is a way to proactively teach children creative problem solving?
    a. Discuss what the client did wrong when resolving conflicts with friends or family.
    b. Talk about conflicts with friends or family and generate a list of potential strategies and responses.
    c. Tell the client that responding with angry or aggressive behavior is never acceptable.
    d. Using consistent, evidence-based discipline.

11. The client's parents have learned to show social skills and problem-solving skills at home without directly instructing the client. What is it called when a person observes the behavior of another and then imitates that behavior?
    a. Reinforcement
    b. Mindfulness
    c. Modeling
    d. Prosocial behaviors

12. What method was the counselor using when they reenacted a recent conflict with the teacher, allowing the student to problem solve and choose a new response?
    a. Role-playing
    b. Social skills training
    c. Play therapy
    d. Anger management

13. What step should you take next when the client's behavior is improving at home but not at school?
    a. Continue to reward positive behaviors at home until behavior improves at school.
    b. Meet with the client and the teacher to discuss in-school behavior.
    c. Remove the client from school until his behavior improves.
    d. Work with the teacher to create a behavioral contract with clear rules and consequences for the client to sign.

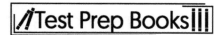
Case Study #11

Part One

Intake

<u>Client</u>

Age: 58

Sex: Female

Gender: Female

Sexuality: Heterosexual

Ethnicity: White

Relationship Status: Married

Counseling Setting: Outpatient—community counseling office

Types of Counseling: Individual

Presenting Problem: Grieving the loss of her father and experiencing the additional stress of taking care of her mother, which is leading to difficulties in her work and home life

Diagnosis: V62.82 Uncomplicated bereavement

Presenting Problem:

Your new client is a 58-year-old schoolteacher who has recently lost her father to a heart attack. She has taken her mother in to live with her and her family. The client and her husband have been married for twenty years and have two teenage sons. The client has expressed great sadness over the loss of her father and is finding it very difficult to work all day and then return home to manage her family's affairs and care for her mother. Her mother has diabetes and requires specialized care with regular medical visits. Her mother does not drive herself, so the client is responsible for taking her to these appointments, the pharmacy, the grocery store, and other outings. As a result, the client has taken several days off from work over the last few months. The client and her husband have been bickering a lot lately over small things, and there is a lot of tension in the house. The client expressed the need to "get her life back on track," and with all the different responsibilities on her shoulders, she doesn't even know where to begin.

Mental Status:

When the client arrived late to the first session, her hair was unkempt, and she appeared to be very rushed. She apologized and explained that she has had so many responsibilities lately that it is difficult to keep up. Along with missing her father and experiencing feelings of sadness, she is also trying to keep up with her job as a schoolteacher, care for her two teenage sons, and assist her recently widowed mother. She stated that she has felt overwhelmed and has had little to no time to herself. The client

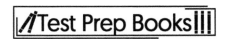
reported feeling shortness of breath, a rapid heartbeat, and difficulty concentrating. She can generally fall asleep with little trouble, but she wakes up several times in the night.

Family History:

The client has been experiencing a lot of changes in her home life and family dynamics recently. She is dealing with the loss of her father and has also allowed her mother to move into her house so she can help care for her. This is also putting strain on the client's relationship with her husband. She feels like she never has time with him, and she is often taking care of her mother or her two teenage sons. She and her husband usually have a great relationship, but lately there has been a lot of tension and small arguments. The client has an older brother who is married with no children. He lives an hour away and said he would come to help with their mother anytime. She admitted she hasn't asked for his help, but she feels like she is in this alone.

1. Feelings of sadness, difficulty concentrating, and sleeping disruption are symptoms of grief and what serious and long-lasting mood disorder?
   a. Bipolar disorder
   b. Major depressive disorder
   c. Generalized anxiety disorder
   d. Social anxiety disorder

2. Besides the loss of her father, what other major life changes may be adding to the client's level of stress?
   a. Caring for her teenage sons
   b. Working full time as a schoolteacher
   c. Becoming a caregiver for her mother
   d. Arguing with her husband more frequently

3. What disorder would you diagnose if the duration of the individual's bereavement lasts at least six months and exceeds expected social, cultural, or religious norms?
   a. Major depressive disorder
   b. Generalized anxiety disorder
   c. Insomnia
   d. Prolonged grief disorder

4. Which of the following is an example of the counselor expressing empathy for the client?
   a. "I understand that you have been feeling overwhelmed lately, and you have a lot of responsibilities on your shoulders right now."
   b. "When I was caring for my elderly mother, I felt very overwhelmed and exhausted too."
   c. "You have too much on your plate right now, and you should ask for help."
   d. "Tell me more about what has been overwhelming for you lately."

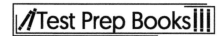

5. Often helpful for individuals experiencing grief and bereavement, what form of therapy is based on the core idea that talking about things that are bothering you can allow you to process what you are feeling and help with emotional distress?
 a. Exposure Therapy
 b. Interpersonal Therapy
 c. Psychotherapy
 d. Psychodynamic Therapy

Part Two

Second session, one week after the initial intake:

The client arrived at the session visibly exhausted and admitted she has not been getting any rest lately. When asked to describe her day-to-day life, she recognized there have been a lot of changes over the past few months. She has been working full time, taking her teenage sons to most of their activities, and taking care of her mother on evenings and weekends. She used to have time to socialize once or twice a week, often attending book clubs and dinners with friends. She said she hasn't had the time or energy for these activities. The disagreements with her husband have become more frequent as well. He is frustrated that she won't ask her brother for help with caring for her mother. He also said he feels neglected since they usually have a date night once a week. After her mother moved in, the client doesn't want to leave her alone on Friday nights. While she wishes she could please everyone, she feels like she isn't pleasing anyone. She reported that she is feeling hopeless, and she doesn't know what to do next. To relate to the client and build trust, you share your personal experience about caring for your elderly mother. You explain how you, too, felt hopeless when trying to handle it on your own until you came to the realization that you needed to ask for help and support from friends and family members.

6. Which of the five stages of grief would you say the client is currently experiencing, with the current symptoms of withdrawing from social activities, feeling overwhelmed, and experiencing trouble sleeping and feelings of hopelessness?
 a. Anger
 b. Depression
 c. Bargaining
 d. Denial

7. What is the condition characterized by physical, mental, and emotional exhaustion typically resulting from an individual neglecting their own physical and emotional health because they are focused on caring for an ill or injured loved one?
 a. Major depressive disorder
 b. Job burnout
 c. Caregiver stress syndrome
 d. Uncomplicated bereavement

8. What is the long-term therapeutic goal for this client?
 a. Reduce levels of stress and teach healthy coping mechanisms
 b. Improve occupational functioning
 c. Improve social functioning
 d. Create a schedule for all her new responsibilities

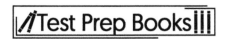

9. What counseling skill was being applied when the counselor shared a personal story about being a caregiver for her mother?
   a. Confrontation
   b. Immediacy
   c. Self-disclosure
   d. Interpretation

Part Three

Fourth session, three weeks after the initial session:

During the last two sessions, you have focused on building a positive therapeutic relationship with the client and working together to set realistic goals for therapy. You have established that while she has been grieving the loss of her father, the cause of most of her stress is becoming a caregiver for her mother while still caring for her children and working full time. The client had a breakthrough last session, where she realized she can't do everything on her own. She recognized that it is okay to ask for help when she needs it. Last session, you created a schedule of weekly responsibilities that she could ask for help with. With your assistance, she identified her husband and her brother as people who want to help. She was happy to report that she completed her homework assignment by asking her husband and brother to divide up some of the responsibilities. Her brother is now going to take their mother to her weekly doctor's visit and on another outing on Friday nights. Her husband is going to take their sons to soccer practice on Monday and Wednesday nights. This will allow the client to have more free time to focus on herself, relax, and de-stress. She expressed surprised that they were happy to help her! While having this support a few times a week is a step in the right direction, the client still feels like she needs additional help. She has trouble falling asleep and staying asleep. She is exhausted, and her performance at work has been suffering. You pull together additional resources and let the client know there are options that may allow her to take a break from full-time work. You also encourage the client to resume some of her normal activities, such as time with friends and date nights with her husband.

10. What is the term that describes when a client has an "aha!" moment in counseling, suddenly becoming aware of a factor in their life that was previously unknown?
   a. Empathy
   b. Insight
   c. Self-awareness
   d. Reflection

11. Which of the following techniques would help the client prioritize self-care, boost their mood, and reduce their level of stress?
   a. Exercise
   b. Mindfulness
   c. Healthy eating
   d. All of the above

12. The client is exhausted and is having difficulty falling asleep and staying asleep. What type of medication would you recommend to the client?
   a. Sedatives
   b. Antidepressants
   c. Analgesics
   d. Stimulants

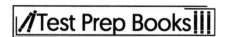

13. Based on the client's concerns with work performance and work life balance, what advice would you give next?

    a. Advise the client to quit her job, so she has more free time and less stress.

    b. Provide the client with information about the Family and Medical Leave Act, through which she could receive up to 12 weeks of unpaid, job-protected leave.

    c. Tell the client to focus on work and stop taking on other responsibilities at home.

    d. Call her employer directly to tell them what she is going through.

Answer Explanations

Case Study #1

1. D: Choice *D* is correct. Binge eating large amounts of food is a unique characteristic of Bulimia. Anorexia typically involves restricting calories, but not binge eating. Choices *A*, *B*, and *C* are incorrect. They are all common behaviors of people with both Anorexia and Bulimia.

2. B: Choice *B* is correct. The severity of Bulimia Nervosa is determined based on the number of binge-eating episodes per week. Since the client has between 4-7 episodes per week, the severity of her diagnosis is Moderate. Choices *A*, *C*, and *D* are incorrect because feelings of guilt, amount of exercise, and being late for other obligations are not taken into consideration when determining severity of diagnosis.

3. C: Choice *C* is correct. Comorbidity is the simultaneous, but independent, presence of two or more medical conditions. For example, a client may have both Bulimia Nervosa and Depression. Choice *A* is incorrect. Codependence is a condition characterized by the need for approval due to low self-esteem. It involves an unhealthy attachment and relationship with another person. Choice *B* is incorrect. Diagnosis is the process of identifying a disease, condition, or injury from its symptoms. Choice *D* is incorrect. Morbidity is the condition of suffering from a disease or medical condition.

4. A: Choice *A* is correct. Major depression is the most common comorbidity with Bulimia Nervosa. Anxiety disorders, such as generalized anxiety disorder, panic disorder, post-traumatic stress disorder, and obsessive-compulsive disorder are also common. Choices *B*, *C*, and *D* are incorrect. Schizophrenia, bipolar disorder, and dissociative identity disorder are not commonly associated with Bulimia Nervosa. Also, the client did not show any specific symptoms of these disorders.

5. D: Choice *D* is correct because being late to school and work are both evidence that the client's eating disorder is affecting other areas of their life. Choices *A* and *B* are incorrect. They are both symptoms of the eating disorder but do not illustrate how it is affecting other areas of the client's life. Choice *C* is incorrect. The client working and attending college are not evidence of the eating disorder or how it is affecting the client's quality of life.

6. C: Choice *C* is correct. The therapeutic alliance, also known as the therapeutic relationship, helping alliance, or working alliance, is one of the most important predictors of success in therapy. All of these terms refer to the relationship between the counselor and their client. The therapeutic alliance is a measure of the relationship and collaboration between the counselor and the client. Choice *A*, *B*, and *C* are incorrect. The mental health diagnosis, the experience level of the counselor, and the ability to follow directions are not main predictors of success in therapy.

7. A: Choice *A* is correct. Cognitive behavioral therapy is the form of psychological treatment that involves recognizing and changing unhelpful ways of thinking and learned patterns of unhelpful behaviors. Individuals experiencing psychological problems can learn better ways of coping through challenging these negative or unhelpful thinking patterns and behaviors. This form of treatment is often utilized for clients with eating disorders. Choices *B*, *C*, and *D* are incorrect because these forms of therapy are not characterized by recognizing and challenging unhelpful thoughts or unhelpful behavior patterns.

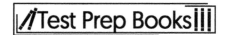

8. C: Choice *C* is correct. If you are not trained in a specific area, it is best to refer the client to another counselor who has the proper training and experience. Choices *A* and *D* are incorrect. While focusing on self-esteem, depression, or other issues may be helpful, it is most important to focus on the primary diagnosis of the client. Choice *B* is incorrect. Researching the topic yourself in order to keep the client is not what is best for the client. Ethically, it is best to refer the client to a counselor who has experience treating clients with eating disorders.

9. B: Choice *B* is correct. This statement is an example of empathic responding. Empathic responding is expressing an understanding of how the client feels and the reason behind that feeling. Choice *A* is incorrect. This is not an empathic response and could come across as negative or judgmental. Choice *C* is incorrect. This is an example of a reflection, not empathy. Choice *D* is incorrect. This is not an empathic response. It is an example of developing discrepancy with the client.

10. D: Choice *D* is correct. Identifying and addressing distorted perceptions about food, learning how to eat healthy portions of food, and managing compulsive behaviors such as excessive exercising are all realistic treatment goals for this client. Through the use of cognitive behavioral therapy, the counselor will address each of the above thought processes and behavior patterns. Choice *A* is incorrect. Different levels of treatment include outpatient, inpatient, or residential counseling. Choice *B* is incorrect. Concurrent treatment refers to the use of two treatments at the same time, for example a client who is in both couples therapy and individual therapy. Choice *C* is incorrect because the goals listed are not barriers to client goal attainment. An example of a common barrier is a difference between counselor and client perspectives on goal setting.

11. A: Choice *A* is correct. Congruence is when a therapist is real, authentic, and genuine with their clients. Congruence refers to the counselor's inner experience matching their outward expression. Congruence is important in therapeutic relationships, as good therapeutic relationships are based on trust and honesty, which is shown through congruence. Choice *B* is incorrect. Empathy is the expression of regard for the client's feelings and experiences. Choice *C* is incorrect. Reflection involves restating or reflecting back the client's thoughts or feelings. Choice *D* is incorrect. Positive regard involves caring for the client and accepting and valuing the client as they are without judgement, criticism, or evaluation.

12. B: Choice *B* is correct. This statement is an example of amplified reflection. In amplified reflection, the idea the client expressed is stated back by the counselor in an overstated or dramatic way. The goal is for the client to be more understanding after hearing this exaggeration of their own feelings. Choice *A* is incorrect. This is an example of an empathic statement. Choice *C* is incorrect. This is an example of reflection. Choice *D* is incorrect. This is an example of an open-ended question.

13. D: Choice *D* is correct. The term *social connectedness* refers to Adler's belief that all people wish to belong and that as humans we need one another. Choices *A* and *B* are incorrect. Introversion and extraversion are personality traits described by Jung. Jung described introverts as being focused more on the internal world of reflection and extraverts as preferring to engage with the outside world of objects. Choice *C* is incorrect. Compensation is a defense mechanism where individuals cover up weaknesses or feelings of inadequacy in one area of life by overachieving in another area of life.

Cast Study #2

1. C: Choice *C* is correct. The severity of alcohol use disorder is determined by the number of symptoms present. The client's case is considered mild if they have 2-3 symptoms present, moderate if there are 4-

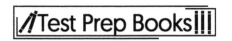

5 symptoms, and severe if there are 6 or more symptoms. Choices A, B, and D are incorrect. While it's important to understand how many drinks a client is consuming, how many months this has been an issue, and the client's feelings about drinking, this information isn't taken into consideration when determining the severity of alcohol use disorder.

2. A: Choice A is correct. In the family history section of the intake, the client revealed that he is having issues with his mother and father due to his drinking. These are social or interpersonal problems cause by the alcohol use. Choices B and C are incorrect. The increased amount of sleep and low mood described in the mental status section of the intake are evidence of symptoms related to depression, not persistent interpersonal problems. Choice D is incorrect. The client explained that he used to drink socially with his father, but this was before it became a larger issue causing interpersonal problems.

3. B: Choice B is correct. Tolerance occurs when a person must drink increasingly larger amounts of alcohol to become intoxicated, or when the same amount of alcohol results in a lower level of intoxication. Choice A is incorrect. Withdrawal is the occurrence of physical and mental symptoms when a person stops drinking or cuts back on the amount they have been drinking. Choice C is incorrect. Binge drinking is when an individual drinks a lot of alcohol within a short time frame. Choice D is incorrect. Persistent social or interpersonal problems caused by alcohol use is a symptom of alcohol use disorder, but this symptom is not defined by how much a person can drink without feeling the side effects.

4. D: Choice D is correct. Counselors use confrontation to point out inconsistencies they observe in the client's words and behavior. Choice A is incorrect. Paradoxical intervention is a technique created by Alfred Adler. It is commonly referred to as reverse psychology. Choice B is incorrect. Active listening is a technique used by counselors that involves listening carefully to a client and questioning when necessary to get an accurate understanding of what the client is both expressing and feeling. Choice C is incorrect. Accurate empathy occurs when a counselor can experience the client's point of view in terms of feelings and cognitions, sensitively and accurately in the here and now.

5. A: Choice A is correct. Lack of motivation, low mood, and sleeping more than usual are all symptoms of major depressive disorder. Choices B, C, and D are incorrect. Although each of these symptoms may be present in people with these disorders, the presence of the three symptoms together are not common indicators of generalized anxiety disorder, post-traumatic stress disorder, or borderline personality disorder.

6. B: Choice B is correct. Denial occurs when an individual refuses to accept or believe the uncomfortable or painful truth about negative events happening in their life. The individual pushes away reality in order to protect themselves from experiencing negative thoughts and emotions. In this case, the client is in denial that his drinking is a serious issue, explaining it away by saying that his friends drink all the time too. Using denial as a coping mechanism interferes with treatment and reaching treatment goals. Choice A is incorrect. Repression occurs when individuals cannot recall certain memories or traumatic situations without the assistance of therapeutic tools like hypnosis. Choice C is incorrect. Compensation is a defense mechanism where individuals focus on overachieving in certain things to make up for failures in other areas of their life. Choice D is incorrect. Sublimation is a defense mechanism in which individuals focus socially unacceptable or other undesirable urges into more acceptable or constructive behaviors.

7. D: Choice D is correct. Interpersonal psychotherapy is a counseling approach that is used with clients who have mood disorders, such as depression, to help strengthen relationships and social interactions

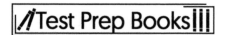

that have deteriorated due to the disorder. This would be a good treatment option for a client who would like to improve relationships with family and friends. Choices A, B, and C are incorrect because these forms of therapy are not characterized by the specific focus on interpersonal and social relationships.

8. A: Choice A is correct. Reflection is the method used when the counselor repeats the client's words back to them. This statement accurately reflects what the client has expressed and shows that the counselor is listening and understands the client's feelings. Choice B is incorrect. Brief invitations to continue speaking, such as "Tell me more," are called encouragers. Encouragers include a variety of verbal and nonverbal ways of prompting the client to continue talking. Choice C is incorrect. While this statement may be accurate, it is not a reflection of what the client is saying. Choice D is incorrect. While the question is important, asking it in this way may be seen as confrontational. If proper trust has not been built, the client may feel defensive in response to the statements in C and D.

9. D: Choice D is correct. A test with true/false answers has dichotomous recognition items. This simply means there are two opposing choices. Choice A, B, and C are incorrect. These types of assessments are not characterized by true/false answers. A multipoint item is when there are three or four forced choices, as seen on multiple choice tests. Free choice is when an examinee can respond in any way he or she chooses. Fill-in-the-blank questions leave a blank to be written in or filled using provided options.

10. C: Choice C is correct. When a counselor states that privileged communication is qualified, this means that exceptions may exist. Some common exceptions to confidentiality include reporting abuse, or if the client intends to hurt themselves or others. Choice A is incorrect. There are limits to confidentiality between the client and the counselor. Choice B is incorrect. In individual counseling, the details of counseling sessions cannot be shared with the client's family members. Choice D is incorrect. There are certain instances where the counselor would have to disclose information discussed in counseling.

11. B: Choice B is correct. Resistance is the client's tendency to fight or challenge the therapeutic process. The client was showing resistance to the process by refusing to do their treatment homework. Choice A is incorrect. Projection is when an individual unconsciously assigns feelings or attributes that are true about themselves to another person. Choice C is incorrect. The defense mechanism rationalization is used to explain unacceptable behavior by giving logical and rational reasons for the behavior. Choice D is incorrect. Collaboration refers to negotiating the goals for counseling and deciding the best steps to reach those goals. Collaboration involves actively participating in the therapeutic process, not resisting it.

12. D: Choice D is correct. Insight occurs when a client suddenly becomes aware of a factor in their life that was previously unknown. This can also be referred to as the "Aha! moment." Choice A is incorrect. Repression occurs when individuals cannot recall certain memories or traumatic situations without the assistance of therapeutic tools such as hypnosis. Choice B is incorrect. Introjection is a method that children use to cope with having parents who are unavailable or absent. Choice C is incorrect. Denial is a coping mechanism where an individual protects themselves by pushing away negative thoughts and emotions and not dealing with negative events.

13. A: Choice A is correct. Active listening is a technique where the counselor listens carefully to a client and asks them questions. The counselor is able to show that they fully understand both the content of the message and what the client is feeling. This statement shows the counselor is listening and clarifying

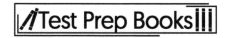

what the client has expressed. Choice *B* is incorrect. Nodding is a gesture that silently lets someone know you are engaged. However, without paraphrasing or asking further questions, it is not active listening. Choice *C* is incorrect. Asking a confrontational question is not a form of active listening. Choice *D* is incorrect. Looking down or writing in a notebook are not characteristics of active listening.

Case Study #3

1. D: Choice *D* is correct. The major life event that may have triggered the client's depression is her recent divorce. Most of her symptoms, including extreme sadness, lack of energy, and loss of interest in life and socializing began after the divorce. Choice *B* is incorrect. While the loss of a job does qualify as a major life event that can trigger depression, the client did not lose her job. She has continued to attend work. Choices *A* and *C* are incorrect. While these are major life events, they occurred decades ago and did not trigger this depression.

2. A: Choice *A* is correct. The fact that coworkers have noticed a change in her mood and appearance (such as appearing tearful) is evidence of a depressed mood that is observed by others. Choices *B, C,* and *D* are incorrect. They are all symptoms of depression but cannot be inferred by her coworker's observations.

3. B: Choice *B* is correct. When determining the diagnosis of major depressive disorder, you must exclude schizophrenia, delusional disorder, and other psychotic disorders. Choices *A, C,* and *D* are incorrect, because these disorders do not need to be excluded when diagnosing depression. Generalized anxiety disorder, obsessive-compulsive disorder, and post-traumatic stress disorder are common comorbidities for people with depression.

4. C: Choice *C* is correct. Based on the information provided in the intake, we can assume that the client's depression is brought on by a combination of genetic and environmental factors. Clients who have family members or parents with depression often have a higher likelihood of experiencing depression themselves. Environmental factors such as the major life event of her divorce also played a role. Choice *A* and *B* are incorrect. Genetic factors or environmental factors alone did not cause the depression. Choice *D* is incorrect because the client does not have a history of substance abuse.

5. A: Choice *A* is correct. The Patient Health Questionnaire-9 is considered a diagnostic test because it is used to diagnose an illness or condition—specifically, depression. It can also be used to determine the severity of depression based on how many symptoms are present and the strength of the client's self-reported answers. Choice *B* is incorrect, because summative evaluations provide an overall picture to decide whether goals and progress standards are met. These are typically used in an educational setting. Choice *C* is incorrect because norm-referenced tests are any assessments in which scores are interpreted in comparison with a norm. For example, an IQ test is a norm-referenced test. Choice *D* is incorrect, because a performance appraisal is a process of setting goals and measuring and enhancing individual and organization performance. This type of test is often used in career development.

6. D: Choice *D* is correct. Sigmund Freud is known as the "father of psychoanalysis." He developed this treatment modality for patients who were not responding to other medical or psychological treatments that were available at the time. Choices *A, B,* and *C* are incorrect. Although they were influenced by the work of Sigmund Freud, they are not credited with the invention of talk therapy.

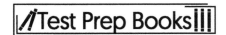

7. B: Choice *B* is correct. Medication-assisted therapy has been shown to be effective with people suffering from emotional or behavioral problems such as depression. Medication in combination with talk therapy has been shown to be more effective than talk therapy or medication alone. Choice *A* is incorrect, because it has been shown to be very effective. Choice *C* is incorrect, because talk therapy alone has similar effectiveness long term. The success of talk therapy is similar if the client sticks with the counseling for a significant period of time. Choice *D* is incorrect, as there is no evidence to suggest that medication interferes with the effectiveness of talk therapy.

8. A: Choice *A* is correct. A support system is a network of people who provide an individual with practical or emotional assistance. When a client feels isolated or alone, developing a support system is an important goal. Choices *B*, *C*, and *D* are incorrect. Family, friends, and the counselor are all critical parts of a support system, but each one alone is not a network. A healthy support system can include all these people.

9. C: Choice *C* is correct. Collaboration is the process of working together with a client to establish treatment goals and objectives. It is about negotiating the goals for counseling and deciding how to reach them. Choice *A* is incorrect because codependence occurs when an individual is focused on the needs of others rather than their own needs. Choices *B* and *D* are also incorrect. The therapeutic relationship, also known as the helping relationship, refers to the relationship between a counselor and client. A therapeutic relationship involves mutual trust, honesty, and respect. Collaboration is a critical part of a good therapeutic relationship.

10. B: Choice *B* is correct. Goal attainment scaling focuses on a time-limited goal and measuring the degree to which that goal has been achieved. Choice *A* is incorrect. Goal setting is one of the first steps of goal attainment and involves identifying and clearly defining goals and pathways to reach those goals. Choices *C* and *D* are incorrect. Resistance and rationalization are both defense mechanisms that can act as barriers to goal attainment.

11. C: Choice *C* is correct. This is an example of self-disclosure. Self-disclosure refers to a counselor's sharing of personal information in order to bond with their clients and show them a different point of view. When used sparingly, it is helpful and reveals similarities between the counselor and the client. Choice *A* is incorrect, as this is an example of reflection. Choice *B* is incorrect because this is an example of amplified reflection. Choice *D* is incorrect, as this is not an example of self-disclosure because the counselor is not sharing a personal experience.

12. A: Choice *A* is correct. The defense mechanism of idealization occurs when individuals focus only on someone's positive qualities and ignore their flaws. Choice *B* is incorrect. Denial is a coping mechanism that is used by individuals to ignore unfavorable circumstances in order to protect themselves from the associated negative feelings. Choice *C* is incorrect. Regression is a defense mechanism in which clients, often children, will suddenly act younger again, "escape" to an earlier stage of development, or revert to past behaviors to cope with trauma or loss. Choice *D* is incorrect. Displacement occurs when individuals experience negative reactions or emotions but redirect these responses to a person or source who is less likely to react negatively than the person or source who actually caused the reactions.

13. B: Choice *B* is correct. Rumination occurs when someone experiences persistent thoughts that focus on negative content. Focusing on these negative thoughts and emotions is often harmful and causes emotional distress. The client focusing on her divorce and what she perceives as past failures every day after work is a form of ruminating. These thoughts are causing her emotional distress and making it

238

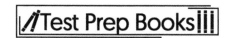

impossible for her to live in the present or future. Choice *A* is incorrect. Repression occurs when an individual pushes away memories, emotions, or thoughts that are causing emotional distress. Choice *C* is incorrect, as introspection is the practice of observing one's own mental and emotional processes, thoughts, and feelings. Choice *D* is incorrect because sublimation is a method to reduce anxiety caused by unacceptable or unhealthy feelings or urges by focusing on more socially acceptable behaviors.

Case Study #4

1. C: Choice *C* is correct. Based on her symptoms, the client has the combined type of ADHD, in which symptoms of both inattention and hyperactivity/impulsivity are present. Choice *A* is incorrect. The inattentive type does not include the symptoms of hyperactivity or impulsivity that she exhibits. Choice *B* is incorrect because the hyperactive-impulsive type does not include the symptoms of inattention that she exhibits. Choice *D* is incorrect because mild is not a type of ADHD. It is a level of severity. ADHD can be mild, moderate, or severe.

2. D: Choice *D* is correct. It is common for children to act out in school when they have a life change such as a new sibling *and* when they have a disorder like autism, ADHD, anxiety, or a learning disorder. Choices *A* and *B* are not the best choices because it is common in both instances. Choice *C* is incorrect because while it is common for children to act out when they have oppositional defiant disorder, this behavior is not exclusive to this disorder.

3. A: Choice *A* is correct. Neurodevelopmental disorders are disorders in which the brain and the nervous system are affected. This can lead to differences in experiencing emotions, thought processes, learning abilities, and memory development. Choice *B* is incorrect. Psychotic disorders cause abnormal ways of thinking, distorted thoughts, and false perceptions. Choice *C* is incorrect. Anxiety disorders are mental health disorders in which symptoms of anxiousness, nervousness, panic, fear, sweating, and rapid heartbeat may be present. Choice *D* is incorrect. Personality disorders are characterized by thoughts, emotions, and behaviors that deviate from the norm and cause problems with functioning in everyday life.

4. D: Choice *D* is correct. Oppositional defiant disorder includes the symptoms of acting argumentative and challenging people and is commonly comorbid with ADHD. Often symptoms in oppositional defiant disorder are more severe, including acting angry, defiant, and violent. Choice *A*, *B*, and *C* are incorrect. These symptoms are not common in anxiety disorder, major depressive disorder, or obsessive-compulsive disorder.

5. B: Choice *B* is correct, because impulsive individuals tend to interrupt others a lot and speak at inappropriate times. They find it difficult to listen to directions and wait their turn. Choices *A*, *C*, and *D* are incorrect. Interrupting is not best explained by characteristics of hyperactivity, lack of attention, or distractibility.

6. C: Choice *C* is correct. Regression is the defense mechanism used when one "escapes" to an earlier stage of development. This includes behaviors like tantrums, sucking the thumb, or carrying comfort items like a blanket or stuffed animal from an earlier age. Choice *A* is incorrect. Repression is when an individual unconsciously chooses to hide negative past experiences or emotions or forgets them entirely. Choice *B* is incorrect. Displacement is a defense mechanism in which individuals who are experiencing negative emotions or reactions direct them onto people who are less likely to respond negatively than the people who actually caused the negative emotions or reactions. Choice *D* is

239

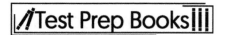

incorrect. Compartmentalization is separating one's life into independent sectors, to protect or block off issues from other parts of their life.

7. A: Choice *A* is correct. Self-regulation is the ability to both understand and control one's feelings, behaviors, and reactions to life events. Choice *B* is incorrect. Separation anxiety is a heightened sense of worry or fear of being separated from family members or other people that an individual is strongly attached to. Choice *C* is incorrect. Cognitive behavioral therapy is a type of therapeutic treatment that helps individuals pinpoint unhealthy or unhelpful patterns of thought and behavior and replace them with healthier and more productive thoughts and behaviors. Choice *D* is incorrect. Social skills are skills uses every day to interact and communicate with others. These include verbal and nonverbal communication, speech, gestures, facial expression, and body language.

8. D: Choice *D* is correct. Parents spending uninterrupted one-on-one time with their child each day helps to facilitate the secure attachment style. This attachment style is characterized by feeling worthy and deserving of love and trusting that their parents will not abandon them. Choices *A*, *B*, and *C* are incorrect. They are not considered healthy attachment styles. Children with these attachment styles do not have a secure attachment or relationship with their parents or caregivers.

9. A: Choice *A* is correct. John Bowlby is the psychologist who came up with attachment style. He was the first to focus on attachment, describing it as "a lasting psychological connectedness between human beings." Choices *B*, *C*, and *D* are incorrect. They are not attachment theorists. Lev Vygotsky focused on the sociocultural theory of cognitive development. Erik Erikson described eight stages of psychosocial development. His theory describes the development of personality throughout these stages, in a specific order, starting at infancy and moving through adulthood.

10. B: Choice *B* is correct. Reasonable accommodations are adjustments made in a system for an individual based on proven need. Examples of reasonable accommodations for children with ADHD include allowing them to stand at their desk, use a fidget toy in class, or get additional time on a test. Choice *A* is incorrect because operant conditioning occurs when an individual learns through the use of rewards and punishments to alter specific behaviors. Choice *C* is incorrect because reinforcement is the process of encouraging or establishing a belief or pattern of behavior by using a reward. Choice *D* is incorrect because a physical outlet can be used to release energy or anxiety, but it is not an adjustment provided within a system based on a proven need.

11. D: Choice *D* is correct. Hyperactivity can be displayed by the failure to sit still when necessary. Choices *A, B,* and *C* are incorrect. Standing and moving around in class are not best explained as characteristics of impulsivity, lack of attention, or distractibility.

12. C: Choice *C* is correct. This statement is a good example of empathy, which involves recognizing and acknowledging the child's feelings and why they are feeling that way. Choices *A* and *B* are incorrect because neither response demonstrates empathy. In both cases, the child's feelings are not understood or validated. Instead, the parent is telling the child not to feel the way they are feeling. Choice *D* is incorrect because this parent is responding by trying to distract the child with an activity to change their mood.

13. A: Choice *A* is correct. Stimulants are the most commonly used medications for the treatment of ADHD when behavioral therapy and parent training do not lessen the child's symptoms. Choices *B, C,*

240

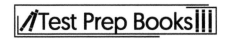

and *D* are incorrect. Antidepressants, depressants, and steroids are not appropriate medications for the treatment of ADHD.

Case Study #5

1. A: Choice *A* is correct. Cultural competence occurs when the counselor has an understanding of their own culture and how it affects their interactions with a client who has their own unique beliefs or is from another culture. Choice *B* is incorrect because a counselor with cultural competence will be more likely to take cultural considerations into account. Some examples of cultural considerations are language barriers, distrust of health care services, personal experiences/past trauma, or religious differences. Choice *C* is incorrect. Culture shock occurs when an individual has feelings of fear, anxiety, homesickness, and isolation while adapting to a new culture. Choice *D* is incorrect because the adjustment stage is one of the five stages of culture shock.

2. C: Choice *C* is correct. Narcissistic personality disorder is not commonly comorbid with social anxiety disorder. Individuals with narcissistic personality disorder often have an inflated ego, are self-centered, and lack empathy for others. Choices *A*, *B*, and *D* are incorrect, as generalized anxiety disorder, avoidant personality disorder, and panic disorder are all commonly associated with social anxiety disorder.

3. B: Choice *B* is correct. The comfort zone is the state of mind where an individual feels calm, comfortable, and in control. In the comfort zone, an individual does not feel anxiety or stress. Choices *A*, *C,* and *D* are incorrect. Personal growth happens between the comfort zone and the danger zone. The danger space is considered the reverse of the comfort zone. It is a place where the individual feels uncomfortable, out of control, and stressed. The learning zone is the mental and emotional space where people step out of their "comfort zone" to learn.

4. D: Choice *D* is correct, because avoiding anxiety-producing social situations and enduring social situations with intense fear and anxiety are both common reactions to the worry that is experienced by those with social anxiety disorder. Choice *A* and *B* are therefore both correct. Choice *C* is incorrect because people with social anxiety disorder are not likely to feel relieved once they arrive at a social gathering that they have been fearing. This is more likely a response of someone without social anxiety, who was just slightly nervous. For example, an individual might be nervous to go on a date, but they feel calmer once they are there and start talking. With social anxiety, the feelings of anxiety or fear would persist.

5. C: Choice *C* is correct. Therapeutic surrender is when a client psychologically allows themself to open up to a counselor from a different culture by sharing their thoughts and feelings. For therapeutic surrender to happen, the counselor must fight barriers to treatment goals, like client resistance. They must also create a positive therapeutic relationship by actively listening, expressing empathy, and gaining the client's trust. Choice *A* is incorrect. Therapeutic alliance is very important to the success of therapy, but it is the collaborative working relationship between the client and counselor. Choice *B* is incorrect. Self-disclosure is the counselor's sharing of personal information during the counseling session. The purpose of this is to strengthen the relationship and build trust. Choice *D* is incorrect. The helping relationship is another name for the therapeutic alliance.

6. D: Choice *D* is correct, cultural norms are the standards we live by, which often are taught or reinforced by parents, teachers, or friends while growing up in a society. These expectations and rules are shared by individuals and guide behavior within social groups. Choice *A* is incorrect, laws are

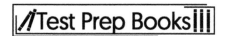

formally written at the state or federal level. When laws are broken there are predetermined consequences and formal punishments enacted. Choices *B* and *C* are incorrect because cultural adjustments and culture shock occur when an individual is adapting to an unknown culture or new environment. They may experience feelings of anxiety, confusion, or uncertainty while they are adapting.

7. C: Choice *C* is correct. Worrying about making other people feel uncomfortable is a symptom of social anxiety often found in Eastern cultures. Choices *A*, *B*, and *D* are incorrect because blushing, overheating, rapid heartbeat, and shaking are all symptoms of social anxiety disorder commonly found in Western cultures.

8. A: Choice *A* is correct. Culture shock occurs when an individual moves to a new culture or unfamiliar environment. They may have trouble adjusting and experience feelings of anxiety or uncertainty. These feelings often include homesickness, helplessness, disorientation, and isolation. Choices *B* and *C* are incorrect because social anxiety disorder, also referred to as Social Phobia, is characterized by feelings of persistent fear and anxiety, and avoidance of social situations. It does not necessarily include symptoms of homesickness or disorientation like culture shock does. Choice *D* is incorrect because the Adjustment Period is one of the stages of Culture Shock.

9. D: Choice *D* is correct. Japan is a collectivist culture. Instead of focusing on independence and the needs of the individual, the culture focuses on the needs of the group or larger community. Choices *A* and *B* are incorrect because Western culture and Eastern culture are terms to describe the differences in cultural and social norms in differing parts of the word. Western cultures like the United States are individualistic cultures, while Eastern cultures are traditionally collectivist cultures. Choice *C* is incorrect because individualistic cultures value a person's independence and autonomy. The needs and wants of the individual are seen as more important than the needs of the group.

10. D: Choice *D* is correct because coping skills are the positive methods a person uses to deal with stressful situations. These skills allow individuals to take action and solve their problems in a healthy way. Choice *A* is incorrect because coping mechanisms are psychological strategies or adaptations that a person relies on to manage stress. Choice *B* is incorrect because reframing is a way of changing the way you are looking at something. In cognitive behavioral therapy, this would be the ability to change one's perspective of events, people, and interactions. Choice *C* is incorrect. Challenging negative self-talk is the ability to create a positive change in perspective by noticing and questioning negative self-talk.

11. B: Choice *B* is correct. During exposure therapy individuals repeatedly confront their fear or anxiety-causing situations. This repeated exposure leads to lessening of symptoms of anxiety or fear over time. For example, when the client goes to the coffee shop each week, she exposes herself to situations that are uncomfortable for her repeatedly, becoming more comfortable over time. Choice *A* is incorrect because positive reinforcement is used to increase the likelihood of a behavior occurring in the future by adding a rewarding stimulus after the desired behavior is performed. Choice *C* is incorrect because negative reinforcement is used to build better behavior by taking away something that is viewed as bad or disagreeable. Choice *D* is incorrect because systematic desensitization is a method for treating phobias. This treatment involves exposing a client to stimuli that trigger fear or anxiety, and teaching relaxation techniques to manage the client's negative reactions or feelings.

12. A: Choice *A* is correct because tangible reinforcers are actual physical rewards. Favorite drinks, pastries, foods, medals, toys, and treats are examples of these. Since rewards like these provide instant

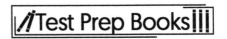
satisfaction, they are effective for encouraging changes in behavior early in the process. Choice *B* is incorrect because social reinforcers are responses or behaviors from other people that express approval. These include pats on the back, clapping, smiles, hugs, and words of affirmation. Choice *C* is incorrect because natural reinforcers are those that are naturally occurring following a behavior. For example, if you are hungry and then you eat a good meal, the natural reinforcer is feeling full and satisfied. Choice *D* is incorrect because token reinforcers involve the collection of smaller reward or tokens, then redeeming them for a larger reward in the future. For example, collecting stickers on a sticker chart and then redeeming these for a toy once a certain number of tokens or stickers have been collected.

13. C: Choice *C* is correct. Individuals are able to identify and change negative thought patterns through cognitive restructuring. Clients can use this skill to both interrupt and redirect thought patterns that are negative or destructive. Choice *A* is incorrect because goal setting is the process of collaborating to set goals and plan the smaller milestones needed to work toward those goals. Goals in counseling should be realistic and specific. Choice *B* is incorrect because self-empathy is the acknowledgement that you deserve understanding and compassion. Choice *D* is incorrect because reflection occurs when the counselor reflects back to the client what they have said. The counselor is reflecting the client's feelings so they can understand them better.

Case Study #6

1. C: Choice *C* is correct. Safety needs represent the second tier in Maslow's hierarchy of needs. This level focuses on safety and security, including job security and an overall sense of stability regarding family, health, and freedom from threats. Choice *A* is incorrect because self-actualization is the highest level of Maslow's hierarchy of needs. It includes the search for self-fulfillment, personal growth, and reaching your full potential. Choice *B* is incorrect because esteem is the fourth level in Maslow's hierarchy of needs, including self-worth, accomplishment, and respect. This level can include pride in oneself as well as desire for attention and recognition from others. Choice *D* is incorrect because love and belonging is the third level of Maslow's Hierarchy of Needs. This level includes the need for close social relationships, including friendships, family relationships, and romantic love.

2. D: Choice *D* is correct. The dual-career family is characterized by both partners having jobs of their own, which they are committed to on a continual basis. This type of family usually has more financial security compared to a traditional family. Choice *A* is incorrect because the traditional family is a family where one partner is the sole earner, and the other partner is a homemaker and caregiver to the children. Choice *B* is incorrect because the term *nuclear family* refers to a couple and their dependent children. Choice *C* is incorrect because it refers to a couple that made the choice to not have children.

3. B: Choice *B* is correct. Underemployment occurs when a worker is engaged in a position which is below his or her skill level. If the client accepted a low-paying position that does not utilize her skills or education, she would be underemployed. Choice *A* is incorrect because unemployment occurs when a person is jobless, actively seeking work, or available to take a job. Choice *C* is incorrect because overemployment occurs when an employee is overworked and wants to work fewer hours. Choice *D* is incorrect because leisure refers to an activity that one engages in for pleasure rather than money.

4. A: Choice *A* is correct because symptoms of insomnia include struggling to fall asleep and waking up often. As many as 75% of people with generalized anxiety disorder have insomnia. Choice *B* is incorrect

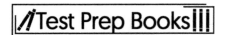
because panic disorder is not a sleep disorder, it is an anxiety disorder. Individuals with panic disorder experience symptoms of anxiety, fear, and panic. They often experience trouble breathing, rapid heartbeat, and chest pain during these episodes. Choice *C* is incorrect because individuals experiencing night terrors often wake up screaming and flailing. When an individual wakes up, they may also experience extreme and unexplainable feelings of fear. Choice *D* is incorrect because sleep apnea refers to a sleep disorder characterized by an irregular breathing pattern or breathing that stops and starts repeatedly.

5. D: Choice *D* is correct. Cultural stigma refers to a collection of attitudes or beliefs within a culture that may have a negative impact on how individuals view themselves or others. The client's mother holds a cultural stigma toward seeking help for mental health. Choice *A* is incorrect because cultural norms often guide individual's behaviors in social situations. They are learned rules and expectations of how individuals should act in any given social situation. Choice *B* is incorrect because an individual can experience culture shock when moving into a new environment or to a different culture. They may feel anxiety, confusion, or nervousness while transitioning and adapting to their new life. Choice *C* is incorrect because social norms are unspoken rules and guidelines that influence how an individual acts in any given social situation.

6. C: Choice *C* is correct. The Generalized Anxiety Disorder Severity Scale collects psychometric data. Psychometrics, also known as psychological measurement, describes participants by assigning numeric values to behaviors, symptoms, and other attributes. Choice *A* is incorrect because qualitative data describes qualities or characteristics. It is often collected using questionnaires, interviews, or observations. Choice *B* is incorrect because nominal data is data that is not a specific numerical value or ranked in order. Examples of nominal data include categories like gender or race. Choice *D* is incorrect because quantitative data is data on a numeric scale that can be counted or evaluated.

7. A: Choice *A* is correct. Major life events often lead to an increase in the severity of a client's anxiety. Based on the client's history, her anxiety was once mild to moderate. After these major life events, her anxiety is considered severe and is interfering with her quality of life. Choice *B* is incorrect because the client doesn't mention any distractions from previous anxiety and instead says she'd like to find ways to control her feelings of worry and anxiety. Choices *C* and *D* are incorrect. Based on the client's report, her symptoms of anxiety have increased rather than lessening or staying the same.

8. D: Choice *D* is correct. Anxiety often is associated with physical symptoms, compromises an individual's ability to function in daily life, and is more persistent than normal feelings of worry.

9. B: Choice *B* is correct. Emotion regulation refers to the ability to control or manage your emotional state. Choice *A* is incorrect because mindfulness is a state of being that is achieved by focusing on the present moment and noticing and accepting current thoughts and feelings. Choice *C* is incorrect because interpersonal effectiveness skills help individuals manage relationships and balance priorities with outside demands or challenges. Examples of these skills include learning how to say "no" or asking for what you need. Choice *D* is incorrect because distress tolerance refers to the capacity to cope with emotional distress.

10. B: Choice *B* is correct. Depressants, more specifically benzodiazepines, are commonly used in the treatment of generalized anxiety disorder. These specific medications reduce anxiety and treat sleep issues as well. Choice *A* is incorrect because antipsychotics are medications that are generally used to treat psychotic disorders. Choice *C* is incorrect because antidepressants are medications used to treat

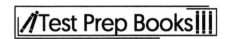

depression. They are sometimes used to treat anxiety disorders, especially if they are comorbid with major depression. Choice D is incorrect because stimulants are medications that are often used to treat attention-deficit/hyperactivity disorder.

11. A: Choice A is correct. Sleep habits are the behaviors surrounding bedtime, which include nighttime routine, drinking caffeine at night, duration of sleep, and schedule for sleep medications. Changing your sleep habits can help a client get into a better sleep routine. For example, they may cut out caffeine after 4:00pm or take a sleep medication at the same time every night. Choice B is incorrect because sleep hygiene is the routine utilized by an individual before bedtime. Examples of good sleep hygiene are going to bed at the same time each night and turning off electronic devices two hours before bedtime. Choice C is incorrect because insomnia is a sleep disorder characterized by the struggle to fall or stay asleep. Choice D is incorrect because sleep disturbances encompass multiple sleep disorders, including insomnia, sleep apnea, and restless leg syndrome.

12. D: Choice D is correct. Dialectical behavior therapy is the specific type of cognitive behavioral therapy being used by the counselor with this client. It is a treatment characterized by the use of the strategies and techniques including mindfulness, distress tolerance, interpersonal effectiveness, and emotion regulation. Choices A, B, and C are incorrect. While they are all forms of cognitive behavioral therapy, they are not focused on the same methods as dialectical behavioral therapy.

13. C: Choice C is correct. Mindfulness refers to the ability to connect with the present moment and notice passing thoughts without being controlled by them. Mindfulness helps individuals focus on the present or "live in the moment." Choice A is incorrect. While mindfulness is the awareness of "something," meditation is the awareness of "no-thing." Meditation is used to clear the mind. Choice B is incorrect because individuals employ self-soothing behaviors to control their emotional state. For example, individuals may self-sooth by listening to music or taking a bubble bath. Choice D is incorrect because active listening occurs when the counselor focuses on both what the client is saying as well as their body language. The counselor listens intently and then provides appropriate feedback.

Case Study #7

1. B: Choice B is correct. Bragging, exaggerating achievements and talents, and expecting to be recognized are examples of a grandiose sense of self-importance. Choice A is incorrect because someone who takes advantage of others and uses them for their own personal gain is being interpersonally exploitative. Choice C is incorrect because this example does not illustrate the client being envious of others. Choice D is incorrect because narcissistic rage refers to flashes of rage in individuals with narcissistic personality disorder. This rage is often triggered by small incidents or frustrations, or for no reason at all.

2. C: Choice C is correct. A sense of entitlement is the irrational belief that all other individuals should automatically agree with your opinions or treat you favorably. Choice A is incorrect because preoccupation with fantasies of extreme power, success, and brilliance is often much more extreme. They may hold false beliefs that they will be the most beautiful or most brilliant person. Choice B is incorrect because lack of empathy is present when someone is not willing or able to recognize or understand the feelings or needs of others. Choice D is incorrect because the symptom of believing one is "special" or unique involves the desire to associate with other high-status people and the need to receive exorbitant amounts of admiration and praise.

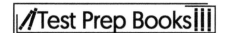

3. D: Choice *D* is correct. Taking out frustrations on others and withdrawing at work are both symptoms of burnout, a work-related stress that is common in those with narcissistic personality disorder. Choice *A* is incorrect because unemployment occurs when a person is jobless, actively seeking work, or available to take a job. Choice *B* is incorrect because a stressful work environment can lead to negative physical and emotional symptoms. This often occurs when an employee has little control over job demands, meeting deadlines, and other work-related stressors. Choice *C* is incorrect because job performance evaluates how well an individual performs their job duties. Job performance can suffer when someone is experiencing burnout.

4. C: Choice *C* is correct. It is NOT true that narcissists often make understanding their partner's thoughts and emotions a priority. Narcissists typically lack empathy. Choices *A*, *B*, and *D* are incorrect answers because they are all accurate descriptions of how a narcissist typically acts in a relationship. They have difficulty loving someone else, they often look for a partner based on whether that person can meet their needs, and their partners often feel ignored, uncared for, and unimportant.

5. A: Choice *A* is correct. In terms of gender, research on narcissistic personality disorder has found that males are 75% more likely to be diagnosed compared to females. Choice *B* is incorrect because females are not more likely to be diagnosed with NPD. Choice *C* is incorrect because research has demonstrated marked gender differences, finding that NPD is much more prevalent in men. Choice *D* is incorrect because there have been a lot of research studies focusing on narcissistic personality disorder and gender.

6. B: Choice *B* is correct. Childhood emotional neglect occurs when parents have limited emotional interactions with their children. These parents are often unresponsive and unavailable, failing to meet their child's emotional needs. This is a common experience in the childhood of those who grow up to have narcissistic personality disorder. Choice *A* is incorrect because childhood trauma is described as adverse childhood experiences including psychological trauma and physical abuse. Choice *C* is incorrect because physical abuse can be classified as childhood trauma, as it involves hurting or causing bodily injury to another individual intentionally. Choice *D* is incorrect because self-preservation is the natural or instinctive tendency to act to protect yourself from harm or death.

7. D: Choice *D* is correct. Low self-esteem is present when an individual doesn't feel confident in themselves or their abilities. An individual with low self-esteem will often feel incompetent, unloved, or inadequate. While it may seem like narcissists have high self-esteem and self-love, the opposite is actually true. They are insecure and have low self-esteem. Choices *A* and *C* are incorrect, although they are symptoms of narcissistic personality disorder. Choice *B* is also incorrect. Although individuals with this disorder expect admiration, absence of admiration is not a term for lack of confidence or feelings of incompetency, being unloved, or inadequacy.

8. A: Choice *A* is correct. The counseling method where you focus on "everything as it is" without making judgements about the accuracy or value of the client's words is known as a nonjudgmental stance. Choice *B* is incorrect because active listening occurs when the counselor focuses on listening to the client's words and closely observing their body language. Then the counselor shows they have been listening attentively by responding and providing feedback. Choice *C* is incorrect because constructive confrontation is a useful counseling intervention that can help clients be more self-aware. If used effectively, the counselor can point out discrepancies in what the client is saying, how they are acting, as well as non-verbal behaviors. Choice *D* is incorrect because accurate empathy refers to the counselor's ability to understand the client's experience in the here and now, both sensitively and accurately.

246

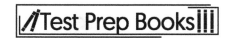

9. D: Choice *D* is correct. Lack of emotional empathy is when an individual is not willing or able to relate to or understand what others are feeling or experiencing. One of the main reasons relationships and friendships are so difficult with those with narcissistic personality disorder is their self-centeredness and lack of empathy. Choices *A, B,* and *C* are incorrect, although they are all common symptoms of narcissistic personality disorder.

10. C: Choice *C* is correct. Victim mentality is the learned behavior where individuals refuse to take responsibility for situations or issues. They blame others for anything negative that is happening to them, without reason. Narcissists often have a victim mentality and fail to take any responsibility for their own behaviors and how they affect their relationships and life circumstances. Choice *A* is incorrect because denial is a defense mechanism characterized by a refusal to accept reality or facts. Choice *B* is incorrect because projection is a defense mechanism characterized by misattributing one's own uncomfortable thoughts and feelings to another person. Choice *D* is incorrect because displacement is a defense mechanism that occurs when individuals focus negative emotions or frustrations on a less threatening person or object. An example is when someone is angry at their boss and goes home and acts angry at their wife. His displaced anger is targeting his wife since she is perceived as less threatening than his boss.

11. B: Choice *B* is correct. Overcompensation is the defense mechanism where someone learns to overachieve in one area to make up for failures in other areas, thus protecting themselves from feelings of inadequacy, insecurity, and unlovability. Choice *A* is incorrect because repression is the defense mechanism characterized by the unconscious choice to hide memories, thoughts, or beliefs that may be painful to reexperience. Individuals often block these thoughts and memories for long periods of time or forget them altogether. Choice *C* is incorrect because compartmentalization is the defense mechanism characterized by the suppression of thoughts and emotions from one area of life to keep them from "spilling over" into other areas of your life. Choice *D* is incorrect because rationalization is the defense mechanism characterized by attempts to justify, describe, interpret, or explain a bad behavior or attitude with logical reasons to make it seems more proper or attractive.

12. D: Choice *D* is correct. Empathy involves the understanding that other people have their own thoughts, feelings, and motivations. Empathy is the ability to understand or relate to what another person is feeling or going through. This is the ability to "put yourself in someone else's shoes." Choice *A* is incorrect because mindfulness occurs when an individual focuses on the present, paying attention to the thoughts and feelings they are experiencing in the moment. Choice *B* is incorrect because compassion is being sensitive to the emotional aspects of the suffering of others. Choice *C* is incorrect because sympathy is the perception of, understanding of, and reaction to the distress of another.

13. A: Choice *A* is correct. Constructive confrontation is the therapeutic method used to help achieve a positive outcome through teaching improved communication, self-awareness, and reduced conflict. Choice *B* is incorrect because authenticity is the practice of being genuine, honest, reliable, and trustworthy. Choice *C* is incorrect because congruence occurs when the counselor expresses themselves genuinely, openly, and honestly. Their inner thoughts and feelings match their outward expression. This is an important aspect for facilitating growth in counseling. Choice *D* is incorrect because de-escalation is an approach to conflict resolution focusing on preventing the escalation of conflicts.

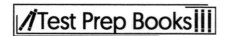

Case Study #8

1. D: Choice *D* is correct. Grief includes strong emotional and physical symptoms after experiencing a loss. Those who are grieving have feelings of sadness and longing to be with the deceased person again. Choice *A* is incorrect because mourning is defined as the social expression of bereavement or grief, which is often formalized by custom or religion. Choice *B* is incorrect because bereavement is the reaction to a loss by death. Choice *C* is incorrect because denial is the defense mechanism that involves ignoring the reality of a situation to avoid anxiety.

2. B: Choice *B* is correct. Major depressive disorder is common following the loss of a loved one and shares many key similarities to prolonged grief disorder. Major depressive disorder can be comorbid with prolonged grief disorder. Choice *A* is incorrect because generalized anxiety disorder is very different from prolonged grief disorder. It is marked by excessive, exaggerated anxiety and worry about everyday life events for no specific or obvious reason. Choice *C* is incorrect because social anxiety disorder includes anxiety and avoidance of social activities that interfere with relationships and daily life. Choice *D* is incorrect because bipolar disorder is defined by extreme mood swings that include emotional highs, called mania or hypomania, and lows, like depression.

3. B: Choice *B* is correct. By constantly mentioning missing his wife and wanting to be with her again, the client is demonstrating intense focus on or preoccupation with the deceased person, a primary symptom of prolonged grief disorder. Choices *A, C,* and *D* are incorrect. Although they are not shown with this example, these are all common symptoms of prolonged grief disorder.

4. C: Choice *C* is correct because counterfactual thinking includes imagining ways in which events in one's life might have turned out differently. This often involves feelings of regret or guilt, like the client is feeling here. Choice *A* is incorrect because wishful thinking is an attitude or belief that something you wish or want to happen will happen even though it is not likely or possible. Choice *B* is incorrect because magical thinking is the belief that one's ideas, thoughts, actions, words, or use of symbols can influence the course of events in the material world. Choice *D* is incorrect because critical thinking is the analysis of available evidence, facts, observations, and arguments to form a judgment.

5. A: Choice *A* is correct. Rumination occurs when an individual has constant, repetitive, or obsessive thoughts about an idea, situation, person, or choice that interferes with normal mental functioning. Choice *B* is incorrect because emotional numbness is the state of being in which a person does not feel or express emotions. This may provide temporary relief from painful feelings. Choice *C* is incorrect because avoidance is a coping mechanism characterized by avoiding difficult conversations or social situations or focus on doing something else as an escape or distraction from negative feelings. Choice *D* is incorrect because acceptance is the fifth and final stage of grief. During this stage, the person is finally able to accept how the loss has changed their life and stop wishing for things to go back to how they used to be.

6. C: Choice *C* is correct. Collaboration refers to the teamwork of the counselor and client when deciding what the counseling goals and the steps to reach those goals will be. This is an important part of the therapeutic process and is proven to be critical for success in goal attainment. Choice *A* is incorrect because the therapeutic alliance is the cooperative working relationship between client and therapist. Collaboration is one important aspect of building that therapeutic alliance. Choice *B* is incorrect because client goal attainment refers to the client's success in reaching their counseling goals. Choice *D* is

248

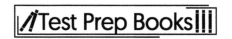

incorrect because treatment plan compliance is the degree to which a client conforms to treatment advice and methods to reach their counseling goals.

7. A: Choice *A* is correct. Reluctance is when a client is hesitant to develop a relationship with the counselor or meet the demands necessary to make changes. This may involve a client who does not participate in goal setting, the therapeutic process, assigned homework, or other critical steps to reach their goals in treatment. Choice *B* is incorrect because reluctance itself is actually a barrier to goal attainment, which is anything that may make it difficult or impossible to reach treatment goals. Choice *C* is incorrect because termination occurs when the goals that are mutually agreed upon by the counselor and client have been achieved, or when the client's symptoms are resolved or at a manageable level. At this point the client does not attend counseling sessions anymore. Choice *D* is incorrect because resistance is any opposition to the therapeutic process, including the client pushing back against suggestions or efforts that could help them.

8. D: Choice *D* is correct. When the client feels like a part of him has died and he doesn't know who he is anymore, this is an example of identity disruption. Identity disruption is common in those with prolonged grief disorder. It is disruption caused by the major life event of losing a loved one. Choices *A*, *B*, and *C* are incorrect. Although suicidal thoughts or actions, sleep disruption, and persistent preoccupation with the deceased are common symptoms in prolonged grief disorder, they are not illustrated in this specific example.

9. B: Choice *B* is correct. Suicidal thoughts or actions are one example of an at-risk behavior that is prevalent in both prolonged grief disorder and major depressive disorder. There is a difference in how these symptoms present in people with each disorder. In prolonged grief, this will often be associated with the wish to be reunited with the deceased. In depression, thoughts of suicide are more commonly associated with a feeling of not deserving to live, a wish to put an end to an intolerable situation, or the idea others would be better off without you. Choices *A*, *C*, and *D* are incorrect. Although they are all examples of at-risk behaviors, these behaviors are not common in both major depressive disorder and prolonged grief disorder.

10. B: Choice *B* is correct. The therapeutic technique that involves challenging unhealthy thought and behavior patterns is cognitive behavioral therapy. Grief-focused cognitive behavioral therapy is an effective form of therapy for those with prolonged grief disorder. Choice *A* is incorrect. Talk therapy may be helpful for clients with grief but after a period of time it is important to address thoughts and behaviors that are not helping the client move forward and heal. Choice *C* is incorrect because dialectical behavior therapy is an evidence-based psychotherapy that is often used to treat personality disorders and interpersonal conflicts. Choice *D* is incorrect because exposure therapy is a psychological treatment that was developed to help people confront their fears through exposure to the situation, object, or event that triggers the anxiety, fear, or panic for them.

11. D: Choice *D* is correct. Cognitive restructuring is the method where the counselor identifies irrational thoughts and feelings, challenges them for accuracy, and helps the client replace these thoughts with more functional and realistic ones. Choice *A* is incorrect because role playing is a technique to allow a person with a fear or phobia to practice new behaviors. Therapeutic role playing can be used to practice confronting a person the client is afraid to confront, like a parent or boss. Choice *B* is incorrect because evocative language refers to the use of tough or harsh words to speed up the process of acceptance, instead of softening the message with more subtle language. Choice *C* is incorrect because reframing is a method to change the way a person looks at something, and therefore, changes their experience of it.

249

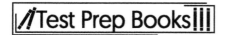

12. A: Choice *A* is correct. Acceptance is the fifth and final stage of grief. This stage of grief involves acknowledging how the loss has changed the person's life and the ability to stop wishing for everything to be exactly as it used to be. Choice *B* is incorrect because denial is the first stage of grief, where the person is coping with a loss through living in a preferable reality instead of actual reality. Choice *C* is incorrect because bargaining is the third stage of grief, where a person may try to make a deal with God or a higher power in return for healing or relief from grief and painful emotions. Choice *D* is incorrect because depression is the fourth stage of grief, where a person begins to realize and feel the true extent of the loss. This stage is characterized by trouble sleeping, lack of energy, poor appetite, and crying spells.

13. A: Choice *A* is correct. Treatment plan compliance is the degree to which a client conforms to the treatment advice and methods to reach their counseling goals. The client is taking steps toward reaching their counseling goals by scheduling time with friends and family. Choice *B* is incorrect because goal setting is the step in the therapeutic process where the client and counselor determine short-term and long-term goals for the client. Choice *C* is incorrect because reassurance is when the counselor gives support and expresses a belief in the client and their ability to reach their goals. Choice *D* is incorrect because collaboration refers to the teamwork of the counselor and client when deciding on counseling goals and the steps to reach those goals.

Case Study #9

1. B: Choice *B* is correct. Borderline personality disorder is also commonly referred to as emotional dysregulation disorder. Emotional dysregulation is a term used to describe an emotional response that is poorly regulated and doesn't fall within the traditionally accepted range of emotional reaction. Choice *A* is incorrect. Although there are many similar symptoms, bipolar disorder is a different mental health condition characterized by extreme mood swings including emotion highs (mania) and lows (depression). Choice *C* is incorrect because oppositional defiant disorder is a disorder in children marked by defiant and disobedient behavior toward authority figures. It does have some similarities to borderline personality disorder, including anger, impulsivity, and self-harm. Choice *D* is incorrect because bipolar disorder is often referred to as manic depression.

2. D: Choice *D* is correct. Borderline personality disorder is often misdiagnosed as bipolar disorder due to some similar symptoms such as mood instability and impulsive behaviors. In some cases, both disorders are present, and the client will have a dual diagnosis of the two disorders. Choices *A, B,* and *C* are incorrect. Narcissistic personality disorder, schizophrenia, and generalized anxiety disorder are not commonly confused with borderline personality disorder.

3. A: Choice *A* is correct. The intense and inappropriate anger associated with borderline personality disorder is referred to as borderline rage. The individual may react to an event that seems small to someone else, such as a misunderstanding or perceived slight, with very strong and unhealthy anger or physical violence. Choice *B* is incorrect because reaction formation is a defense mechanism where emotions and impulses that produce anxiety or are perceived as unacceptable are expressed by a directly contrasting behavior. Choice *C* is incorrect because passive-aggressive people often exhibit resistance to requests or demands from family or friends by procrastinating, expressing sullenness, or acting stubborn. Choice *D* is incorrect because assertiveness is the ability to speak up for yourself in a way that is honest and respectful.

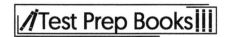

4. D: Choice *D* is correct. Disagreements, separations, and rejections are all common triggers for anger and violent outbursts in those with borderline personality disorder. Small slights or perceived rejections can lead to very strong and unhealthy anger or even physical violence for these individuals.

5. C: Choice *C* is correct. Fear of abandonment is common in individuals with borderline personality disorder. This fear of abandonment can lead to being overly sensitive to criticism, having difficulty trusting others and making friends, and taking extreme measures to avoid rejection or separation. Choice *A* is incorrect, fear of social situations is often associated with social anxiety disorder. Choice *B* is incorrect, fear of negative evaluation is very common in social anxiety. This fear may result in individuals with social anxiety avoiding social situations altogether. Choice *D* is incorrect, fear of failure is experienced by most people at one time or another.

6. B: Choice *B* is correct. Commonly seen as a symptom of bipolar disorder, pressured speech occurs when someone has the extreme need to share their thoughts, ideas, and comments. The speech will come out rapidly, does not stop at appropriate intervals, and is often erratic. Choice *A* is incorrect because interrupting occurs when an individual speaks over others or disrupts the conversation. Choice *C* is incorrect because narcissistic monologue occurs when someone uses incessant talking to monopolize the conversation and keep the attention focused on themselves. Choice *D* is incorrect because hyperverbal speech refers to fast, increased speech or talking quickly to get out everything you have to say.

7. C: Choice *C* is correct. Hypersexuality is the dysfunctional preoccupation with sexual fantasies, urges, or behaviors that are difficult to control. This is common in individuals in borderline personality disorder, along with other impulsive behaviors. Choice *A* is incorrect because impulsivity refers to a problem with emotional or behavioral self-control. Choice *B* is incorrect because sexual dysfunction is a problem that can happen during any phase of the sexual response cycle, preventing a person from experiencing satisfaction from sexual activity. Choice *D* is incorrect because lack of sexual desire refers to when a person is not interested in sex, has low or no sex drive, and it bothers them.

8. A: Choice *A* is correct. Disappearing for days, excessive spending, and risky sexual behaviors are all evidence of an individual experiencing a manic episode. Choice *B* is incorrect because symptoms of a depressive episode in bipolar disorder may include anxiety, feeling hopeless, frustration, fatigue, or loss of interest in things once enjoyed. Choice *C* is incorrect because hyperactivity refers to constant activity, being easily distracted, an inability to concentrate, and aggressiveness. Choice *D* is incorrect because common risky behaviors include alcohol use, illegal drug use, reckless driving, violence, and self-injurious or risky sexual behavior.

9. D: Choice *D* is correct. Borderline personality disorder involves a long-standing pattern of abrupt, moment-to-moment swings in moods, relationships, self-image, and behavior. Choices *A* and *C* are incorrect. Distinct episodes of mania or depression lasting days or weeks are common in bipolar disorder. Individuals with borderline personality disorder may experience ups and downs within a single day. Choice *B* is incorrect because changes in mood in borderline personality disorder *are* usually triggered by conflicts with other people.

10. C: Choice *C* is correct. Dialectical behavior therapy is the therapeutic technique being utilized with the client. This involves core mindfulness, interpersonal effectiveness, emotion regulation, and distress tolerance. Dialectical behavior therapy is the most commonly recommended therapy for borderline personality disorder, and it is known to help manage crisis behavior, suicidal behavior, and self-harm.

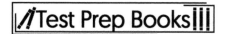

Choice *A* is incorrect because psychotherapy, or talk therapy, is a way to help people with a broad variety of mental and emotional difficulties. Choice *B* is incorrect because cognitive behavioral therapy is a psychosocial intervention technique that is most often used for individuals with anxiety or depression. Choice *D* is incorrect because transference-focused therapy focuses on revealing underlying causes of a client's condition and building a new, healthier way for the patient to think and behave.

11. B: Choice *B* is correct. Emotion regulation is the ability to exert control over one's own emotional state. This involves learning skills and strategies for enhancing control over personal emotions. Individuals with emotion regulation skills are able to control their urges to engage in impulsive actions such as physical aggression, reckless behavior, or self-harm during times of emotional stress. Choice *A* is incorrect because distress tolerance refers to an individual's ability to manage actual or perceived emotional distress. Choice *C* is incorrect because interpersonal effectiveness skills are intended to help the client become aware of how their behavior affects personal relationships and make positive changes. Choice *D* is incorrect because coping skills are methods an individual uses to deal with stressful situations.

12. D: Choice *D* is correct. Mindfulness is a strategy for coping with impulsive and emotion-driven behavior in dialectical behavior therapy. Clients are taught both "what" skills and "how" skills. The "what" skills teach individuals to observe, describe, and participate fully in the present moment. The "how" skills teach individuals to be present in the moment with a nonjudgmental mindset and focus on one thing at a time. Choice *A* is incorrect because emotional detachment is defined as being disconnected or disengaged from the feelings of other people. Choice *B* is incorrect because emotion dysregulation refers to an emotional response that is poorly regulated and does not fall into the traditionally accepted range of emotional reaction. Choice *C* is incorrect because psychosocial skills are the abilities for adaptive and positive behavior that enable individuals to deal with the demands and challenges of everyday life effectively.

13. A: Choice *A* is correct because nonsuicidal self-injury is the deliberate, self-inflicted destruction of body tissue without suicidal intent. This type of self-harm is common in individuals with borderline personality disorder. However, suicidal behaviors are also a common symptom, so counselors should be diligent when looking for these behaviors. Choice *B* is incorrect because high-risk behaviors encompass a broader category of acts that increase the risk of disease or injury, which can subsequently lead to disability, death, or social problems. Choice *C* is incorrect because suicidal behavior is defined as any behavior involving self-harm that includes suicidal ideation or intention. Choice *D* is incorrect because suicidal ideation or suicide thoughts involve thinking about or planning suicide.

Case Study #10

1. C: Choice *C* is correct, the client's refusal to cooperate or comply with small requests from his teacher and mother show that he meets the criteria for the symptom of often actively defying or refusing to comply with requests from authority figures. Choices *A, B,* and *D* are incorrect. While these are each symptoms of oppositional defiant disorder, the behavior in the example does not prove the client exhibits these symptoms.

2. A: Choice *A* is correct. Based on the client's history, you can deduce that genetic factors may be linked to his diagnosis of oppositional defiant disorder. In his family history, it is noted that his uncle has been diagnosed with antisocial personality disorder. It is common for those with oppositional defiant disorder to have a close family member with oppositional defiant disorder, conduct disorder, or antisocial

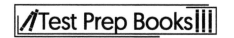
personality disorder. Choice *B* is incorrect. Although environmental factors can be linked to oppositional defiant disorder, there are no known environmental factors mentioned in this client's history. Choices *C* and *D* are incorrect because there is no history of a biological defect or brain injury with this client.

3. D: Choice *D* is correct. Oppositional defiant disorder can lead to conduct disorder if parents are unable to get their child's behavior under control. Conduct disorder is often found in teens and young adults, with symptoms including aggression toward people and animals, destruction of property, deceitfulness, and theft. Choice *A* is incorrect because borderline personality disorder is not commonly associated with oppositional defiant disorder. It is a mental disorder characterized by unstable moods, behaviors, and relationships. Choice *B* is incorrect. Although children with oppositional defiant disorder may develop antisocial personality disorder, this is a mental health condition in which the individual has a long-term pattern of manipulating, exploiting, or violating the rights of others. Choice *C* is incorrect because bipolar disorder is not a commonly associated with oppositional defiant disorder. This is a mental health condition characterized by extreme mood swings that include emotional highs and lows.

4. B: Choice *B* is correct. Attention-deficit/hyperactivity disorder is almost always comorbid with oppositional defiant disorder, meaning most children with oppositional defiant disorder also have attention-deficit/hyperactivity disorder. Choice *A* is incorrect because sensory processing disorder is a condition that affects how an individual's brain processes sensory information. This can be common with those with ADHD. Choice *C* is incorrect because conduct disorder is often found in teens and young adults, with symptoms including aggression toward people and animals, destruction of property, deceitfulness, and theft. Oppositional defiant disorder in a child may progress to conduct disorder in teens or young adults without the proper treatment. Choice *D* is incorrect because a large percentage of children with autism spectrum disorder exhibit symptoms of oppositional defiant disorder. Autism spectrum disorder is a neurological and developmental disorder that affects how individuals interact with others, communicate, learn, and behave.

5. D: Choice *D* is correct. Although clients are most commonly diagnosed with oppositional defiant disorder between the ages of eight and twelve, and are significantly more likely to be male, these are not required to diagnose an individual with oppositional defiant disorder. Choices *A, B,* and *C* are incorrect because each of these are true when diagnosing an individual with oppositional defiant disorder.

6. C: Choice *C* is correct. Parent management training involves teaching parents techniques to help their children improve behaviors and learn new social and problem-solving skills. This is found to be the most successful treatment when treating children with oppositional defiant disorder, decreasing aggression, defiance, and oppositional behavior in children and adolescents. Choice *A* is incorrect because cognitive behavioral therapy is a treatment method that aims to reduce symptoms of various mental health conditions, primarily depression and anxiety disorders. Choice *B* is incorrect because dialectical behavior therapy teaches individuals how to live in the moment, develop healthy ways to cope with stress, improve relationships, and regulate their emotions. Choice *D* is incorrect because psychotherapy, or talk therapy, can help eliminate or control symptoms so an individual can function better and increase well-being, health, and quality of life.

7. B: Choice *B* is correct. Cognitive behavioral therapy is very successful for those with oppositional defiant disorder, especially when it is combined with parent management training. Cognitive behavioral therapy focuses on identifying and replacing unhealthy thoughts and behaviors with more productive and healthy thoughts and behaviors. Choice *A* is incorrect because social skills training is a behavioral

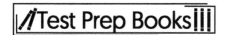

approach to teach age-appropriate social skills, communication, and problem solving. Teaching social skills is often included in the treatment of those with oppositional defiant disorder. Choice *C* is incorrect because mindfulness-based interventions are helpful to effectively reduce some symptoms of comorbid attention-deficit/hyperactivity disorder and oppositional defiant disorder. Mindfulness is the practice of focusing on the present moment and noticing what you are sensing and feeling. Choice *D* is incorrect because play therapy is therapeutic technique where children can express themselves through play. This may include art, toys, or storytelling.

8. A: Choice *A* is correct. Correcting and replacing all negative, defiant, or uncooperative behaviors is an unrealistic goal for a child with oppositional defiant disorder. It is best to choose which behaviors are the most disruptive and focus on changing those, while determining which behaviors to ignore. Choices *B, C,* and *D* are incorrect because all of these are realistic therapeutic goals for a child with oppositional defiant disorder. These are all excellent goals for the client.

9. D: Choice *D* is correct. Positive reinforcement is the use of rewards to increase repetition of a desired response or behavior. Choice *A* is incorrect because negative reinforcement is used to build better behavior by taking away something that is viewed as bad or disagreeable. Choice *B* is incorrect because punishment refers to the consequences that are enforced in response to disagreeable behavior, with the intention of keeping that behavior from ever happening again. Choice *C* is incorrect because extinction refers to the gradual weakening of a conditioned response that results in that behavior decreasing or disappearing.

10. B: Choice *B* is correct. Talking about conflicts with friends and family and generating a list of potential strategies and responses is an effective way to proactively teach children creative problem solving. Choice *A* is incorrect because only discussing what the client did wrong would not teach them problem solving skills. Choice *C* is incorrect because telling the client that responding with angry or aggressive behavior is never acceptable does not teach them problem solving skills. You can point out what behaviors are not acceptable, but it is important to discuss replacement behaviors and strategies as well. Choice *D* is incorrect. While using consistent, evidence-based discipline is important when working with children with oppositional defiant disorder, it is not an example of teaching children creative problem solving.

11. C: Choice *C* is correct. Modeling is a type of observational learning or social learning where direct instruction is not needed. In this case, the child can observe the behavior of their parents and imitate that behavior. Choice *A* is incorrect because reinforcement is the process of encouraging a pattern of behavior, often through encouragement or reward. Choice *B* is incorrect because mindfulness is the practice of focusing on the present moment and noticing what you are sensing and feeling. Choice *D* is incorrect because prosocial behaviors are behaviors which can benefit others, including helping, cooperating, comforting, and sharing. These are important skills for those with oppositional defiant disorder to learn to improve their interpersonal relationships.

12. A: Choice *A* is correct. The counselor was using role-playing to teach the student creative problem solving. Role-playing is an educational tool that is used to practice different ways of handling a situation. Choice *B* is incorrect because social skills training is a behavioral approach to teach age-appropriate social skills, communication, and problem solving. Teaching social skills is often included in the treatment of those with oppositional defiant disorder. Choice *C* is incorrect, because play therapy is a therapeutic technique where children can express themselves through play. This may include art, toys, or storytelling. Choice *D* is incorrect because anger management teaches relaxation techniques,

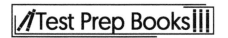

effective problem-solving, and recognition of consequences. This is important for children with oppositional defiant disorder who struggle with emotion regulation and controlling their anger.

13. D: Choice *D* is correct. Working with the teacher to create a behavioral contract with clear rules and consequences for the client to sign is the best option. This has been shown to be very effective for students with oppositional defiant disorder. Choice *A* is incorrect because this method will continue to help with behavior at home but might not translate to better behavior at school. Choice *B* is incorrect because you should not meet with the teacher to discuss the behavior in front of the client. It is best to meet with the teacher separately to plan next steps. Choice *C* is incorrect because removing the student from school will not improve the client's in-school behavior.

Case Study #11

1. B: Choice *B* is correct. Feelings of sadness, difficulty concentrating, and sleeping disruption are all symptoms of grief that are also common in major depressive disorder. There was a grief exception in the DSM until recently, and now it is recognized that grief and the more serious condition of major depressive disorder can coexist. Choice *A* is incorrect because bipolar disorder is not commonly triggered by grief. The symptoms of bipolar disorder include extreme mood swings that include highs (mania or hypomania) and lows (depression). Choice *C* is incorrect because generalized anxiety disorder is marked by excessive, exaggerated anxiety and worry about everyday life events. Choice *D* is incorrect because social anxiety disorder is a type of anxiety disorder that causes extreme fear in social settings.

2. C: Choice *C* is correct. Based on the client's symptoms, the major life change that may be adding to her level of stress is becoming the caregiver for her mother. Her mother moved in with her recently as well. Caregiver stress and burnout is more common among those who live with the relative they are caring for, as they do not get a break. Choices *A* and *B* are incorrect. She was already caring for her teenage sons and working full time as a schoolteacher, so these are not likely causes for her recent increase in stress. Choice *D* is incorrect because arguing with her husband more frequently is likely caused by the recent increase in stress. Grief can lead to an increase in irritability, and becoming a caregiver can be very stressful as well.

3. D: Choice *D* is correct. Prolonged grief disorder is diagnosed when the duration of an individual's bereavement lasts at least six months and exceeds expected social, cultural, or religious norms. Choice *A* is incorrect because major depressive disorder is diagnosed when there is a persistent feeling of sadness or loss of interest. This can also lead to a range of behavioral and physical symptoms such as changes in sleep, appetite, energy level, concentration, or self-esteem. Choice *B* is incorrect because generalized anxiety disorder is marked by excessive, exaggerated anxiety and worry about everyday life events. Choice *C* is incorrect because insomnia is a sleep disorder characterized by trouble falling asleep or staying asleep. Sleep issues are common in individuals experiencing grief and depression.

4. A: Choice *A* is correct. This is a good example of an empathy statement. In counseling, empathic responding is when a therapist reflects both what the client is feeling and why they are feeling that way. Choice *B* is incorrect because this statement is an example of self-disclosure. The counselor is relating to the client by sharing a personal story or experience. Choice *C* is incorrect because this is an example of giving advice (to ask for help), but it does not show that the client is understanding what the client is feeling. Choice *D* is incorrect because this is an example of an open-ended statement or question that encourages the client to elaborate.

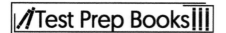

5. C: Choice *C* is correct. Psychotherapy is the form of therapy that is based on the core idea of talking about things that are bothering you. This form of therapy is helpful for those experiencing grief and bereavement, as it can allow them to process what they are feeling and help them manage their emotional distress. Choice *A* is incorrect because exposure therapy is a psychological treatment that was developed to help people confront their fears. This form of treatment is often used for individuals with anxiety disorders. Choice *B* is incorrect because the main goal of interpersonal therapy is to improve the quality of interpersonal relationships and social functioning. Choice *D* is incorrect because psychodynamic therapy is a form of psychoanalysis, with the primary focus on revealing the unconscious content of a client's psyche.

6. B: Choice *B* is correct. The client is likely in the depression stage of grief, based on her symptoms of withdrawing from social activities, feeling overwhelmed, having trouble sleeping, and experiencing feelings of hopelessness. Choice *A* is incorrect. During the anger stage of grief, the individual often experiences feelings of anger and a sense of isolation, and they may be seen as unapproachable by others. The anger is masking the more vulnerable feelings or sadness. Choice *C* is incorrect. During the bargaining stage of grief, individuals often bargain with or give requests to a higher power to alleviate the pain. This could include making promises in exchange for feeling less emotional pain or wishing for the person you love to come back. Choice *D* is incorrect because denial helps people minimize the overwhelming pain of a loss. As individuals process their emotional pain, they may unconsciously choose to live in a state of denial and not accept the current reality they are living in.

7. C: Choice *C* is correct. Caregiver stress syndrome is a condition characterized by physical, mental, and emotional exhaustion typically resulting from an individual neglecting their own physical and emotional health because they are focused on caring for an ill or injured loved one. Choice *A* is incorrect because major depressive disorder is diagnosed when there is a persistent feeling of sadness or loss of interest. This can also lead to a range of behavioral and physical symptoms such as changes in sleep, appetite, energy level, concentration, or self-esteem. Choice *B* is incorrect. Job burnout is a type of work-related stress, a state of physical or emotional exhaustion that can lead to individuals becoming easily frustrated or struggling at the simplest tasks. Choice *D* is incorrect because uncomplicated bereavement is a condition experienced after the loss of a loved one. Deep sadness, irritability, and sleep disruption are all common symptoms.

8. A: Choice *A* is correct. Reducing levels of stress and teaching healthy coping skills are both excellent long-term therapeutic goals for this client. Choices *B* and *C* are incorrect. While they are good goals for the client, they are not specific enough. Reducing levels of stress and teaching healthy coping skills will help the client improve both her social and occupational functioning in the long run. Choice *D* is incorrect because creating a schedule that includes all her new responsibilities will not solve the problem. She cannot handle all these responsibilities on her own. Asking for help from others and practicing self-care are critical.

9. C: Choice *C* is correct. Self-disclosure is the technique where a counselor shares a personal story or experience from their life to connect with the client. Choice *A* is incorrect because confrontation is a direct technique in which the counselor challenges clients to face themselves or a situation realistically. Choice *B* is incorrect. Immediacy refers to when the counselor briefly and appropriately discloses their immediate responses about the client to the client. Choice *D* is incorrect. Interpretation is a skill that relies on self-disclosure, as the counselor must disclose their interpretation of what the client is saying.

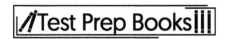

10. B: Choice *B* is correct. Insight occurs when a client has an "aha!" moment in counseling, suddenly becoming aware of a factor in their life that was previously unknown. Choice *A* is incorrect because empathy is the ability to understand and share the feelings of another person. Choice *C* is incorrect because self-awareness is the conscious knowledge of an individual's own character, feelings, motives, and desires. Choice *D* is incorrect because reflection is a skill where the counselor repeats the client's words back to them. It is called reflection since it allows the client to see themselves and their words as if reflected in a mirror, thus understanding themselves better.

11. D: Choice *D* is correct. All of these options are effective methods of self-care, shown to improve mood and reduce levels of stress. Caregivers often neglect themselves and need to learn to prioritize self-care and healthy habits.

12. A: Choice *A* is correct. Those who are grieving often have difficulties sleeping or experience insomnia. Prescribing sedatives or sleeping medications on a temporary basis will help the client with sleep issues, allowing them to get more rest. Choice *B* is incorrect. Antidepressants would be prescribed if the symptoms of depression are the main concern. Choice *C* is incorrect because analgesics are pain relief medications. Choice *D* is incorrect because stimulants are medications that can boost alertness and keep an individual awake. The client needs something to help with sleep, not something to help with wakefulness.

13. B: Choice *B* is correct. Providing the client with information about the Family and Medical Leave Act is the best choice. Sharing this information will let the client know she has the option to take job-protected leave if she needs a break. Choices *A* and *C* are incorrect. Advising the client to quit her job or to focus solely on work are not the best options. Offering advice can hinder the client's growth. It's best to give the client options and resources and allow them to determine the best decision for them. Choice *D* is incorrect because it is a breach of confidentiality to call the client's employer and share personal information.

Index

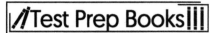

Elisabeth Kubler-Ross, 97

Emic, 145

Emotional Abuse, 122

Emotional and Dependency Issues, 23

Emotional Cutoff, 145

Emotional Detours, 177

Emotional Dysregulation, 124, 221, 223, 250

Emotional Proximity and Distance, 139

Emotional Regulation, 151

Emotional Responses, 104

Empathic Responding, 178, 234, 255

Empathy, 164, 177, 187, 214, 231, 234, 247

Empowerment, 153

Empty Chair Technique, 165

Empty Nest Syndrome, 145

Encopresis, 62

Encryption, 32

End Stage, 170

Enmeshed, 139

Entry Phase, 30

Enuresis, 62

Ethical Dilemmas, 20

Ethnic

    Group, 143

Ethnicity, 46, 93, 184, 189, 193, 198, 202, 206, 211, 216, 220, 224, 228

Ethnocentrism, 145

Ethnocide, 145

Ethnology, 145

Etic, 145

Evaluation, 19, 88

Excoriation, 58

Existential Crisis, 110

Experimental Quantitative Research, 13

Exploration of Feelings and Definition of Problem, 31

Exposure and Response Prevention (ERP), 102

External Boundaries, 147

External Stress, 110

External Validity, 13

Eye Movement Desensitization and Reprocessing (EMDR), 11

Families, 93, 111, 139, 144, 147, 148, 166

Family Dynamics, 149

Family Hierarchy, 139

Family in Later Years, 148

Family Life Cycle Theories, 148

Family Projection Process, 144

Family Systems Theory, 144

Family Therapy, 115

Family With Adolescents, 148

Family With Young Children, 148

Fear, 80, 94, 121, 251

Feeding and Eating Disorders, 61

Five-Point Scale, 84, 89, 98

Fluid Intelligence, 91

Focus Groups, 12

Follow-Up Session, 134

Formal Observation, 78

Forming, 169, 171

Four D's of Abnormality, 49, 74

Functional Analysis, 78

Functional Roles, 168

Furthering, 182

Gambling Addiction, 106

Gender, 16, 21, 43, 47, 49, 64, 65, 78, 83, 95, 96, 121, 140, 146, 153, 165, 173, 174, 179, 213, 244, 246

Gender Dysphoria, 49, 64, 65, 96

Gender Fluid, 96

Gender Identity, 95, 173

Gender Queer, 96

Gender Schema Theory, 145

Generalized Subtype, 64

Generativity Versus Stagnation, 102

Genetic Theory of Addiction, 111

Genito-Pelvic Pain/Penetration Disorder, 64

Genogram, 83

    Genograms, 168

George Engle, 41

Gerald Caplan, 158

Gerald Corey, 170

Gerard Egan, 154

Gerontology, 90

Goal-Attainment Scaling, 89

Gottman Method, 119, 157

Grief, 97, 217, 248, 249, 255

Group Counseling, 33

Group Work, 139

Guided Imagery, 154

Guidelines, 18, 24, 155

Hallucinations, 113, 114

Hamilton Depression Rating Scale (HAM-D), 98

Happiness, 153

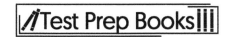

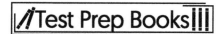

Dear NCMHCE Test Taker,

We would like to start by thanking you for purchasing this study guide for your NCMHCE exam. We hope that we exceeded your expectations.

Our goal in creating this study guide was to cover all of the topics that you will see on the test. We also strove to make our practice questions as similar as possible to what you will encounter on test day. With that being said, if you found something that you feel was not up to your standards, please send us an email and let us know.

We would also like to let you know about another book in our catalog that may interest you.

NCE

This can be found on Amazon: amazon.com/dp/1628458615

We have study guides in a wide variety of fields. If the one you are looking for isn't listed above, then try searching for it on Amazon or send us an email.

Thanks Again and Happy Testing!
Product Development Team
info@studyguideteam.com

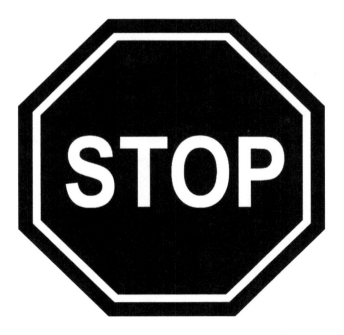

FREE Test Taking Tips Video/DVD Offer

To better serve you, we created videos covering test taking tips that we want to give you for FREE. **These videos cover world-class tips that will help you succeed on your test.**

We just ask that you send us feedback about this product. Please let us know what you thought about it—whether good, bad, or indifferent.

To get your **FREE videos**, you can use the QR code below or email freevideos@studyguideteam.com with "Free Videos" in the subject line and the following information in the body of the email:

- a. The title of your product
- b. Your product rating on a scale of 1-5, with 5 being the highest
- c. Your feedback about the product

If you have any questions or concerns, please don't hesitate to contact us at info@studyguideteam.com.

Thank you!

CPSIA information can be obtained
at www.ICGtesting.com
Printed in the USA
LVHW062350180723
752684LV00009B/814